Transforming Your Lifestyle One Belief at a Time

christopher
SASHA

Notice

The information given here is designed to help you make informed decisions about your health and body. The suggestions for specific foods, nutritional supplements and exercises in this program are not intended to replace appropriate or necessary medical care. Before commencing any exercise program and/or nutritional supplements, always consult your primary physician. If you have specific medical symptoms, consult your primary physician immediately. If any recommendations given in this program contradict your primary physician's advice, be sure to consult your physician before proceeding. Mention of specific companies, organizations or authorities in this book does not imply endorsement by the publisher, nor does mention of specific companies, organizations or authorities imply that they endorse this book. The author and the publisher disclaim any liability or loss, personal or otherwise, resulting from the procedures in this program. Internet addresses and telephone numbers given in this book were accurate at the time it went to press.

Additional copies of this book are available at special quantity discounts to use as education, premiums and training programs.

Contact Christopher Sasha directly with the number of books required and your shipping address.

E-mail: sasha@fitbodiesbysasha.com Website: http://www.fitbodiesbysasha.com

First Edition, March 2012

Photographs: Dan DuVerney
Photograph page 3 courtesy @ Christopher Sasha and Brian McCabe
Photograph page 278 courtesy @ Christopher Sasha and Sheila
Charapata (photographed by Aaron Miller)
Illustrations: Peter Wilstermann
Page design, layout and typography: Aaron Miller
Cover design: Aaron Miller

Library of Congress Cataloging-in-Publication Data

Sasha, Christopher
    Transforming Your Lifestyle / Christopher Sasha
    ISBN-13: 978-0-9845134-4-4
    ISBN-10: 0-9845134-4-2
    1. Reducing Diet. 2. Exercise. 3. Healthy Living.

Dedicated to all
who are committed
to being proactive
in helping prevent
obesity-related diseases.

Most of all for me, to Greg Houseton.
Your spirit lives on!

Acknowledgments i

Preface iii

Introduction xi

PART I
SECRETS FOR TRANSFORMING YOUR LIFESTYLE

Chapter 1 WINNING THE WAR ON HEALTH MANAGEMENT . 3

Strategy 1: Understandeth that not all grams are created equal 6

Strategy 2: Thou must burn more calories than thou consumes. 6

Strategy 3: Thou shalt not lose more than one or two pounds per week.
Avoideth rapid weight loss diets 7

Strategy 4: Honour exercise to sustain a healthy weight 11

Strategy 5: Thou shalt always make time for breakfast 12

Strategy 6: Increaseth thy number of meals per day whilst
decreaseth the calories per meal 13

Strategy 7: Thou shalt not ban foods 15

Strategy 8: Thou shalt not forget that forgotten calories add up quickly 16

Strategy 9: Thou must learn to read Food Labels 17

Strategy 10: Thou must form new habits to implement a maintenance
plan to keep unwanted weight off 18

Let's consider habits in a little more detail 20

Chapter 2 FOOD LABELS 23

Anatomy of a Food Label 25

Nutrients Recommended by the FDA 34

Think You Can Beat the Experts? 46

Chapter 3 DAILY CALORIC REQUIREMENT 49

Body Mass Index (BMI) 50

Waist Circumference 50

Metabolism 53

From Obese to a Healthy Weight 61

Chapter 4 LEARN TO EAT AT FAST FOOD RESTAURANTS . . 71

McDonald's. 73

Wendy's 84

Burger King 94

PART II
NUTRIENTS FOR TRANSFORMING
YOUR LIFESTYLE

Chapter 5 CARBOHYDRATES **111**

Complex Carbohydrates 113

Simple Carbohydrates 120

Types of Sugars 121

Sugar Addiction 132

Net Carbohydrates. 134

Chapter 6 FATS **137**

The Bad Fats 138

The Good Fats 143

Spot Reduction 148

Chapter 7 PROTEIN **151**

Amino Acids 152

Immune System 152

Enzymes 153

Zinc. 156

Iron 156

Vitamin B-12 157

Lean Meats 158

Deli Meats 163

Whey Protein 166

Protein Overload 170

Chapter 8 HYDRATION **173**

    Drink More Water 174

    Coffee & Soda Thwart Weight Loss 176

    How Much Water 177

    Dehydration 179

    Hyponatremia 180

    Tap Water vs. Bottled Water 182

PART III
ESSENTIALS FOR TRANSFORMING
YOUR LIFESTYLE

Chapter 9 ABDOMINALS **191**

    Health Benefits 192

    Abdominal Anatomy 193

    Erector Spinae 195

    Genetics 196

    Fast- and Slow-Twitch Muscle Fibers 197

    Periodization 198

    Detailed Ab Periodization Program 201

    Focus and Form 208

    Abdominal Exercises 209

    Lower Rectus Abdominis (illustrations) 211

    Obliques (illustrations) 220

    Upper Rectus Abdominis (illustrations) 229

    Erector Spinae (illustrations) 238

    Transverse Abdominis (illustrations) 242

Chapter 10 CARDIOVASCULAR **245**

    Benefits of Cardio 246

    Aerobic vs. Anaerobic 247

    Maximum Heart Rate (MHR) 248

    Estimated Calories Burned per Hour 253

    Cardio Before or After the Workout? 253

Human Growth Hormone. 254

Intensity Levels 255

Timing and Duration. 257

Does Cardio Metabolize Muscle? 257

Rehydrate 259

Chapter 11 SLEEP AND REST 261

Immune System 262

Human Growth Hormone (hGH). 263

Three Ways to Increase hGH 264

Sleep Deprivation 267

How Much Sleep Do I Need? 268

PART IV
PUTTING IT ALL TOGETHER

Chapter 12 MY MEALS. 273

Changing My Eating Habits 274

Kiss Method 276

Five Days Following Me Around 281

My Main Foods That Keep My *Transforming Your Lifestyle* Physique 293

Chapter 13 HOW I LOST 31 POUNDS OF FAT WITHOUT FAT BURNER PILLS 299

Miracle Drug or Miracle Waste of Money? 301

Losing Weight Without Thermogenics 303

Tactics Used by Fat Burner Advertisement Photos 308

christopherSASHA

Acknowledgments

First, I want to take a moment to mention the people I don't want to thank. Like my senior year high school English teacher who never gave me a grade higher than a D+. But seriously… WOW! What a ride. This book endeavor has been a tremendous roller coaster with a plethora of obstacles to overcome. There were as many disappointments as there were overwhelming triumphs. I was utterly fortunate to have an army of faithful souls who contributed to my efforts because they believe as much as I believe that this book you're about to read will help you live a healthier, happier, longer life. It's also my belief that it will make an impact on our current obesity epidemic. This book is a 13-year collaboration of health questions and concerns from all my clients (past and present), friends, other personal trainers and their clients, and anonymous people on trains, planes, buses and social events. They are the true authors. I'm merely the vehicle to deliver the organized product – *TRANSFORMING YOUR LIFESTYLE.*

To my mother, Gail, my brother and sisters – Scott, Kim, Pam and Dawn – you're my pillar of strength. You continuously remind me that nothing is impossible.

To Jo-Ann Oleksy for truly teaching me by example that life is a gift and a joy. And there is no greater power in this world than love.

Profound thanks to all of my friends, especially Christine Clausen and Danny and Marie Lena for being a citadel filled with unconditional love and wisdom that has gotten me through extremely trying times.

I would like to bestow special thanks to Jim Gordon for guiding me through some of life's most arduous times, picking me back up, brushing me

christopherSASHA

off and constructively suggesting that there are always other options to obtain personal goals. He is truly a giant in my life with an unfaltering shoulder to lean on.

A serene hug to Rosemarie Dias for helping me understand the importance of creating a calmness within while still living in a chaotic world.

A very special thanks to David Maize whom I've never personally met yet took a tremendous amount of time reading my first draft manuscript and offered organizational suggestions to put order to my thoughts. Thank you for getting this horse out of the gate.

To friends, family and clients, especially Dr. Thomas Carlson, Kathy Sommer, Ken Griffin, Peter Shull, Dick Elden, Rod Keith, Rick Shoemaker, and Kyle Petersen all of whom in one way or another made a significant contribution toward the birthing of this book. I am terribly grateful to them all.

Special thanks to Debbie Manning, who as my editor, skillfully guided me through the production process. Debbie, as you know, writing a book can be an intense experience, but you made it a wonderful memory. I'm so grateful for your countless hours reading and proofing the manuscript. Thank you for your support with this endeavor.

To Aaron Miller for the layout design and book cover, thank you for paying attention to the details and the numberless ideas you brought on board to make this book more aesthetically pleasing.

A magnitude of humble thanks to Carlos Dias, author of *Strategic Value Innovation*, who has been an incredible mentor to me. I'm eternally appreciative for your constant offerings of getting me in contact with organizations to get this book to the market. Your enthusiasm in your work energizes my aspirations to greater accomplishments. Many thanks for your 30-plus years of business experience lessons you have passed on to me to help me make better future business decisions.

To a lifelong friend, Dr. Phillip Zinni III, DO, FAOASM, MS, ATC, Co-Medical Director, Health Link Medical Center for Regenerative Interventional Orthopedics (I know that was a mouthful). My utmost gratitude for your time and effort crossing the t's and dotting the i's, assuring me that my explanations for the biochemical processes I mention were thoroughly clear for the reader to easily understand.

To all of my clients, past and present, I've learned much from you. To the Uber-Mind, which goes by many names, I offer my gratefulness – every day.

christopherSASHA

Preface

Since the beginning of time, our bodies have dealt with the inconsistent availability of food by storing excess calories as fat. Until recently life was either feast or famine! Our bodies stored excess calories from the feast, which converted into fat. During the times that we didn't eat, our bodies would slow our metabolism down to a screeching halt – to protect fat and save it as energy to survive until the next feast.

Food availability has drastically changed in the past 100 years. Our relationship with food has also changed, including the way scientists increase shelf life and optimize food appearance. In general, we no longer wonder when the next feast is going to be. Food is readily available and we rarely get to the point where our bodies need to utilize fat as a main source of energy.

This is where many dieters lose sight of the big picture. They think that if they just eat a minute amount of food, they'll lose weight. In the short term, they're absolutely correct – *but only in the short term*. Because they're trying to survive on small amounts of calories, odds are they'll be in a constant state of hunger, which jeopardizes their hard work dieting. They're trying to do the right thing, but approaching it in the wrong way. With this style of dieting – being hungry all the time – the body slows its metabolism, enabling it to adapt and survive on fewer calories.

But then, when the typical dieter finally attains the desired weight, odds are they dump the diet and go back to their old eating habits. At this point, the body has learned to function on fewer calories, so when the dieter increases his/her caloric consumption, the weight comes right back. Furthermore, the weight a sedentary person loses through diet alone is between 25-50% muscle. When that person regains the lost weight, it's not muscle that's gained back – it's mostly fat. This makes the sedentary person fatter proportionally, making it harder to lose weight and easier to gain more weight.

> Between 25-50% of weight loss is muscle tissue, which slows your metabolism.

To lose weight and keep it off, you must combine exercise with a slight reduction in calories. If you drastically reduce calories, your body will think it's in starvation mode and slow your metabolism, enabling you to gain more fat. You must never be hungry, particularly while losing weight. Therefore, we need to be thinking not in terms of a diet, but rather in terms of a *lifestyle*.

christopherSASHA

Since 1985, obesity has become the number 2 American health problem, next to health risks associated with tobacco. The definition of overweight and obesity is a Body Mass Index (BMI) of 25 and 30 respectively. According to the Centers for Disease Control and Prevention in the *2005-2006 National Health and Nutrition Examination Survey*, 67% of American adults over the age of 20 were overweight with 34.3% being obese and 5.9% "extremely obese". This was the first time obese Americans actually outnumbered the merely overweight, which accounted for 32.7% of Americans. However, the *2007-2008 National Health and Nutrition Examination Survey* indicates that obese and extremely obese American adults are becoming more aware of their weight because these percentages have dropped to 33.8% and 5.7% respectively. Unfortunately, though, 18.1% of American adolescents (aged 12-19) are obese with the rates for children who are obese approximately quadruple what they were in 1980. This increase affects all race and gender groups. Statistics show that overweight children become overweight adults, especially if being overweight starts before the age of eight. Obese children and adolescents have higher risk factors for diseases like high cholesterol, high blood pressure, type 2 diabetes, stroke, gallbladder disease, sleep apnea, respiratory problems, and coronary heart disease. Americans notoriously eat too much, have poor eating habits, exercise too little, and lack improved health literacy.

2010 State Obesity Rates

State	Rate	State	Rate	State	Rate
Alabama	32.3%	Kentucky	31.3%	North Dakota	27.2%
Alaska	24.5%	Louisiana	31.0%	Ohio	29.2%
Arizona	24.3%	Maine	26.8%	Oklahoma	30.4%
Arkansas	30.1%	Maryland	27.1%	Oregon	26.8%
California	24.0%	Massachusetts	23.0%	Pennsylvania	28.6%
Colorado	21.0%	Michigan	30.9%	Rhode Island	25.5%
Connecticut	22.5%	Minnesota	24.8%	South Carolina	31.5%
Delaware	28.0%	Mississippi	34.0%	South Dakota	27.3%
District of Columbia	22.2%	Missouri	30.5%	Tennessee	30.8%
Florida	26.6%	Montana	23.0%	Texas	31.0%
Georgia	29.6%	Nebraska	26.9%	Utah	22.5%
Hawaii	22.7%	Nevada	22.4%	Vermont	23.2%
Idaho	26.5%	New Hampshire	25.0%	Virginia	26.0%
Illinois	28.2%	New Jersey	23.8%	Washington	25.5%
Indiana	29.6%	New Mexico	25.1%	West Virginia	32.5%
Iowa	28.4%	New York	23.9%	Wisconsin	26.3%
Kansas	29.4%	North Carolina	27.8%	Wyoming	25.1%

Source: Centers for Disease Control and Prevention

According to the Archives of Internal Medicine, only 3% of American adults are at a healthy weight, consume 5 or more fruits and vegetables a day, don't smoke, and exercise regularly.

On April 30, 2010, the *Washington Post* headline read, ***"The Latest National Security Threat: OBESITY."*** A study conducted by Army researchers found that 27.1% of the 18-year-olds who applied to join the military in 2006 were overweight – up from 22.8% in 1993. When the United States military has to reject individuals because they're 50-100 pounds overweight, there's a problem with the standard American diet (SAD). According to the Centers for Disease Control and Prevention, only 6% of 18- to 34-year-olds were obese in 1987. By 2008, 23% of that same age group was considered obese. That's almost a 400% increase! According to the latest Pentagon figures, 35% of the roughly 31.2 million Americans aged 17-24 are unqualified for military service because of physical and medical issues. According to the Pentagon's director of accessions, the major component of this is obesity.

Obesity related diseases cost Americans $147 billion in 2008.

Before World War II, the government had to "beef up" soldiers so they would have the strength and endurance to fight. Back then, most of the soldiers came from farms and worked outside all day. They were thin – obviously a little too thin. After World War II the government even published nutritional guidelines to combat malnutrition. We went from one extreme to the other. Now obesity is a major epidemic, costing billions and billions of dollars in the healthcare arena each year. In 2008, the U.S. spent an estimated $147 billion on the direct and indirect costs of American obesity. Obesity is associated with almost 112,000 premature deaths annually in America.

According to an August 2009 article in the *American Journal of Medicine*, 62.1% of bankruptcies in the United States in 2007 were caused by medical bills – up 50% from 2001.

If just 10% of adults began some type of moderate-intensity physical activity (such as walking) on a regular basis, Americans could save $5.6 billion in costs related to heart disease. (*Critical Pathways in Cardiology*, December 2004)

We spent $58.6 billion on weight loss products and diet books in 2008 according to Marketdata Enterprises. The Calorie Control Council survey reported that 29% of U.S. adults were on a diet in 2007. But what's even more amazing is that for those individuals who lose weight, 95% regain their lost

95% of dieters regain their lost weight - and then some - within 1-5 years.

weight – and then some – within 1 to 5 years, according to the American Dietetic Association. *DIETS ALONE DON'T WORK!* We live in an instant gratification society – we want what we want – now.

Many of us are notorious for not eating all day and realizing late in the day that we're hungry. We're not educated enough about nutrition and diets to know that our metabolism slows down by mid-afternoon, making it even worse to start eating late. Because we're hungry now, we want to eliminate that uncomfortable feeling – instantly.

So what do we do? Because we want instant gratification, we thrive on fast food joints. So, we pull up to a drive-thru and order a bunch of "processed" food. We ignore the fact that the more the food is processed, the more fattening it becomes. And we fail to consider that this processed food will spike our insulin levels. The roller coaster effect is that when the insulin level is high, the metabolism slows down and the circumference around our waists (belly fat) increases.

Then we wonder why we're gaining weight! We only ate once all day!

In 1960, the average woman had a 30 inch waist, according to the Centers for Disease Control and Prevention. A 35 inch waist is an indicator for obesity in women. Today, the average woman has a 37 inch waist! In 1950, the average woman's dress size was an 8. By 2002 it had increased to a size 14.

If you eat only once all day, your body tells itself to store the excess calories as fat because it doesn't know when it's going to be fed again. Your body thinks it now has extra fuel, just in case it's not going to eat for a while. That time never actually comes, though, because you're sure to eat at least once the following day. Your body repeats this process daily, and, before you know it, you've gained 10 pounds within a year.

In fact, all variables remaining constant, if 95 calories per day were added to your diet, in 1 year you would gain 10 pounds! That's approximately 2 Oreo cookies a day. (For 1 pound of body fat, there are 3,500 calories, and 95 calories x 365 days = 34,675 calories, or 10 pounds.)

Also, consider that as early as our mid-20s inactive people lose about one half of a pound of muscle each year. As you'll see later, muscle loss slows the metabolism even more. Compared to fat, the same amount of muscle utilizes calories at a faster rate as energy to survive because muscle tissue is much more metabolically active. The more muscle mass you maintain in your body composition, the more calories you burn. This means you don't have to do anything. Just sitting reading a book or sleeping, you'll burn more calories to feed your muscle. This is one reason why it's imperative to maintain muscle tissue. As we age, we gradually lose muscle tissue, so we need fewer calories, also making it easier to gain weight.

> Your metabolism is responsible for up to three-fourths of the calories you burn.

People who eat once or twice a day are training their bodies to survive on less energy and to store extra calories as fat, according to scientists at Georgia State University. When meals are skipped, blood sugar levels get thrown into disarray.

We have to change our beliefs about our food consumption. Instead of eating 1 or 2 times per day, we need to decrease our portion sizes and eat 5 or 6 smaller meals per day. Ideally we should eat 3 meals with 2 or 3 snacks between them. Reducing our portion sizes and increasing the number of times we eat (every 2 or 3 hours) will help prevent a drop in blood sugar. Frequent eating helps maintain muscle mass, thereby accelerating our metabolism and maintaining our energy levels throughout the day.

As we age, we gradually lose muscle tissue and our resting metabolic rate (RMR) and human growth hormone (hGH) decrease, all contributing to weight gain.

American portion sizes have gotten way out of control. This is due in part to the fascinating marketing concept of the Super Size menu at fast food chains. USDA statistics indicate that in the last 20 years the average daily caloric intake has risen from 1,854 calories to 2,002. On the average person that's about an extra 15 pounds every year. It's no wonder that airplane and movie theatre seats have increased in size. It's not just because engineers for the airlines and movie theatres want their loyal customers to feel comfortable – they'd be losing money on that strategy. It's because the average American can't squeeze their rears into the seats anymore. *Instead of fixing the problem, we're accommodating the problem.*

According to the *American Journal of Preventative Medicine*, the increase in America's average weight caused airlines to spend an extra $275,000,000 on fuel in 2000.

Compare dinner plates from the 1940s and today. The dinner plates from the '40s were approximately the size of modern salad plates. In the 1970s, the standard restaurant dinner plate was 9 inches – today they average 12 inches. If we keep this pace, in 50 years, we'll be using our current dinner plates as salad plates and our current salad plates as butter plates. Our dinner plates will be the size of garbage can lids. The bigger the plate, the more food it holds, and the more we eat.

Portion size is paramount to weight control – it's three-fourths the battle. In fact, my belief is that the next diet craze is going to be based on portion sizes. I see it already. Snacks like Oreos, Pringles chips, and Wheat Thins are packaged in smaller bags that contain one serving equal to 100 calories. Coca-Cola has 8 ounce cans equaling 100 calories. This marketing ploy will solve only half the problems we currently have with obesity. The fact is, most Americans consume way too many calories. None of the products I listed offers much nutrition. They're referred to as empty calories. At least downsizing the product's calorie content is a step in the right direction. In general, a portion size is 3 ounces, or the palm of your hand (excluding basketball player Shaquille O'Neal); for boxers, it's the size of a fist; and gamblers might relate to a deck of playing cards.

To get a true sense of how obese America has become, visit any airport, shopping mall, movie theatre, zoo, or any other public place. You'll see it firsthand. Why have we become uncontrollably fat? First, because we're eating too much! Everybody has different amounts of fat cells, in different shapes and sizes, distributed in different areas. Generally, men store more fat in their upper body, including their midsection and women store more in their lower body, including their hips and thighs. Body fat in women also plays a crucial role in normal menstruation.

As body fat is gained, the fat cells get larger. As body fat is reduced, the fat cells decrease in size. IT'S THAT SIMPLE! Now here is the controversy: some experts believe that fat cells can only grow so large. So what happens when the adipose tissue grows to maximum size? New fat cells form from preadipocytes, which are tiny stems that have the ability to transform into fat cells if you eat too much. The good news is that if you lose fat *slowly*, over six months or so, the *number* of fat cells will decrease. In fact, some will actually die, and some will go back to their preadipocyte form. So when you exercise, your fat will decrease as long as you're burning more calories than you're consuming.

> New fat cells form from preadipocytes, which are tiny stems that have the ability to transform into fat cells if you eat too much.

Another reason why we gain fat is due to the "bad" carbohydrates we eat. These are the highly processed carbohydrates in foods like baked goods, snacks, and "refined" or "enriched" breads and pastas. When these types of carbs enter the body, the pancreas quickly releases a hormone called *insulin*, the function of which is to process fats and sugars. Insulin is the gatekeeper that allows the sugars into the organs where needed, or else puts them in storage for future use. The problem is that when sugars are absorbed quickly, the blood sugar rises rapidly and a balanced amount of insulin is required. This high level of insulin causes the blood sugar level to plummet so we start to get cravings … for more carbohydrates.

These new cravings usually demand quick fixes. We grab the most easily-available carbs we can find – in our desk drawer, at the convenience store, or in the first fast food drive-thru we see. We replenish our body with more – you guessed it – bad carbohydrates. And the vicious cycle continues. Have you heard Albert Einstein's definition of insanity? It's doing the same thing over and over and expecting a different result.

We need to stop being one-trick ponies and start changing our beliefs about our diets. We need to slow the increases and decreases in blood sugar levels by learning to eat the right kinds and amounts of foods. I truly believe that this process needs to start earlier than you might think – while in the womb. The pregnant woman should start her child's eating habits while the child is in the womb by learning to eat the right kinds and amounts of foods herself. Results from the latest National Health and Nutrition Examination Survey (2005-2006) indicates 11% of children between the ages 2 and 5 are overweight. Some children are already having a problem with their weight before they start school.

christopherSASHA

This generation of American children could be the first to live shorter lives than their parents.

Compound poor eating habits at home with the unhealthy food choices in school lunch programs and you have a recipe for early obesity. Schools have some of the worst food settings… vending machines stocked with sugary snacks as well as Taco Bell, McDonald's, Pizza Hut, and more. To make matters worse, fewer than 25% of U.S. elementary schools provide daily physical education, according to the National Center for Education Statistics. If the foods in schools don't become healthier, children will most likely have to deal with serious health conditions. *This could quite possibly be the first generation of American children to live shorter lives than their parents.*

Forget about fat-free this and low-carb that – moderation is the key. Learning the difference between good fats and bad fats and good carbs and bad carbs is equally important. Obesity isn't the result of eating fats and carbohydrates. It's mostly the result of consuming too many calories and exercising too little. Whether the excess calories come from fat, carbs, or protein doesn't matter. Obesity is generally caused by the consumption of too many calories (especially sugars), poor eating habits, lack of improved health literacy, and not enough exercise!

"An ounce of prevention is worth a pound of cure!"   ~Benjamin Franklin

Negative Beliefs Sabotage Goals
(An Introduction)

Recently, a man and his wife went to the Bahamas for their anniversary. The man went for an early swim and encountered a shark 20 feet from shore. He tried to swim back, but the shark attacked, biting through the man's left leg and dragging him out into the ocean. The shark pulled him down so deep, the man soon found himself enveloped in total darkness. Then the shark started shaking him violently, like a rag doll. The man knew he was going to die. But instead of giving into that possibility, he pushed through his fear, picturing in his mind where the shark's jaws of death might be and then prying the jaws open and freeing his leg. The shark swam away as the man headed for shore. Unfortunately, there was no hope of saving the leg. But that man now speaks for the company that made his new prosthetic leg, and he encourages others who have lost a limb to try to accomplish a little more each day – in small intervals. His motto is "You can't even imagine what you can do if you take baby steps."

> You can't even imagine what you can do if you take baby steps.

From a man who faced death comes reassurance that each of us can overcome anything we put our minds to. If, that is, we want it badly enough. For why do some of us achieve greatness, while others settle for mediocrity? How, for example, did Arnold Schwarzenegger, barely able to speak English, come to America, marry into the iconic Kennedy family, and become the governor of the fifth largest economy in the world? What drove him? What helped him overcome the fears he must have had of the obstacles that lay before him?

The fact is, every human being has fears. But every day, ordinary people force themselves to work through their fears and push themselves further than what they believe are their own capabilities. Every one of us has the power to conquer obstacles in our path to achieve our goals.

All we need is the desire.

christopher SASHA

Winners Never Quit
And Quitters Never Win!

Growing up in the suburbs of Chicago, I was a scrawny, nearly emaciated kid. My self-respect level was exceptionally low. Insecurity issues? Absolutely. Confidence? Zero. Positive attitude towards neighborhood kids? No way. I was *always* the last kid to be picked to play in any of the sports played by the neighborhood boys. Even then, it was only if they couldn't find any girls sitting around to fill the position. I mostly sat on the sidelines wondering what it would be like to be a naturally gifted athlete. I wanted to be the one everybody wanted to be like.

After the death of my mother, when I was 8-years-old, the government placed my brother and three sisters and me into foster homes until my father could prove he was stable enough to be a decent single parent to 5 children. It seemed like I was moved to a different foster home every 6 months. As soon as I would be on the cusp of making friends, it would be time for me to move to another home. Finally, I just stopped trying to make friends. I started to develop an even lower level of self-respect and a dangerously negative attitude towards life.

> I started to develop an even lower level of self-respect and a dangerously negative attitude towards life.

After a year or so, my father regained custody of my brother and sisters and me. But he was a blue collar guy who just didn't have the means to take care of 5 kids. We moved into a government-subsidized complex in Carpentersville, Illinois where all of the neighboring families were just as poor as we were. Here I had to learn to defend myself. It seemed there were older, bigger kids everywhere, bullying the smaller kids like me. In school, the more fortunate students would taunt me because they knew my clothes came from the Salvation Army.

When I was 10, my father met Gail. She was educated, cultured, and definitely not from a low-income background. We eventually moved out of the projects and into her two-bedroom apartment. It was cramped, but somehow we made it work. Gail bought us new clothes, introduced us to spirituality, and dragged us out of the Hell we had been living in. She made sure we were fed and that we went to school. She even tried teaching us proper etiquette, albeit with mixed results.

Soon, my father married Gail and she adopted all of us. We moved into a Victorian home in Elgin, Illinois, when I was 12. Things were beginning to move quickly in all of our lives.

It wasn't long, however, before things started going sour. Gail didn't know how to deal with a bunch of obnoxious kids and my father couldn't seem to understand why. Very rarely did we all get along. Meanwhile, I detested school, rarely attending, thinking I would never need any kind of education for what I assumed would be a career in a factory somewhere.

I detested school, rarely attending...

To get away from the troubles at home and school, I joined a local theatrical group that met every Tuesday and Thursday night. It was my haven, my escape from reality. I could focus on learning a new tap dance or song for the next show. The people of the theatrical group were very welcoming, which was completely different than what I had ever experienced. They hugged one another and everybody always asked everybody else how they were doing. My own family, on the other hand, would just as soon whack you as ask how your day was going.

I befriended the director of the group, a Roman Catholic priest who was fond of theatre. He often had tickets to local plays and would invite groups of kids to enjoy the performances with him. I soon became a regular attendee at these plays. Weekend events at the priest's house became more frequent and I enjoyed the group's kindness and generosity.

One evening, I was invited to go to a play that didn't end until after midnight. We all went back to the priest's house afterwards and crashed in sleeping bags on the floor. I hadn't told my father or Gail how late I was going to be, so I assumed (maybe out of spite) that it was all right to sleep over with all the other kids and go home in the morning. That turned out to be a big mistake. When I got home, my father and I got into an argument that escalated into a fist fight. In the end I was banished from my father's house. I was all of 13 years old.

With nowhere else to go I went back to the priest and told him what had happened. We filed child abuse charges against my father. In time, the priest adopted me and enrolled me in a Catholic high school. I made new friends and I would sometimes go to their homes for dinner and observe how each family member interacted with the other family members. I would marvel at how wonderful it must have been to talk with – to be friends with – your father, your mother, your brothers, and sisters. I dreamed that if I were to ever have a family, this is how it would be.

I enjoyed my new life and being around loving people, but still, I loathed school. I never opened a book or did any homework. I received low grades and it became evident to everyone by my senior year that I was the principal's biggest troublemaker. Two weeks before graduation I was expelled for writing a belligerent letter to a teacher – and having the audacity (or stupidity) to sign my name to it. I had to beg and plead with the school directors to let me back so I could graduate. In retrospect, I think they allowed me back in to avoid having to deal with me the following year. I graduated with a 1.1 grade point average. At the age of 18, I was essentially illiterate. My classmates voted me "most likely to be in prison the rest of his life." It turns out, they weren't too far off.

At the age of 18, I was essentially illiterate.

I suppose I had some street smarts, but my lack of book smarts got me into trouble right off the bat. In a job interview, the hiring manager asked me when I would be ready to make the transition into the offered position. When I had to ask him what "transition" meant, the interview essentially concluded. Needless to say, I never heard from him again.

Eventually, my father, with whom I had begun speaking again, found me work as a janitor, right alongside of him. One night after work my father took me to one of the bars he and his colleagues would frequent. As the smallest one in the group usually does, I tried to drink more than everyone else to prove I could keep up. And, as what usually happens, the smallest one failed. One of my father's friends drove me to his house where I fell asleep on the couch. I was later awakened by him and his girlfriend arguing. Needing fresh air, I ventured out, not paying a whole lot of attention to which apartment I had left. When I returned, I ended up knocking on several doors, staggering into three of them before realizing they were the wrong ones. Eventually, someone must have called the cops because before I knew it I was handcuffed and poured into the backseat of a squad car. I was charged with 3 counts of breaking and entering along with an array of other charges.

I was subsequently kicked out of the priest's house and, with nowhere else to go, went to live with my oldest sister who had, by then, been living with her boyfriend and her son. My other two sisters and my brother had moved out of my father's house by then, too, and had also moved in with my older sister. There we all were – seven of us, living in a one-bedroom apartment.

I continued to get in trouble with the law. I was in a virtual no man's land, without a clue as to what I was going to do with my life. Then I saw the movie *Top Gun* and had an epiphany. Thinking it would be cool to be in the Navy, I enlisted, imagining the life of heroic glamour and excitement that I had seen on the screen. Of course it was nothing like that. Instead, they had me doing push-ups until I vomited. But if there's one thing I owe the military, it's learning the meaning of discipline. The company commanders didn't let anyone quit anything. I would later learn to appreciate that.

After my naval excursion, I moved back in with my adopted priest father, promising that I would become serious about getting into the local community college and get my life on track. But I failed miserably on the entrance exam and was forced to take remedial classes to bring me up to a college level in mathematics and English. The only thing I got right on the ACT was my name, even though I think I even misspelled my last name.

The fact is, I was nervous. At age 20, I had a 9th grade education in math and an 8th grade level in reading. Since I did slightly better in math, I determined to get a degree in accounting. Unfortunately, the whole debit/credit thing threw me off and the mock companies in my classroom exercises always ended up making zillions because I just kept adding all the numbers together. "I'd like to invest in a company of yours," my instructor told me sarcastically. "I'd be a zillionaire, too!"

After one semester, I was bored out of my mind with the whole educational system. I couldn't find an area of study that interested me – at least not until I got involved with the theater department. There's something about people who are drawn to theater; they're all misfits in some way. Perhaps that's why I've always gravitated towards theater.

My theatrical instructor, Jerry Mathis, seemed to think I had talent and worked hard to get certain emotions out of me. At the time, I was dating a super outgoing girl who was ambitious and going places in her life. She, along with Jerry, tried encouraging me to take risks and push myself beyond what I thought my capabilities were. But I wasn't willing to take the risk of straying outside of my comfort zone. My excuse was that I wasn't good enough to do the things they thought I could do. That was always my excuse. It all went back to my low self-esteem, the negative critic I had been nurturing in my head my whole life, constantly telling me *I wasn't good enough*. Eventually, they both got discouraged working with me and my girlfriend broke up with me, telling me that she just didn't think I'd ever be capable of taking the necessary risks one needs to take in order to grow.

> At age 20, I had a 9th grade education in math and an 8th grade level in reading.

christopher SASHA

Maybe that was the catalyst I needed to take my first real leap into the unknown. I put everything I had in me into entering the modeling world, thinking that I could use modeling as a stepping stone to acting. People were always asking if I was a model anyway, so how hard could it be? My first test shoot was with a local photographer who had an artistic eye. I was so nervous my knees were uncontrollably shaking. She suggested a glass of wine to calm myself. That glass turned into almost two bottles. Needless to say, I was beyond calm, close to comatose. But the shoot went well and the next day I called every modeling agency in Chicago, trying to make appointments to get signed on.

...the negative tape-recorded message in my head... controlled me.

When the very first agency I visited rejected me, the negative tape-recorded message in my head returned – as always – telling me to throw in the towel. But I decided to try another agency. Before the booker even looked me in the eye, she rejected me, too. I left that agency and saw a park nearby. I schlepped over to one of the benches and sat for a long while, wondering why I was such a big loser and why I was putting myself through all of this hardship.

Again, I was thinking, *"I'm not good enough."* As with the rest of my life to that point, I was allowing cognitive dissonance to control me. The mental critic that perpetually annihilated my every goal paid me another visit. But should I be upset with the critic? After all, it was only trying to save me from rejection and adversity. I eventually stood up and began walking to my car, wondering along the way what the real purpose of all of this was. Wasn't I just kidding myself? Did I truly expect everyone to drop what they were doing and exalt me as the new Calvin Klein underwear model?

As I thought harder about it, I began to understand that I needed to overcome my fears and push myself beyond what I thought my capabilities were. I needed to move outside of my comfort zone. Challenging my ego's warnings of rejection, I turned around and went to the next agency. Again, I was rejected. The next agency turned me away too. But after 10 different bookers from 10 different modeling agencies tore my looks and physique to shreds, I met Elite's men's department booker, Brad. He broke me down a little, too, but he saw that I could work in the Chicago modeling market and was willing to take a chance on me. I was proud of myself and learned a valuable lesson. I stood up against my inner critic, and proved to myself that maybe I *am* good enough.

Had I walked to my car after that first rejection, I would have never signed a year contract with Elite Modeling Agency – the same agency where Cindy Crawford got her start. Since that turning point, I have come to discover that most of the time, when I push myself beyond my comfort zone, I find I can accomplish my goals and learn more about myself. Sure, sacrifices sometimes need to be made, but the lesson is that if you think the end result is worthwhile, you can overcome amazing obstacles and discover your inner spirit. It's astonishing what you can overcome if you push yourself beyond what you think your limits are. You can accomplish anything you set your mind to. The only limits are those you create for yourself, and those limits are usually caused by ignorance about what your possibilities really are.

The average sedentary person loses about 6 pounds of muscle every 10 years.

When I signed my modeling contract, I had just turned 21. I put my higher learning objectives on the back burner which, at the time, didn't bother me one bit. I was still skinny, but my booker told me I had to start watching what I ate and begin a workout regime. I couldn't quite grasp why he wanted me to do this because I was always able to eat whatever I wanted without gaining an ounce. He explained to me that even though I weighed the same and looked the same on the outside, as I had for the past several years, my body was changing on the inside. The average sedentary person loses about 6 pounds of muscle every 10 years. Yet that person may still weigh the same. This means that the body changes its composition from muscle to fat. The human body is amazing at maintaining homeostasis, keeping itself, in other words, in a consistent state. So if 6 pounds of muscle is lost, 6 pounds of fat will be gained.

I embarked on an exercise plan and cut out ice cream, French fries, and pizza. But to my surprise, I started gaining weight. I couldn't squeeze into my tight T-shirts anymore. I thought I was getting fat! What I didn't realize was that I was gaining important muscle that was denser and therefore weighed more than fat. But all I knew at the time was that there was an apparent connection between my exercising and my weight gain, so I stopped exercising. The end result was that, because I refused to get my body in better shape, my booker stopped working with me and I eventually lost my contract.

Our beliefs, attitudes, and behaviors are just some of the responsibilities of our subconscious minds.

I later learned that losing my modeling contract was just one time, out of many, when my subconscious mind didn't agree with my conscious mind. And when there is a disagreement between the conscious mind and

christopher SASHA

subconscious mind, the subconscious mind always wins.

Our beliefs, attitudes, and behaviors are just some of the responsibilities of our subconscious minds. I made a positive affirmation that I was good enough to earn a contract with Elite Modeling Agency. The positive affirmation was done at the conscious level. I only said it once. More importantly, I actually only said, "*Maybe* I am good enough." In the end, my subconscious mind didn't believe my conscious mind. My underlying belief that "I'm not good enough" was still on high alert and I ended up sabotaging my own efforts.

Without modeling, and not wanting to go back to school, I started working in bars as a bouncer and getting in trouble again. This was another subconscious behavior that reinforced my belief that I wasn't good enough. It was a vicious cycle. Low self-esteem is a breeding ground for negativity. Quantum physics has scientifically proven thoughts to be energy. According to the laws of attraction, negative thoughts attract negative energy. At this point in my life, I was living the theory.

One night, working the front door of a bar, a drunken customer blind-sided me with a right hook to my eye because I wouldn't let his friend in the club. Instinctively, I punched him, knocking him out cold. Another guy, with his girlfriend, enthusiastically waiting in line to get in, gave me $100 for getting the drunken guy away from them. This led to a downward spiral into corruption. I started fighting on the streets for money. I wasn't making enough as a bouncer and I didn't have the education to get a real job. A group of guys, including the one who gave me $100, would start trouble with anyone. When someone would defend himself, the guys would bet him that he couldn't beat me to a pulp. Drunken guys always fell for this trick. There seems to be liquid muscles in beer.

> The only limits and barriers we have are the ones we create for ourselves.

I was at a low point in my life and it didn't matter to me how I was paying the bills. Most of the time the police were called before the fight was over and I would be arrested and brought to the police station.

At the time, I lived with a corrupt police officer who would come get me and would ask the arresting officers to drop everything. That saved me many times, but not every time. The last fight I had, I was arrested and had to stay 24 hours in a cell before they let me out on an "I-Bond," an Individual Bond that promised I would show up in court on the set date. I was given court supervision for 6 months and ordered not to get in trouble during that time.

Being locked up in the cell gave me time to think. It was in that jail cell that I realized I was quickly going nowhere. I promised myself that I would go back to school and finish getting my degree in something. Once again, I moved back in with my adopted priest father, swearing to God that this time I would finish my education.

I kept that promise. I studied day and night to bring my competence level up to where the average 23-year-old should be. I was accepted to Southern Illinois University at Edwardsville. St. Louis was only 10 minutes away from campus, which meant that I could get back into modeling to help pay for my education.

While attending Southern Illinois, a friend of mine tried to talk me into applying to DePaul University in Chicago, a private university that costs a small fortune to attend. The financial aspect was only part of the problem. The bigger part of the problem came from my fear-based inner voice, already whispering, *"You're not smart enough to get accepted."*

After months of waffling on the idea of transferring to DePaul, I decided that I wouldn't know unless I tried. I set an appointment to take the entrance examination and crossed my fingers. A couple of weeks later, I received a call from one of DePaul's representatives. He told me that because I was 24-years-old at the time, I was eligible to be accepted in a new program they were offering for adults. I would be on probation my first year and then they would re-evaluate. My heart stopped. I couldn't believe I was being accepted into a business school whose part-time MBA program has been ranked in the top 10 in the country for the previous 11 years.

My first year at DePaul, I would get to the library before the sun came up and stay until the sun went down. All my hard work paid off. I made the Dean's List, was taken off probation, and became an A-B student. And for no other real reason than because I was apparently better at math than English – 9th grade level versus 8th! – I decided to get a degree in finance. While earning my degree, I got back into modeling for Elite and this time I was determined to make it work for me. I did everything my booker told me to do including working out.

> I made the Dean's List, was taken off probation, and became an A-B student.

I joined a gym and met the most incredible person, Greg Houseton. He was a strong advocate of working out and staying fit. He was more active and in better shape than anyone in the gym. I needed to get in shape quickly so I could start doing underwear modeling again and he was the one to get me there. I followed him around like a lost puppy. Greg competed as a

bodybuilder and had a natural body that could have given Schwarzenegger
a run for his money. I worked out with him religiously
for 3 years and eventually competed with natural amateur
bodybuilding myself.

Competitive bodybuilding forced me to focus, taught
me how to compete and exposed me to new people.
Because of Greg, I got my physique in the best shape of
my life. He taught me the right foods to eat, how much to
eat, and when to eat. I also learned how to diet properly
so I wasn't always on some yo-yo weight gain/weight loss
program. I got my body fat down to 3.9% and weighed in at a cool 198 pounds.
I finally had confidence in front of the camera and the desire to be one of the
best fitness models in Chicago. I did a tastefully nude photo shoot for the
front of my composite card, the calling card models leave with photographers
hiring for the shoot.

Sylvester Stallone has been my physique hero since I was 13-years-old. I
wanted to compare my body to his. I replicated a photo he did for the cover
of *Vanity Fair* in 1993. It was extremely risqué for Chicago, but it rewarded
me many times over. I got a plethora of auditions because of that shot and a
deluge of fashion shows. Thank you, Sly, for inspiring the shot.

> Sylvester
> Stallone has
> been my
> physique hero
> since I was
> 13-years-old.

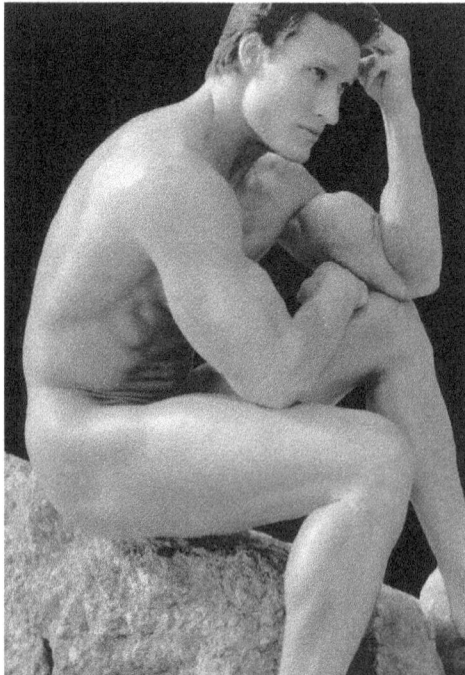

christopherSASHA

I graduated DePaul and landed a job as an internal auditor for Chicago Title and Trust. I had a huge student loan and had to get a part-time job at night and on weekends to help pay it off. An old friend of mine introduced me to a guy who was looking for someone to help him part-time as a personal trainer. The only experience I had was training for competitions, but he gave me a shot at the position, which was my first step into the exciting world of fitness and nutrition.

...my deep subconscious belief that I'm not good enough, or smart enough, or strong enough.

It was a little rocky at first because training for competitions and training weekend warriors are two entirely different animals. I was used to pushing people through their physical barriers and what they thought were the confines of their capabilities. Now I had to get myself to relax in the gym by not pushing the client too hard, but hard enough to at least break a sweat. I often found myself wondering how my clients could have the drive and determination to own and operate their own companies when they gave up so easily in the gym. When things got tough, they would quit and then complain that they weren't losing weight or gaining muscle.

I was working in corporate America and personal training for a little over a year when Chicago Title and Trust merged with Fidelity. When the merger was finalized, my team was laid off and I had my first encounter with corporate perfidiousness. I was disappointed, embarrassed, humiliated and felt betrayed after all the long hours and sacrifices I had made to work my way up the corporate ladder.

I had embarked on a road of interviews to find another finance position when my boss at the gym asked me to work full-time as a personal trainer while he laid the groundwork for a new company he was starting. The deal was that I would lead his personal training division while he focused on the start-up. We agreed that I would handle all the personal training affairs and give him one year to get the company up and running, then I would slide into the chief financial officer position and relinquish the training to a new hire. Finally, my professional career had taken off.

At least, that's what I thought. After 6 months of this arrangement, everything fell through. He was constantly borrowing from his investors to pay bills until he was in over his head. He stopped coming to the office and eventually disappeared with a huge sum of investors' money. Again, I was made to realize how treacherous corporate America could be and determined that the only way I could prevent myself from falling victim to this situation again was to be my own boss. But what a frightening thought. And there it

christopher SASHA

was again: my deep subconscious belief that I'm not good enough, or smart enough, or strong enough. I was at the end of the plank with pirates jabbing me with their daggers. It was time to jump into the unknown, the depths of the deepest oceans, and either sink or swim.

I didn't have a clue as to what I was doing. But I starting thinking about how I accomplished all the things in my life that I didn't initially think I could do. All the things I attained, when I thought the goal was impossible, happened because I slowly changed my subconscious belief that *I'm not good enough* to *I am good enough*. Coupling my new belief that *I am good enough* with everything I learned in the gym helped me become successful in the fitness and nutrition business. In the gym, I learned determination and hard work. I learned how to focus and set both short-term and long-term goals. I learned how to overcome my fears and how to struggle to progress to the next level. From the gym, I already had every tool I needed. And I had created a new belief. Now it was just a matter of organizing and setting short-term goals.

In the end, I came from the dregs of society and cultivated and positioned myself amid some of the most prominent business people in America through physical fitness. There were many times I questioned if I was doing my part to make this world a little better place to live. After years of being a personal trainer, I have met some of the most incredible people who have taught me that it's not what you do for a living, but rather how you contribute to the lives of others. I now realize that I make my clients happier and healthier one hour at a time.

> "If you think you can or think you can't.... you're right."
> ~ Henry Ford

Never give up on your goals and aspirations, and know that you can accomplish anything you set your mind to because you ARE good enough.

President Franklin D. Roosevelt famously stated that, "The only thing we have to fear is fear itself." Push yourself through what you might think are your limits and I promise you will find that you are capable of much more than what you expect. Always remember that the only limits and barriers we have are the ones we create for ourselves.

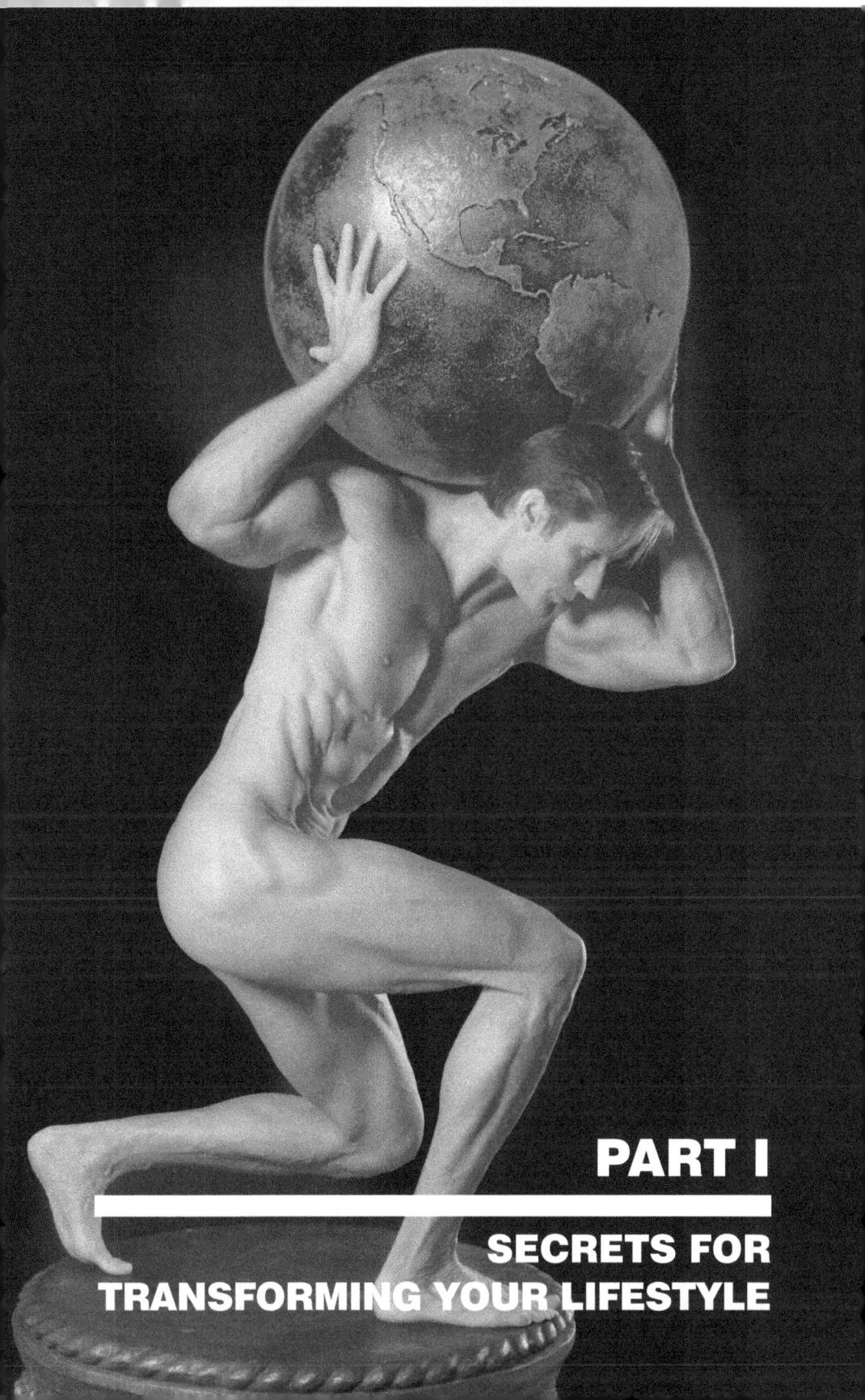

PART I

**SECRETS FOR
TRANSFORMING YOUR LIFESTYLE**

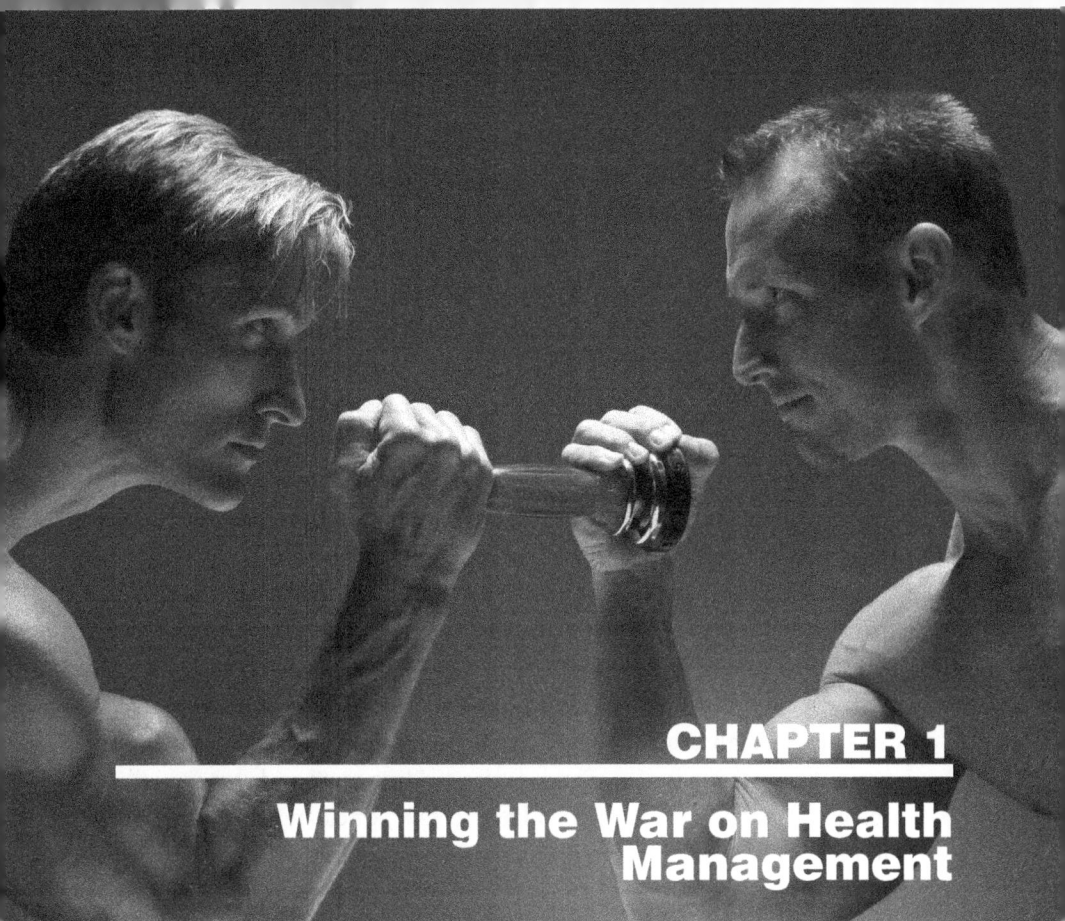

CHAPTER 1
Winning the War on Health Management

The ancient poet and philosopher Virgil said, "The greatest wealth is health." It seems most people are so worried about their *wealth* management that they put their *health* management on the back burner. They lose their health to make money... then lose

"The greatest wealth is health."

~ Virgil

their money to restore their health. In the end, we come to the realization that health and wealth go hand-in-hand.

Almost everyone I know has a retirement plan. They know exactly how much money they have in their checking account, money market account, 401(k) – right down to the penny. And they have budgets and know exactly how much money they need to cover their expenses. Yet almost none of them can recite their cholesterol levels or blood pressure readings, or even remember the last time they had a physical. If people would put a fraction of their efforts towards health management as what they put into wealth management, heart attacks, chronic illnesses, and obesity would not be at the epidemic proportions they currently are in the United States.

The thing is, our monetary aspect of life is elementary when you stop and think about it. It's a simple equation. You have to have enough green stuff in your account to pay your bills. Whatever remains after that makes your account fat. Well, if you start thinking about calories like money and your body as the bank, you'll find that losing and/or managing weight is also a simple system. Just as you know how much money you need to pay your bills, you should know how many calories your body requires to achieve and/or remain at a healthy weight. Earning more dough than what you owe your creditors makes your bank account overflow the same as consuming more calories than your body can utilize results in an overflowing waistline. Get the picture?

...planning time for exercise and what to eat and when to eat is our plan of attack.

No war has ever been won without a plan of attack. Most people use a financial planner to get their retirement plan rolling. The financial planner uses strategies and a plan of attack to assist in building a nest egg for your future. Your wealth management plan is to save enough money so that you will have enough to enjoy your much deserved retirement when the time comes. My question is, if so many of us are willing to set aside time to talk with a financial planner, adjust our budgets to save, calculate compound interest on an annual basis and watch our wealth grow, then why don't we spend a fragment of that time learning a few tactics to plan exercise and calorie intake to achieve and/or maintain a healthy body? After all, if you don't have your health, all that cash you've been saving isn't going to go towards your retirement. Assuming you survive long enough, it's probably going to be spent on doctor and hospital bills.

Losing weight usually doesn't just happen. So allow me to be your health management coach. Just like with financial planning, you need to think and prepare, especially at the beginning. Here are the main criteria I follow to maintain a *Transforming Your Lifestyle* body, outlined on the following page:

10 Transforming Your Lifestyle COMMANDMENTS...

1. Understandeth that not all grams are created equal.

2. Thou must burn more calories than thou consumes.

3. Thou shalt not lose more than one or two pounds per week. Avoideth rapid weight loss diets.

4. Honour exercise to sustain a healthy weight.

5. Thou shalt always make time for breakfast.

6. Increaseth thy number of meals per day whilst decreaseth thy calories per meal.

7. Thou shalt not ban foods.

8. Thou shalt not forget that forgotten calories add up quickly.

9. Thou must learn to read Food Labels.

10. Thou must form new habits to implement a maintenance plan to keep unwanted weight off.

Obesity and chronic disease is our war, and planning time for exercise and what to eat and when to eat is our plan of attack. Permanent weight control is linked to a few healthy habits:

1. Understandeth that not all grams are created equal.

Calories come from our three macronutrient sources – protein, carbohydrates, and fat. One gram of protein and carbohydrate each equals 4 calories, whereas one gram of fat equals 9 calories. Try to use fats (including monounsaturated and polyunsaturated) sparingly so you don't spend too many of your daily calories on this food source. Concentrate on eating proteins and complex carbohydrates. Our daily goal is to keep our macronutrients as close as possible within the range of 30% fats, 30% protein, and 40% carbohydrates. Many of my clients seem to think that they can eat as much as they want of a food as long as it's healthy. What they're forgetting is that even healthy foods have calories – from fats, proteins, and carbohydrates. Portion control is essential.

> One gram of protein and carbohydrate each equals 4 calories, whereas one gram of fat equals 9 calories.

2. Thou must burn more calories than thou consumes.

An individual may devour 3,000 calories per day and only burn off an average 2,750 calories per day. Though this might sound inconsequential, when you add up the numbers at the end of a month, this person will have gained a little over 2 pounds. This is how most people gain unnoticeable weight. Then they wonder how they packed on 24 pounds in a year and can't fit into their clothes anymore.

Weight gain is usually a slow, steady process. Throughout the day, a few extra calories are eaten here and a few extra calories are eaten there. One daily Oreo cookie has 50 culpable calories which translates to over 5 unwanted pounds each year. Fortunately, the opposite is also true. If an individual eats 2,000 calories per day and metabolizes 2,250 calories, that individual will theoretically lose a little over 2 pounds every month. The problem that most dieters have a hard time accepting is how long it takes to lose weight the correct and healthy way. They fail to realize that

> One Oreo cookie per day translates to over 5 unwanted pounds per year.

they didn't become overweight or obese overnight. And that leads us to our third strategy.

3. Thou shalt not lose more than 1 or 2 pounds per week. Avoideth rapid weight loss diets.

According to the Prevention Research Center at Yale University School of Medicine, the progression from lean to overweight to dangerously obese occurs one pound at a time. We can also regress from dangerously obese to overweight to lean one pound at a time. Cutting back a few calories each day leads to a lot of lost calories by the end of the year. Getting to your desired weight doesn't happen overnight, just like becoming overweight didn't happen overnight.

The problem is that we live in a society of instant gratification. When we finally get the courage to lose weight, we're gung-ho at the beginning, trying to lose 10 pounds in a single week, looking for that quick fix. We want *rapid* weight loss and won't settle for anything less! No wonder you see advertisements for weight loss pills everywhere you look – in magazines, commercials, billboards, busses – all with mind-boggling promises of "melting" 30 pounds in 30 days.

But the fact is, if you're losing more than a pound or two a week, you're probably losing more water and muscle than fat. For every 3 pounds of total body weight lost, an average of one pound will be muscle. If you're extremely overweight, you could very well lose an extraordinary amount of weight very quickly. But let's take a closer look at the weight that you'd be losing. On the outside, you might see a slimmer and sexier person. But the inside is a different story. With a rapid weight-loss program, your new body will most likely be the result of the loss of water and muscle and, unfortunately, very little fat.

Cutting your calories drastically slows your metabolism to a screeching halt, sending a signal to your body directing it to store fat for future energy in what it perceives to be an impending famine. When you radically cut your calories, your body simply learns to live on fewer calories. The more extreme you are, the more your metabolism will slow down and the more you will undermine your own efforts to lose weight. Your best bet is to *slightly* cut back calories.

Most people don't know how many calories they're consuming on a daily basis, so they don't know how many calories they can safely cut out of their diet without metabolic interference. This is why food diaries (Chapter 3) are essential. To record your food diary more efficiently, go to my Electronic Food Journal on my website at www.fitbodiesbysasha.com.

Plateaus

Researchers from the National Heart, Lung and Blood Institute recommend a combination of a reduced caloric intake with an increase in physical activity as the best method to achieve *steady and healthy* weight loss. For example, if you cut back 250 calories per day while burning an additional 250 calories exercising, you should lose one pound of weight per week.

An Electronic Food Journal is available on my website at www.fitbodiesbysasha.com.

But you can expect weight plateaus. They're just par for the course. Whatever diet you choose, you will inevitably hit a plateau. One reason might be that the amount of daily calories you consume will eventually equal the amount of calories you burn during the day. At this point, you will neither lose weight nor gain weight – your caloric consumption and caloric expenditure will be at equilibrium. Therefore, a plateau will occur. When you lose weight, your metabolic rate slows down and your body requires fewer calories. Once that happens, you'll need to slightly reduce your caloric intake again to start losing weight again. This is where a food diary becomes your ally.

Start a food diary for the next two weeks to see where you can shave a few calories. Remember: if you cut back on your calories *too* much, your metabolism will slow down, possibly causing a plateau in your weight reduction efforts. In the weight management world, slow and steady always works for the long haul.

Another reason you might confront a plateau is water retention. Your body retains water for various reasons. You might have too much sodium in your system, for example. This can be reversed by increasing your water consumption to dilute the sodium already in your body. Or try lowering your sodium intake. Some medications can also cause water retention. Believe it or not, the muscle you've gained from exercising will also make you weigh more. Don't fret! This is "good weight." It will keep your metabolism revving and your fat perishing. Muscle is over 4 times more dense than fat, which means that, given the same amount of space, muscle weighs more. If your clothes are getting droopy and you still weigh the same, you're doing everything right.

The scale can't determine if the weight loss is fat or lean muscle mass.

Most fad diets, and in fact any diet that requires you to practically eliminate whole food groups, may result in a quick-fix weight loss, but will more than likely fail you in the long term. And when whole food groups are essentially eliminated, certain nutrients are lost. When carbs are eliminated, for instance (or even greatly reduced to the 20-60 grams per day recommended by your average "low-carb" diet), fiber is lost. Fiber helps control blood sugar levels, reduces levels of serum cholesterol, and reduces the risk of colon cancer by quickly carrying waste products through the digestive tract.

Most diet books these days promise you will "lose 10 pounds in one week," "lose belly fat first," "lose weight without exercising," or "never have to count calories." If these diets delivered what they promise, why, according to the Center for Disease Control and Prevention, are more than 67% of adult Americans over the age of 20 overweight, of which 34.3% are obese? Furthermore, 18% of American adolescents (ages 12-19) are overweight and obese. These figures are steadily increasing each year. Why are there more than 112,000 premature deaths associated with obesity each year in the United States, second only to deaths related to smoking?

67% of American adults are overweight… fad diets don't deliver what they promise.

Americans spend billions of dollars on diet products yet, according to a government review, two-thirds of U.S. dieters regain all the weight they lose within a year, and 95% regain it within five years. According to IRS Ruling 202-19 (April 2, 2002), "Obesity is medically accepted to be a disease in its own right." That's right – obesity is no longer considered the catalyst. It's actually the disease.

95% of American dieters regain all their lost weight within 5 years.

Clearly fad diets are, at best, short-term solutions to long-term problems. Remember, overweight or obese individuals don't become that way overnight. It takes effort to reverse the condition, and time. But if you're serious about losing weight and keeping it off, I promise that it gets easier. I won't promise you that you'll lose 10 pounds in a week – or even that you'll lose one pound per week. I won't promise you that you won't feel hungry at first. Your body is accustomed to 'x' amount of calories per day and when it doesn't get it, you'll suffer hunger pangs (which usually subside within 20 minutes). It'll take a little while for your body to adjust and the hunger pangs to abate.

But what I *will* promise you is that, just like anything else, you'll get out of the *Transforming Your Lifestyle* program what you put into it. You'll learn to constantly evaluate calories to make better food decisions, something which will get easier in time because you'll start remembering how many calories are in a certain food. In time, it will become a habit, which is one of the many responsibilities of your subconscious mind. It will become your new belief. And after a while, you'll find that you won't be checking the clock constantly to see how long it's been since your last meal.

Recently I did a little experiment of my own. For two days I consciously counted how many times I thought about the calories in the foods I was about to consume to adjust for upcoming meals and my caloric requirements for the day. And I counted how many times I looked at my watch to see how long it had been since I'd last eaten. The results didn't surprise me. I thought about the calories in my meals as often as Joan Rivers has plastic surgeries (zillions). But I looked at my watch just once, after a three hour meeting. You might be thinking that I've lived a healthy lifestyle for quite some time so these results might be expected. That's the point! In time, you'll have this mindset as well.

In the beginning, when I decided to do everything within my power not to become a statistic of heart disease, type 2 diabetes, hypertension, gallbladder disease, prostate cancer or colon cancer (and so on), it was a laborious undertaking to count calories and to compute my daily caloric intake. But as time passed, it became easier. I made a basic framework for my diet. I wrote down all the foods I like and broke down each macronutrient in each one. Then I created a daily meal plan to meet my calorie requirements for the day. I stay close to this plan, with little tweaks here and there, and I always end at or a little under my recommended daily calories. Today, I do it subconsciously, making basic calculations with food choices and allowing my body to tell me when to eat. Brave through the blast-off phase and I pledge that a healthier lifestyle will become more manageable with each day.

4. Honour exercise to sustain a healthy weight.

A balanced fitness program consists of resistance training, cardio activities, and stretching.

If you're not doing resistance training while dieting, you're going to lose a lot of muscle. The muscle you lose while dieting is gone forever unless resistance training is a part of your daily activities. This is why diets alone don't work. As early as our mid-twenties, we begin to lose muscle mass. Sedentary people will have a slower metabolism than what they had in their teens, and they accumulate more fat from calories consumed. Muscle burns about five times more calories (even in a resting state) than fat because it's more metabolically active than fat. Resistance training and cardio increase your metabolism, burning calories not only while you exercise, but also *after* your workout, called afterburn. In order to keep the weight off long term (longer than a year), weight must be taken off slowly and a strength training regimen must be implemented.

During these physical activities (weight lifting, kick boxing, tennis – I recommend a combination of both resistance and cardio training), try to keep your average heart rate between 70-75% of your maximum heart rate, discussed in Chapter 10. This will increase the amount of calories burned. Also in Chapter 10, we'll discuss three intensity levels, each producing different results. If you're fine-tuning and want to specifically burn body fat, low-intensity cardio will burn a higher percentage of fat from total calories. If you're trying to lose weight in general and you're in good physical shape, the medium-intensity level might be best for you. The more intense and vigorous your workout, the more calories will be expended.

Gaining muscle seems to be a problem with many of my female clients. They'll notice their bodies getting larger, become alarmed, and stop any and all resistance training. These women start with a certain amount of body fat and a lesser amount of muscle. Then, as they embark upon their weight training program, they gain muscle, making their bodies appear larger. They now have their original body fat *coupled* with the added muscle mass. What they fail to understand is that the new muscle will help their metabolism run faster and will help burn fat in their bodies. This phase is actually only temporary. The body fat diminishes with diet, resistance training, and cardio activities.

> Muscle burns about 5 times more calories than fat.

christopherSASHA

If you feel like your body is getting bigger initially, bear with it through this short phase. I can assure you that you won't be disappointed with your results. Remember, muscle is denser than fat, making it take less space and making your body smaller. When the percentage of your body fat dwindles – and it will – you'll see a much more svelte, sexier you, both inside and out.

5. Thou shalt always make time for breakfast.

I'm sure you've heard the old adage, "Eat breakfast like a king, lunch like a prince, and dinner like a pauper." Your body slows down its metabolism (burns less calories) as a defense mechanism to conserve energy when it hasn't been fed in a few hours. When you wake up, not having eaten anything since your last meal the night before, your body will be in a catabolic (breaking down) state, meaning that your body is consuming muscle tissue, getting the fuel it needs to get you up and running. While you're asleep your body goes through a biochemical process called gluconeogenesis. Your body takes amino acids (protein) from your muscle tissue and transports them to your liver where they're converted to glucose, the only thing your brain can use for energy. Since you haven't eaten for a few hours, your body is low on stored glucose (glycogen) and needs to get it from somewhere to keep your brain fed and operating, so it steals from your muscles, taking the amino acids and converting them into energy. This is why the first macronutrient you need to replenish in the morning is protein, which will stop the cannibalization. I start my day with a whey protein shake because it's a fast-acting protein that gets into the bloodstream quickly, stopping my body from eating my hard earned muscle. I also have a bowl of whole-grain cereal to get the carbs and fiber my body needs to keep my blood sugar level steady and to keep me in control of my appetite for the rest of the day.

> Skipping breakfast lowers the metabolism by 5%.

According to Dr. Wayne Callaway, an obesity specialist at George Washington University, skipping breakfast lowers the metabolism by 5%. Yet I continually hear my clients saying, "If I don't eat breakfast, I'll save myself from some calories." Wrong!

A recent Harvard study found that those who regularly eat breakfast are less likely to become obese. Studies indicate that most people who skip breakfast tend to binge in late morning because they're starved and start to get the jitters due to low blood sugar levels. By the time they eat, their metabolism is even slower than it was when they first woke up. They ignore portion control and gorge on too many calories – usually high-fat, high-density foods which lead to more weight gain.

The National Weight Control Registry (NWCR) was created in 1994 to investigate the characteristics and behaviors of individuals who have been successful at achieving weight loss and keeping the weight off long-term. Participants in the study must have lost at least 30 pounds and must have kept it off for at least a year. Most participants, however, have lost over double that and they've kept it off for over 6 years. Of these members, 90% have one thing in common: they eat breakfast at least 4 days per week.

And if you think a doughnut, Cap'n Crunch, or even a "healthy" breakfast bar is considered breakfast, think again. These types of foods are loaded with sugar which causes your blood sugar level to drop shortly after you eat them. Then you feel sluggish and you're more likely to grab another high-sugar, refined food as a "pick me up." All the while, you're consuming more and more calories, and packing on more and more undesired weight. The body will only utilize the calories it needs to perform its functions. The rest gets either stored as body fat or excreted as waste.

> All the while, you're consuming more and more calories, and packing on more and more undesired weight.

Realize, too, that a cup of black coffee or tea isn't breakfast either. These are essentially calorie-free liquids and will eventually lead to a mid-morning energy crash.

6. Increaseth thy number of meals per day whilst decreaseth thy calories per meal.

Eating more meals consisting of 40% carbs will help calm both you and your appetite. If you continue to eat small meals, your body will perpetually burn calories to digest the foods you're eating. This, in turn, increases your metabolism. The operative words here are "small meals." As you decrease the amount of calories per meal, make certain each meal is well balanced with protein and good fats and carbohydrates. I wouldn't recommend anything less than 1,500 calories per day in order to meet all your daily nutrient requirements.

Here's something you might not know...

The bigger your dish, the more food you'll put on it. When we have large dinner plates, we tend to fill them with food. Needless to say, most of the time we eat it all. If you use a smaller plate, you'll probably still fill the plate, but you'll eat less and you'll still feel satisfied with the smaller portion. Portion size is crucial. Go ahead and give it a try. Use smaller dishes with your children or significant other (without telling them, of course) and see if they go for seconds or if they're satisfied with their initial portion. We live in a world of "super-size" and "more is better" – partly why Americans have become overweight and obese.

When I was competing in amateur bodybuilding, I would read all the muscle magazines which would instill in my mind that I needed to gorge to build muscle. I later learned that it's not the amount of food one eats, but the quality and timing. I learned to eat less and at the right times. I lost more body fat and gained more calorie-burning muscle with nutrient-dense, high quality food. Not only did I lose body fat and gain muscle, but I wasn't hungry like I thought I would have been by eating less.

How many calories you need depends on many factors – age, gender, muscle mass, activity level, height, weight, etc. Determining how many calories you need on a daily basis will be discussed in Chapter 3. I try to eat every 2-3 hours to avoid entering a catabolic state and to keep my blood sugar levels steady. If you wait much longer between meals you'll force your metabolism to slow down and drastically increase the chance of hunger pangs which can lead to binge-eating. Entering a catabolic state forces muscle tissue to be used as energy and you need to avoid this stage at all costs. I have three main meals (breakfast, lunch, and dinner) and a few small snacks in between. When you skip out on your meals, your body's calorie-burning furnace slows down. Eat enough calories to get you through the next 2-3 hours. If you're not very active, you'll need fewer calories and vice-versa. Remember, whatever calories your body doesn't utilize get stored as fat or disposed as waste.

7. Thou shalt not ban foods.

Eating healthy is about planning and making better decisions, not about deprivation. When foods are banned, bingeing is usually right around the corner. The more you ban, the more deprived you feel and the stronger the cravings. By the time you finally give in to your cravings, odds are you'll eat a lot more than you would have had you satisfied the craving earlier. Instead of forbidding yourself from eating something, allow yourself a *small portion* to help manage the agonizing cravings. Don't feel guilty. Just resume your well-balanced diet for the rest of the day. Portion control is imperative with foods you just can't live without because they're usually not very healthy. If chocolate is your vice, try having a few bites of dark chocolate.

Caution: if you are a binge eater struggling with self-control, you might want to avoid this tactic. Sometimes "out of sight, out of mind" may be your best strategy.

It's so much easier when you don't fight food cravings…

Cravings are an enigma for researchers who have a hard time trying to define what a craving actually is. There's no scientific proof for *why* we have cravings for specific foods. It's a popular myth that cravings are triggered because our bodies are low on a particular nutrient. Instead, cravings are usually associated with positive experiences from our past, indicating they're a cognitive behavior. Most dieters curse addictions to certain foods for sabotaging their weight-loss efforts, but it's not the craving that has led them astray. It's the overindulgence when the dieter finally gives in.

It's important not to ban foods or be monotonous with the foods you do eat while you're learning new, healthy eating habits. The more restrictive you are and the more you deny your cravings, the more regular and fierce your cravings will become. Unless you're restricting foods for medical reasons, experts suggest that you don't fight your cravings. You'll risk allowing them to get worse, maybe even uncontrollable. *Portion control* is your only defense at this point. Allow yourself to be guilt-free about – but conscious of – the few bites of whatever it is you crave. And recognize that these cravings will dwindle over time.

christopherSASHA

If you do choose to have a little chocolate to settle your craving, remember to deduct those calories from another food in your diet for the day. I know one serving of my favorite dark chocolate (Organic 73% Cocoa Super Dark by Trader Joe's) has 180 calories. So on the days I crave chocolate, I eliminate something in my daily diet that has at least 180 calories (mainly from fat and sugar) to balance my caloric and macronutrient percentage intake for the day. And I prefer dark chocolate because I know that it has less sugar, more fiber, and twice the amount of antioxidants than milk chocolate, making it a healthier choice. Also, research suggests that milk negates the positive effects of antioxidants. Provided you're not a binge-eater, I assure you the cravings will dissipate when you allow yourself small portions of these foods.

> Eating healthy is about planning and making better decisions, not about deprivation.

With some diets, like the low-fat and low-carb fad diets in the '80s and '90s, it's recommended that you practically eliminate whole food groups. But in reality, the people who are most successful at keeping weight off don't eliminate any of the macronutrients – protein, carbohydrates, and fats. Rather, they practice portion control and exercise about an hour a day, expending an average of 2,800 calories per week. In fact, they burn almost a pound of body fat per week through exercise alone – not including calorie reduction. According to the Division of Nutrition and Physical Activity at the Centers for Disease Control and Prevention, physical activity combined with reduced calorie consumption can lead to the 5-10% weight loss necessary to achieve remission of the obesity-associated complications.

8. Thou shalt not forget that forgotten calories add up quickly.

We already know about the calories packed in the hypercaffeinated marketed Starbucks Latte and the 10 teaspoons of sugar in a can of Coca-Cola, but what about a handful of popcorn or a few M&Ms every now and then? These unnoticed bites and sips add up to a lot of forgotten calories. Only 50 extra calories each day will result in 5 unwanted pounds a year if all other variables remain constant. For parents, those bites taken to 'sample' your child's food can add up. Even Tic Tacs and breath-freshening Altoids can be culprits for weight gain. One client of mine, wanting to keep her breath bearable for fellow colleagues while speaking to them at meetings all day, would pop Tic Tacs … all day long. Those little oral revitalizers might only be

1.9 calories a piece but when you eat an entire box throughout the day – *every* day – those innocent breath mints are capable of packing on over 7 pounds per year. Altoids are even bigger offenders.

Most people completely forget about the calories hidden in condiments, too, like ketchup, sauces like Hollandaise and A1, or butter and mayonnaise. One tablespoon of Kraft Regular Mayonnaise has 100 calories of pure fat. Also, remember what you drink can have a substantial impact on your daily caloric intake. Again, maintaining a food diary for a couple of weeks here and there throughout the year is essential for losing and/or maintaining a healthy weight.

9. Thou must learn to read Food Labels.

The FDA regulates food manufacturers' nutritional facts placed on the back of every packaged food. The most important fact on the label is the number of servings. Food manufacturers are remarkably cunning with their marketing and they know that most people are trying to become more health conscious about calorie consumption. Products like Coca-Cola and Oreo cookies are now being sold as "100 calorie" foods because the serving size of the food or beverage is limited to only 100 calories within that particular package. It doesn't mean it's any healthier; it just means that there's less food or beverage in the package.

Manufacturers list the amount of calories per serving, but some include 1½ or 2 servings per package where the consumer thinks the package contains only a single serving! Consequently, the innocent consumer ends up ingesting twice as many calories as they had intended. If this happens often enough, it can thwart even the best dieter's efforts.

And don't forget all the fancy pseudo names food manufacturers concoct to hide the fact that their products contain sugar. High-fructose corn syrup, dextrose, maltodextrin, organic cane juice, etc. are all *sugar*. By law, the label must list the ingredients in order of amount, so if you see any of those pseudo names listed with the top ingredients, you know you're getting mostly sugar. In Chapter 5 we'll discuss the popular types of sugars.

Most of our cravings are for some type of potato chip or chocolate, which are obviously not healthy food choices. Have you ever seen anyone not able to satisfy their cravings for cauliflower? Food scientists manufacture chemicals to make a food taste good and it's usually one or more of these types of sugars that is used to supersede the real taste of these foods. With these sugars come extra calories and extra weight. Portion control is essential.

Short-term diets generate short-term results.

christopherSASHA

10. Thou must form new habits to implement a maintenance plan to keep unwanted weight off.

According to Merriam-Webster's Collegiate Dictionary, *diet* is defined as "food and drink regularly provided or consumed." Whether low-fat, high-protein, low-carb, or any of the other hundreds of different diets that are out there, a diet is a diet. Many people associate the word "diet" with hunger pangs, but a true lifestyle diet isn't based on deprivation. Changing old habits doesn't mean banning foods. It just means that we need to take a different view as to what we eat and how much our bodies require to remain at a healthy weight for life.

Successful weight loss requires long-term commitment to sensible eating, moderation, determination, and exercise.

If you think you can keep weight off by spending a few weeks on a fad diet and then going back to your old eating habits, think again. Short-term diets generate short-term results. Each year, millions and millions of Americans diet and lose weight. Some even lose over 100 pounds. Obviously, getting the weight off isn't the problem – it's *keeping* the weight off that's the problem. If you don't have a maintenance plan, you'll gain your weight back again. After all that diligent work, feeling better both inside and out, and, of course, looking better, why throw it all away? Why have to start all over again? A lifetime of healthy weight maintenance requires long-term commitment to sensible eating, moderation, determination, and exercise.

For over 95% of dieters, the end result is that, ultimately, they weigh more than their pre-diet weight, resulting in feelings of guilt, shame, and failure. Some of the main reasons dieters regain their weight include unrealistic weight loss goals, lack of daily physical activity, and returning to their old eating habits once they reach their desired weight. It seems as though the vast majority of dieters think of dieting like a race to lose as much weight as they can in the shortest amount of time. When they reach their desired weight, they think the race is over and go back to their old habits. But fighting obesity is a race that will last for a lifetime.

In my 13 years of wellness coaching, I've seen people in the gym almost every day claiming that they need to lose weight for various reasons, but I have never heard anyone say that they want to lose weight to become healthier. It's always because of an upcoming event of some description – their wedding day, swimsuit season, a vacation, a class reunion, or maybe just to lose the weight they gained during pregnancy. Of course we all want to look aesthetically appealing, but that's just a bonus of losing and maintaining a healthy weight. Our real goal should be to ward off disease and live a full, happy, healthy life.

But no matter what the reasons, the people I see in the gym trying to lose weight typically get off to good starts. They set goals, they have motivators to reinforce their goals, and they have rewards in mind for achieving their goals. Some of the most successful clients I have had, for example, are women trying to lose weight in order to look sexy in their wedding dresses. Every marrying woman I know starts counting off days to her wedding. Couple this with the fitting of the dress, the arrangements for the dinner, the band, the cake and all the details involved in planning a wedding, and you can see the presence of constant reminders of both the upcoming wedding and the ongoing weight-loss program.

Impending events are great as effective initiatives to start losing weight. They provide excellent short-term goals and constant reminders to stick with a healthy lifestyle. But your program should not stop once you reach your desired weight. To be truly successful at keeping the weight off long-term we need to form new habits. We need to perpetually

- create new short-term attainable goals,
- reward ourselves for attaining these goals, and
- mold this thought process into our daily lives.

Habits are when your brain runs on auto-pilot and behaviors become almost involuntary. As anyone who has ever tried to break one or create one knows, it's not easy to do either.

It's commonly known that it takes 21 days to create a habit. So, since most diets have a beginning phase that lasts anywhere from 30 days to 12 weeks, why do more than 95% of dieters regain their lost weight? If a dieter is diligent well beyond the 21-day threshold, why is he or she so often unable to convert the dieting into habit?

Often times, we develop habits without even noticing them. For example, when I chew gum, I chomp, sounding – I am told – like a grazing cow. I know, I know … it sounds disgusting. The thing is, I don't even realize I'm doing it and every time it's brought to my attention, I make a conscious effort to change the way I chew. But the habit didn't just "happen" overnight. It was formed over a long period of time. My best guess is that it goes back to when I was a kid and I would want to annoy my brother and sisters with the chomping. Now that I'm an adult, it's obviously not so cute.

Reward yourself… there's a close relationship between rewards and learning.

Six months ago I began to get serious about trying to break this annoying habit, and I'm still learning not to loudly chomp my gum. Now, I'm able to catch myself chomping from time to time, so the doctor in me says that I'm getting much better.

The point is, learned habits are hard to instill in your brain because you have to make a conscious effort to repeatedly do the behavior you're trying to make into a habit. When you continuously repeat the behavior, it eventually becomes programmed into your subconscious and becomes a new habit. My arduous struggle to chew gum like a normal person takes effort on my part. I have to consciously chew rather than chomp. Only through repetition of conscious chewing will it be programmed in my brain to chew and not chomp my gum.

Learned habits require your brain to create a new path of action in order to eventually develop the new behavior. And because my brain is unique, and your brain is too, you and I will not form a habit at the same pace; it will take me either more time or less time than you to form a particular habit. Consequently, there is no single blueprint or schedule for how long it will take any given person to form a given habit.

It's not learning the new habit; it's unlearning the old that keeps most falling back to their old ways. Forming new habits requires work. Some pointers to help form new habits might be to …
- Be as specific as possible about the habit you are trying to form.
- Realize that forming new habits takes time.
- Be as consistent as possible to retrain your brain to put this new habit into autopilot.
- Reward yourself whenever you do your new habit because there's a close relationship between reward and learning.

Let's consider habits in a little more detail.

First, be precise as to what habit you are trying to establish. Instead of saying that you want to lose 50 pounds, try saying that you are going to cut back 250 calories per day and will do cardio on the elliptical for 30 minutes (keeping your heart rate between 70-75% of your maximum heart rate – we'll discuss your maximum heart rate in Chapter 10) every Monday, Tuesday, Wednesday, Thursday, and Friday morning at 6:30 a.m. For most people setting a goal of losing 50 pounds would be unrealistic. But cutting back 250 calories per day and doing 30 minutes of cardio every weekday morning *is* realistic.

Second, patience is essential when trying to instill a new behavior. From my experience with clients, people manifest feelings of failure if they don't automatically adjust to the new habit they are attempting to form. Realize that most successes come about as the result of many previous failures. With failure comes the opportunity to learn what went wrong. For many years the Wright brothers had countless crashes, but from each unfortunate crash they learned. Eventually successful flight was born! The crucial point to remember when and if you fail, is to get right back up and continue your endeavor. I promise if you keep repeating your new healthy habits over and over again, they *will* become automatic.

Third, be consistent where and when you make conscious decisions affecting your new healthy habit. For example, when I grocery shop and try a different food that I've never had before, I automatically read the nutritional value label on the back of the package. I do quick nutritional calculations and I read the Ingredient List. Another habit I've developed is that every morning at 5:30 Monday through Saturday, I go to the gym for my cardio. That way nothing interferes with my getting those 30 minutes of exercise for the day.

Finally – the best part! – reward yourself every time you consciously act to embed the new healthy habit into your life. Research at the Massachusetts Institute of Technology (MIT) indicates that rewards actually prompt changes in the group of nuclei in the brain known as basal ganglia. Basal ganglia are associated with functions like motor control, emotions, and learning. The MIT study shows that reward signals can positively influence these functions.

Diets don't work for permanent weight loss.

Rewards don't have to be expensive or elaborate. They can be simple, as long as they're something you enjoy. The point is to establish a positive feeling when you deliberately introduce a new healthy behavior to your brain. Steer clear of using food and/or alcohol as a reward, though, as you may begin to associate them with pleasure, comfort, and a sense of accomplishment which would undoubtedly cripple your weight loss goals. Try to choose something healthy and fun. When one of my clients met the half-way point to his desired weight, he and his wife went on a weekend getaway, hiking the Grand Canyon. Imagine … exercise as a reward! Another client bought a sleek black dress that was a size too small as her reward, and as extra motivation to lose another five pounds.

Focus on the positives of what you will gain rather than what you will lose when you incorporate new healthy habits into your life. The long-term gains you'll enjoy for the rest of your life by living a healthy lifestyle are

christopherSASHA

immeasurable – especially compared to the possibilities of chronic illness and premature death.

Let's make a commitment to lose weight and keep it off – always. Let's commit to weighing in once a day (the same time each day) – in the morning. That will help keep the pounds from creeping back and will keep us motivated. Weigh yourself every morning as soon as you wake up and use the bathroom, using the same scale, naked. Little weight increases can then be fixed by making adjustments before weight gains interfere with your entire healthy lifestyle. Don't become obsessed with weighing in several times per day; weight differentiation in short periods of time will likely be due to water retention or food passing through the digestive system.

Let's not become statistics. Let's not gain back all our lost weight. Let's learn a new lifestyle and eat our way to a healthy weight, warding off diseases and premature death. Let's not look at this as a diet but rather a lifestyle. We've seen that with traditional diets after reaching our desired weight we go back to our old habits. History has proven time after time that diets don't work for permanent weight loss. Change your history by changing your *beliefs* about food and exercise. Set reasonable and attainable short-term goals and reward your achievements.

Are you now ready to begin the journey to Transforming Your Lifestyle*?*

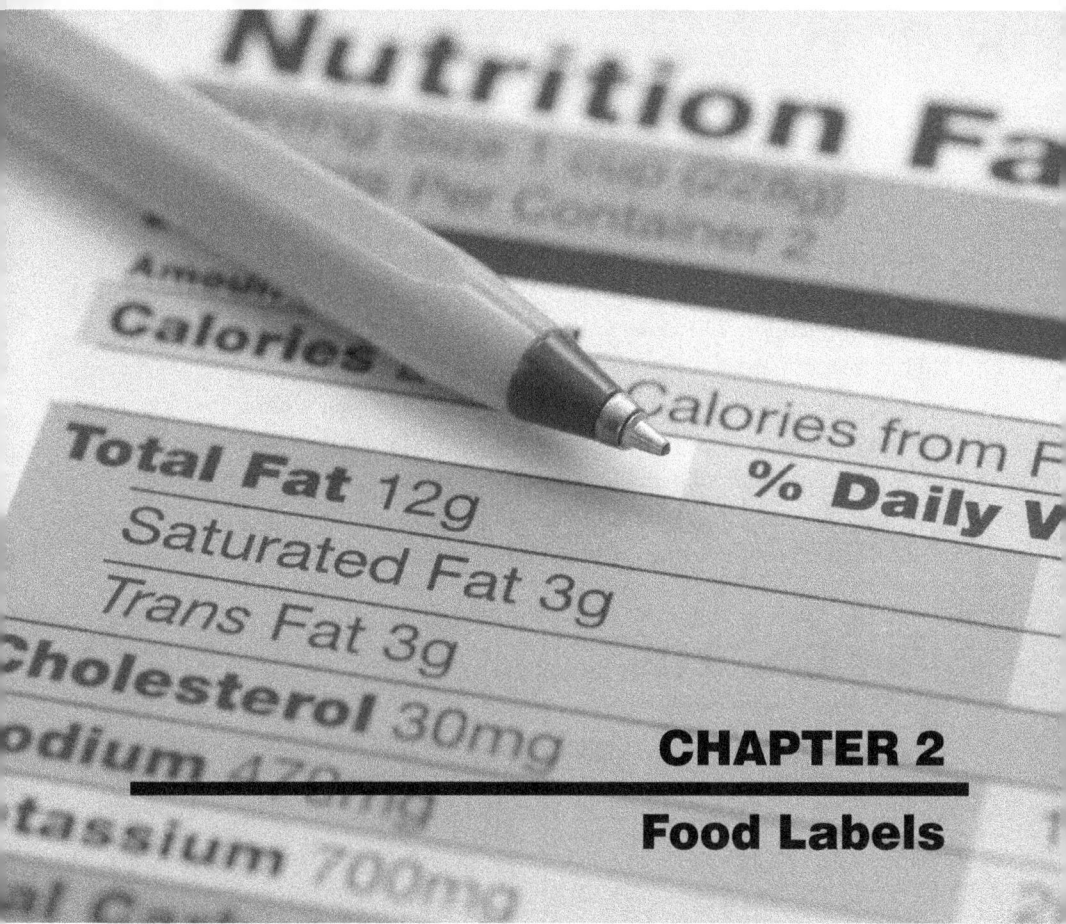

Food Labels, or Nutrition Facts Labels, originated much earlier than most people assume. It's only been a few decades that consumers have utilized these important information notices to make healthier food choices. In 1938, the Federal Food, Drug and Cosmetic Act (FDCA) was passed, requiring every processed and packaged food container to display such information as the name of the food, its net weight, a list of ingredients, etc. Today, the FDA continues to strive to inform consumers about macronutrients (carbohydrates, fat, and protein), and micronutrients (vitamins and minerals) to encourage healthier food choices.

The nutrients currently listed address today's health concerns – diabetes, hypertension, heart disease, cancer, and obesity. These nutrition labels perpetually change as health concerns change with results from the latest studies. Trans fat and food allergens, for example, were required to be listed as of January 1, 2006, after research alerted us to their health dangers. Fats and foods that tend to be

Macronutrients are carbohydrates, fat, and protein; micronutrients are vitamins and minerals.

allergenic, such as milk, eggs, fish, crustacean shellfish, tree nuts, peanuts, wheat, and soybeans are recent additions.

There are many requirements as to what nutrients need to be listed and in what order. Beyond the required nutrients, most of the remaining information on the Nutrition Facts Label is volunteered by the individual food manufacturer. The order is based on the importance of the most current dietary recommendations.

Most people have a very limited understanding about the information on nutrition labels, yet it's imperative to learn how to break down these labels to help you make the choices you'll need to make in order to take control of your diet. At first it may seem a bit daunting, but once you begin learning how to read labels, you'll quickly be able to determine if a food is healthy or not.

Nutrition Facts

Serving Size 1 oz. (28g/about 13 chips) (1)
Servings Per Container 2.5

Amount Per Serving

Calories 140 (2)	Calories from Fat 70
	% Daily Value*
Total Fat 7g	11%
Saturated Fat 1g	5%
Trans Fat 0g (3) (5)	
Cholesterol 0mg	0%
Sodium 105mg	4%
Total Carbohydrate 17g	6%
Dietary Fiber less than 1g (4)	0%
Sugars 0g (3)	
Protein 2g	

Vitamin A 0% (4)	Vitamin C 25%
Calcium 0%	Iron 2%

*Percent Daily Values are based on a 2,000 calorie diet. Your daily values may be higher or lowerer depending on your calorie needs: (6)

		Calories:	2,000	2,500
Total Fat	Less than		65g	80g
Sat Fat	Less than		20g	25g
Cholesterol	Less than		300mg	300mg
Sodium	Less than		2,400mg	2,400mg
Total Carbohydrate			300g	375g
Dietary Fiber			25g	30g
Calories per gram:				
Fat 9		Carbohydrate 4		Protein 4

1	SERVING SIZE / NUMBER OF SERVINGS
2	CALORIES AND CALORIES FROM FAT
3	NUTRIENTS TO RESTRICT
4	NUTRIENTS TO INCREASE
5	PERCENT DAILY VALUE* (%DV)
6	FOOTNOTES

PERCENT DAILY VALUE* (%DV)

5% or less is LOW
6% - 19% is MODERATE
20% or more is HIGH

INGREDIENTS: Potatoes, Corn Oil, Salt.

Source: *Kruncher's - Kettle Cooked Potato Chips (Original Flavor). Individual package.*

Anatomy of a Food Label

1. One of the most important items on the label is the SERVING SIZE / NUMBER OF SERVINGS.

The required nutrition facts are standardized to help make comparisons with similar foods easier, but most people overlook the number of servings in individually-packaged snack foods like chips and candy bars. This can lead to extra calories. Some junk foods contain more than one serving per package, increasing the amount of other nutrients as well as calories. For example, a single bag of Kruncher's Kettle Cooked Potato Chips (Regular Flavor), has 2.5 servings included in what appears to be a one-serving package! If you eat the whole bag, you'll eat two and one-half times the ingredients listed on the nutrition label, resulting in the consumption of 350 calories (140 calories per serving x 2.5 servings). It's an easy mistake to make. You think there are 140 calories, just like the label indicates, but neglect to note the fact that there's more than one serving in the bag. Not only do the calories increase, but other nutrients increase as well. Total fat hits over 17 grams (17g), not the 7g that a cursory look at the Food Label indicates.

Some foods contain more than one serving per package, increasing the amount of calories and nutrients.

This is important because we don't want to ban foods from our diet, but at the same time, we need to manage calories to maintain a healthy weight. Because of this one potential oversight, you might exceed your caloric intake, leading ultimately to significant weight gain over the course of a year.

2. CALORIES AND CALORIES FROM FAT, as you may guess, tells you how many calories are in a food per serving and how many of those calories come from fat.

Calories, the first part of the listing, are a measurement of energy from food – the energy your body needs to produce new blood, transmit messages from your brain to the rest of your body via neurotransmitters, breathe, blink, and everything in between. This information helps those who are trying to count calories.

The other part to this caloric listing, dealing with the amount of calories from fat, indicates just that – the number of calories derived from fat in that particular food. But the problem with the way this information is presented is that people have to stop and *calculate* the percentage of fat calories with respect to the amount of total calories. I believe the percentage itself ought to be displayed. For instance, a food product with 250 total calories might contain 110 calories from fat. But what does that mean? If the percentage was listed, one could tell at a glance that the product is 44% fat.

I know that for me personally, this would have a much bigger impact on my decision as to whether to purchase the food. I already know that I want to keep the total percentage of fat calories around 30% of my daily total caloric intake. At 44%, this food would be out of my range. Or, if I decide I want to eat the food, I know I'll have to choose another food sometime throughout the day with comparable calories, but with almost no calories coming from fat so as to counterbalance the fat from this food.

3. NUTRIENTS TO RESTRICT from our diets because we tend to overeat these "bad" nutrients.

Fats and sodium make foods taste better. The downside is that too much fat, saturated fat, cholesterol, and sodium may increase the risk of cardiovascular disease, hypertension, certain types of cancer, and other chronic diseases. Experts suggest no more than 300 milligrams (300mg) of dietary cholesterol per day no matter how many calories are consumed. In Chapter 6, we'll see how just one large egg yolk contains approximately 210mg of cholesterol.

4. NUTRIENTS TO INCREASE in our diets because we tend to skimp on "good" nutrients like dietary fiber, vitamins A and C, calcium, and iron.

Of course, there's always a possibility of getting too much of these micronutrients.

However, studies indicate that, on average, Americans don't consume enough of them. Calcium is responsible for absorbing fat and building stronger bones, decreasing the risk of osteoporosis. Dietary fiber aids in the flushing of our digestive tracts, which may reduce the risk of colon cancer. Iron helps deliver oxygen throughout our bodies. I don't know about you, but I find that these facts compel me to add more of these micronutrients to my diet.

5. PERCENT DAILY VALUE* (%DV) is the percentage of the listed nutrients from one serving based on a 2,000 calorie diet – not a 1,600 calorie diet, not a 3,500 calorie diet.

I usually consume between 3,000 and 3,500 calories a day, so these percentage values aren't accurate for me. Nonetheless, they do make it easier for me to figure my own values for the amount of daily calories I personally consume. For labeling purposes, 2,000 calories was chosen because many health experts say it approximates the daily required calories for the group at highest risk for excessive intake of calories and fat – postmenopausal women.

Also, it makes it easier for individuals to calculate personal nutrient requirements because it's a round number. Like most people, you might not have a clue as to how many calories you consume on a daily basis. At the very least, you can use these percentages as an educated guess. In Chapter 3 I'll show you how to calculate how many calories you should consume to either lose weight, maintain weight, or to put on quality weight. Or, you may visit my website at www.fitbodiesbysasha.com for all my calculators guiding you to your personal healthy weight. Whatever the case, you'll learn to be as aware of calories as you are with the money in your bank account.

2,000 calories was chosen because many health experts say it approximates the daily required calories for the group at highest risk for excessive intake of calories and fat – postmenopausal women.

Trans Fat

All the calculations for each nutrient, excluding trans fat, sugar, and protein, are done for you on the Nutrition Facts Label. Again, the percentage values are based on 100% of the daily requirements for each nutrient in a 2,000 calorie diet. As for the daily recommendations for trans fat, scientific reports have established how perilous trans fat can be, but no report has yet recommended an amount the FDA can use to determine a % Daily Value. Therefore, trans fat is listed only on the Nutritional Facts Label with the amount of grams per serving until further research is conducted. Trans fat is a bigger health threat than saturated fat because it not only increases LDL

christopherSASHA

28 » Transforming Your Lifestyle

("bad" cholesterol) but it also decreases HDL ("good" cholesterol), and increases the risk of heart disease.

Also, be wary of foods that use hydrogenated oil, whether partially hydrogenated or fully hydrogenated, because this means there is trans fat in the product even though the Nutritional Facts Label might state otherwise. Always vet the Ingredient List for partially hydrogenated oil, hydrogenated oil, or vegetable shortening. If you see any of these pseudo names for trans fat, stay away and find an alternative. This is why it's imperative to read both the Food Label *and* the Ingredient List.

Peanut butter labels (excluding natural peanut butter) are notorious for claiming they have no trans fat. But trans fat is commonly used to prevent oil separation. So how are they able to claim they contain none? They have a little asterisk (*) stating there is **no trans fat per serving**. The FDA allows food manufacturers to claim zero trans fat in their product if there is less than ½ gram of trans fat per serving.

> Read both the Food Label and Ingredient List to get the full story of exactly what's in the foods you eat.

Nutrition Facts

Serving Size 2 Tbsp (32g)
Servings Per Container 14

Amount Per Serving

Calories 190   Calories from Fat 140

% Daily Value*

Total Fat 16g	**25%**
Saturated Fat 3g	**15%**
Trans Fat 0g	
Cholesterol 0mg	**0%**
Sodium 150mg	**6%**
Total Carbohydrate 7g	**2%**
Dietary Fiber 2g	**8%**
Sugars 3g	
Protein 7g	

Vitamin A 0%	Vitamin C 0%
Calcium 0%	Iron 4%
Niacin 20%	Vitamin E 10%

*Percent Daily Values are based on a 2,000 calorie diet.

Ingredients: Roasted Peanuts, Sugar, Hydrogenated Vegetable Oils (Cottonseed, Soybean and Rapseed) To Prevent Separation, Salt.

Source: *Skippy - Creamy Peanut Butter*

Sugars

Sugars are listed on nutrition labels without a %Daily Value because no recommendations have been established for the total intake of sugars per day. However, I strongly advocate keeping sugar intake as low as possible. Unfortunately, on labels, all sugars, whether naturally occurring or added to the food, are categorized in one lump sum. As we'll discuss in Chapter 5, some sugars are worse than others. Fructose, for example, is a natural sugar that comes from fruits the government encourages us to eat. Lactose is a sugar found in the milk products we're urged to consume for our daily requirements of calcium. The sugars we should be more concerned about are the "empty calorie" refined sugars that offer little or no nutrients. These are the sugars that need to be limited.

I strongly advocate keeping sugar intake as low as possible.

On August 3, 1999, the Center for Science in the Public Interest (CSPI) petitioned the FDA to establish a Daily Reference Value for "added sugars" to help consumers better understand the types of sugars they are consuming. Until the FDA mandates nutrition labels to distinguish "natural sugars" from "refined sugars", the only way we can determine if the sugars in a particular food are counterproductive to weight management is to make a special effort to inspect the Ingredient List. By law, this is where food manufacturers must account for everything added when creating the food. The ingredients are listed in descending order by weight, meaning that the most abundant ingredient is listed first. Any preservatives, nutrients, fats, sugars, or color additives that have been added must be listed. This is especially important for individuals who may be allergic to certain ingredients or are trying to reduce certain ingredients… like sugar.

Now that we know where to look for "hidden" sugars, we need to know all the names food manufacturers have concocted to confuse the health conscious consumer. Items like high fructose corn syrup, brown rice syrup, evaporated cane juice invert syrup, maltose, maple syrup, corn syrup, fructose, lactose, glucose, galactose, sucrose, dextrose, fruit juice, organic cane juice, molasses, honey, barley malt, maltodextrin, turbinado, and sorghum are *all sugars*. Again, if you're trying to shave off sugar calories, try avoiding foods that list any of these ingredients at the beginning of the list.

Protein

Protein is the final nutrient with no established % Daily Value. According to the Harvard School of Public Health, adults need a daily minimum of 1 gram of protein for every kilogram of body weight (2.2 lbs.) to help keep the body from slowly breaking down tissue. Beyond that, there's relatively little solid information on the ideal amount of protein in the diet, a healthy target for calories contributed by protein, or the best kinds of protein. However, some people have allergies to certain proteins that come from foods like milk, eggs, fish, crustaceans, tree nuts, peanuts, wheat, and soybeans, which may mean havoc for these individuals when they consume protein from these types of foods.

Another potential problem with protein is what might happen if too much is ingested. Calcium is required to neutralize acids our bodies release during the digestion process, and when large amounts of protein are devoured, an exceptional amount of calcium is required. This means that over long periods of high-protein intake, if you're not getting adequate calcium, your body may excrete calcium from bones, possibly leading to osteoporosis later in life.

Finally, it would be wise to pay attention to drawbacks in some protein choices, such as saturated fat in red meats. If you just can't live without red meat and dairy products, at the very least try selecting lean cuts of meats and skim or low-fat milk products such as ones we'll discuss in Chapter 7. Trust me, your heart will thank you for it.

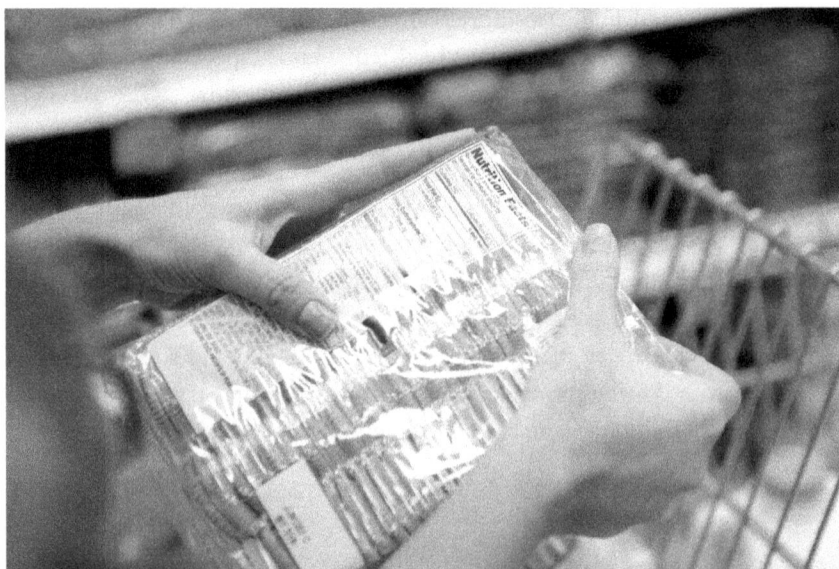

Here's something to make healthy food choices a little easier…

The values in the Percent Daily Value* (%DV) section can be used as a "Quick Guide" to determine if the food item is healthy or not. You can also use the percentages to compare foods. This guide shows you which nutrients have a "low content," "moderate content", and "high content" for a particular food.

- A value of **5%DV or less is LOW.**
- A value **between 6%DV and 19%DV is MODERATE.**
- A value of **20% or more is HIGH.**

When comparing fat, saturated fat, trans fat, cholesterol, sodium and sugar, it's best to choose the products that contain the *lowest percentage values and to consume no more than 100% of the daily value in each of these nutrients*. Dietary fibers, vitamins A and C, calcium, and iron should have *higher percentage values to at least meet 100% of the daily value for these nutrients*.

The important factor to remember when using these numbers is to consider the number of servings in each food package. For instance, look to see whether a package contains a single serving or more. Let's say the package contains 2 servings instead of just 1. Although the quick guide may suggest that each serving contains 14% fat (categorizing this food as having a "moderate" amount of fat per serving), if you ate the whole package, you'd have to double the percentage value, which translates to 28% of your daily value of fat. That would make this food a "high" fat food for a one-time meal/snack. You can still redeem your diet by trading other foods that are low in fat to balance your daily diet. This way, you don't have to forbid yourself from eating foods you enjoy, which will increase your success in *Transforming Your Lifestyle*.

6. FOOTNOTES are at the bottom of nutrition labels.

They state "Percent Daily Values are based on a 2,000 calorie diet. Your Daily Values may be higher or lower depending on your caloric needs." An asterisk (*) after the Percent Daily Value* heading refers to this footnote that is required on all food labels.

There is an additional lower part of the footnote that is not required if the size of the label is too small. This section shows the number of total grams of each nutrient. Some labels show these numbers for a 2,000 calorie diet only, while others provide numbers for both a 2,000 calorie diet and 2,500 calorie diet. When this additional footnote is displayed, these numbers will always be the same no matter what the food product because they're based on public health experts' dietary advice for everyone. Looking closely, you'll notice the only two nutrients that remain constant in both the 2,000 calorie diet and the 2,500 calorie diet are cholesterol and sodium. The cholesterol and sodium numbers don't change because public health experts recommend the upper limit for these two nutrients be less than 300mg and 2,300mg respectively, no matter how many daily calories are consumed. The other nutrients increase as total caloric intake increases.

Some footnotes may even include a "Calories Per Gram" section that lists the macronutrients – fat, carbohydrate, and protein. The purpose of this additional information is to tell the consumer that each gram of protein equals 4 calories, each gram of carbohydrate also equals 4 calories, but each gram of fat equals 9 calories. When you multiply the total amount of protein and carbs by 4 and the total amount of fat by 9, then add the sum of these numbers, it should equal (approximately, due to rounding) the amount of total calories listed in the first section of the Food Label.

Deceptive Claims...

Claims like 85% Fat-free on premium ice cream and 96% Lean/4% Fat on extra lean ground beef are currently flooding supermarkets, erroneously duping the average consumer into believing that he/she is getting a low-fat food. Don't be outfoxed by the food industry! The FDA allows claims like these to be printed on the front label of certain meat and milk products. The only way to protect yourself from these big, bold-print, fallacious claims is to learn how to read and understand the information on the Nutrition Facts Label.

Here's an example label for an extra lean ground beef product I bought at my local supermarket:

96% Lean/4% Fat | Extra Lean Ground Beef

Nutrition Facts
Serving Size 4 oz **(113g)**
Servings Varied

Amount Per Serving

Calories 150	Fat Cal. 45

	% Daily Value*
Total Fat 5g	8%
Sat. Fat 2.5g	13%
Trans Fat 0g	
Cholest. 70mg	23%
Sodium 75mg	3%
Total Carb. 0g	0%
Fiber 0g	0%
Sugars 0g	
Protein 24g	

Vitamin A 0%	Vitamin C 0%
Calcium 2%	Iron 15%

*Percent Daily Values are based on a 2,000 calorie diet.

Source: *Trader Joe's - Butcher Shop*

This product claims to be "extra lean" and "96% lean with only 4% fat". According to regulations, "extra lean" is less than 5g of fat, less than 2g saturated fat, and less than 95mg cholesterol per 100 gram serving. This product contains 5g of fat and 2.5g of saturated fat, so it still qualifies as "extra lean" because the serving size is 113g, which exceeds the 100g serving. Also, there's 70mg of cholesterol, which is less than 95mg suggested by the regulations. The extra lean claim might be hard to dispute.

The second claim, however, is more questionable. The manufacturer claims that this ground beef is only 4% fat. When you convert the fat grams into calories you get 45 fat calories (5g fat x 9 calories = 45 calories) just like the label indicates. But let's put this into a percentage form so we can compare apples with apples. If we divide 45 fat calories by 150 total calories, we don't get the 4% fat that the label professes. We get instead, a whopping 30% fat! (45/150 = .3 or 30%).

You might wonder how the food company gets away with this type of misrepresentation. The answer is they come up with 4% fat based on the weight of the food item. There's 5g of fat per serving and 113g of total weight per serving; when you divide 5g by 113g you'll come up with the same 4% as the food company (5/113 = .0442 or rounded to 4%). Remember, not all grams of macronutrients are the same. There are only 4 calories for each gram of protein and carbohydrate, while each gram of fat carries 9 calories. This means foods are not evenly distributed with macronutrients because more calories are coming from fats than proteins and carbs.

> It's no wonder Americans are getting fatter and fatter with so many loopholes in the regulations for food manufacturers and Nutrition Fact Labels.

This claim should not be allowed on the label. The label should read "70% Lean/30% Fat Ground Beef."

On July 26, 2001, the CSPI petitioned the FDA to prohibit misleading ingredient claims on the front of packages. When there are so many loopholes in the regulations the food industry must follow when labeling their products, it's little wonder that Americans are getting fatter. When health conscious consumers spot claims in bright bold print that a food is 96% lean, they're likely to purchase the product, mistakenly thinking they're getting a lean food. Until the FDA puts stricter, easier to understand regulations on Food Labels, you'll have to guard yourself by understanding the information on the current nutrition labels.

Nutrients Recommended by the FDA

While we're on this topic, let's go over nutrients required on the label and a few I think are worth mentioning. Based on a 2,000 calorie diet, the "current" Daily Values are based on the National Academy of Sciences' 1968 Recommended Dietary Allowances. The amount of each nutrient was originally established to prevent nutritional deficiency in 97.5% of Americans, excluding pregnant and breastfeeding women.

On June 15, 2010, the 2010 Dietary Guidelines Advisory Committee released its preliminary report on its recommendations for the 2010 Dietary Guidelines. The official report was unveiled to the general public on January 31, 2011. The 2010 Dietary Guidelines for Americans in an official report that is *"the federal government's evidence-based nutritional guidance to promote health, reduce the risk of chronic diseases, and reduce the prevalence of overweight and obesity through improved nutrition and physical activity."* Really? If Americans are following the suggestions of this report (which hasn't changed much through the years), why are 67 percent of American adults overweight and obese with obesity-related diseases on the rise? And that's not even mentioning anything about the skyrocketing surge in adolescent obesity.

The 2010 Dietary Guidelines for Daily Values of the more important nutrients are as follows:

NUTRIENT	AMOUNT
Cholesterol	less than 300 milligrams (mg)
Sodium	less than 2,300mg
Fiber	at least 25 grams (g)
Vitamin A	700 micrograms (mcg) for females, 900mcg for males
Vitamin C	at least 75mg
Calcium	1g (1,000mg)
Iron	18mg for females, 8mg for males
Vitamin D	600 IU (15mcg)
Potassium	4,700mg
Magnesium	320mg for females, 420mg for males

Cholesterol

According to health organizations like the American Heart Association, National Research Council of the National Academy of Sciences, and the National Cholesterol Education Program of the National Institutes of Health, you should try not to exceed 300mg of cholesterol per day, no matter how many calories you consume. High amounts of dietary cholesterol are largely found in meat and dairy products. These products raise LDL (bad) cholesterol levels, which may cause plaque build-up in arteries leading to possible heart disease or stroke. Cholesterol is made in our liver, so there's actually no need to consume additional amounts. When comparing foods, opt for the product that contains 5% or less cholesterol in the % Daily Value column.

Sodium

The recommended amount of 2,300mg (approx. 1 tsp.) per day is targeted for the general U.S. population. According to the 2010 Dietary Guidelines for Americans, a much lower amount (no more than 1,500mg per day) is strongly advised for individuals who have hypertension (high blood pressure), individuals who are pre-hypertension, African-Americans, the middle-aged, and the elderly. The exceptions make up 70% of the American population. In general, the higher your salt intake, the higher your blood pressure, putting you at risk for heart disease, stroke, congestive heart failure (CHF), and kidney disease. When reading Food Labels, try to choose foods that are 5% or lower in the % Daily Values section or less than 140mg per serving. Also, beware of processed foods, fast foods, and restaurants (even the expensive restaurants).

Dietary Fiber

According to recent USDA surveys, the average intake of dietary fiber by men 19-50 years of age is about 17g and about 12g for women in the same age range. As you can see, the average American adult consumes about half the recommended amount of fiber on a daily basis. Also note that as your caloric intake increases, so should your dietary fiber intake. Health professionals at UCLA suggest 14g of dietary fiber for every 1,000 calories consumed.

> The average American adult consumes about half the daily recommended amount of dietary fiber.

Humans can't digest fiber because we don't have the enzyme to break it down into energy. Therefore, it passes through our intestines and binds with nutrients like cholesterol for excretion and passes harmful carcinogens (cancer-causing substances) from the intestinal walls helping prevent colon cancer. According to a Harvard study of over 40,000 male health professionals, high total dietary fiber intake was linked to a 40% lower risk of coronary heart disease, when compared to a low fiber intake. Another Harvard study of female nurses produced similar findings.

When reading the Ingredient List you may see names like cellulose, pectins, polysaccharides, and gums. These are also names for fiber. Other foods high in dietary fiber include beans (navy, kidney, black, pinto), split peas, bran cereals (Kashi GoLean, All-Bran, 100% Bran), raisins, raspberries, sweet potatoes, and cabbage. Always try to exceed the recommended 100% Daily Value of dietary fiber by selecting foods with at least 10% in the % Daily Value line. I choose foods that contain at least 3g of fiber to make sure I get enough fiber in my diet. To minimize the side effects of increasing your fiber intake, do it slowly to avoid bloating, abdominal cramps, diarrhea, or intestinal gas. These symptoms usually subside when you become used to a high-fiber diet. Finally, increase your water consumption because fiber absorbs water.

Vitamin A

This is the vitamin that helps with night vision, healthy skin, helps our bodies fight infections, and aids in bone development. Men require slightly more vitamin A than women – 900 micrograms (900mcg) of RE (Retinol Equivalents) and 700mcg of RE per day respectively. There are two types of vitamin A – retinol and beta-carotene. Vitamin A remains in our system for a while because it's fat-soluble and is stored if not used, making it possible to have it in excess. Taking more than double the recommended amount on a regular basis can be toxic and result in problems like headaches and dry skin, or major problems like nerve or liver damage.

More than likely you're getting enough vitamin A, so I wouldn't recommend supplements of this particular vitamin (as always consult with your doctor before taking supplements of any kind). Sources of retinol include egg yolks, meats, and milk products, which the body will utilize immediately. Beta-carotene is found in yellow, orange, and green leafy veggies, which the body will convert into vitamin A.

Vitamin C (a.k.a. Ascorbic Acid)

A water-soluble vitamin that's required every day because it can't be stored. Your body uses what it needs and eliminates the excess. If you have too much vitamin C in your system, it's excreted in urine. Urinating excess vitamin C isn't a complete loss because it protects against urinary tract infections (UTIs) by decreasing harmful bacteria that might be in the urinary tract. However, if you do overdo this vitamin (approximately 2,000mg or more), you may experience symptoms like stomach pain, nausea, diarrhea, and intestinal gas, which should go away once your body discharges whatever amount it doesn't need.

An insufficient amount of vitamin C causes scurvy, a disease most recognized by bleeding gums, bleeding under the skin, and general weakness. Scurvy isn't very common in the United States these days. Manufacturers add vitamin C to all sorts of foods and so it's easily obtained. Vitamin C helps manufacture collagen, a substance found in bones, cartilage, tendons, and the connective tissue that holds our bodies together. It also helps protect against infections by maintaining white blood cells (infection fighters), and helps the body absorb nutrients like iron from the foods we eat.

Debates continue as to the benefits of consuming high doses of vitamin C. When it comes to fending off colds and enhancing the immune system, some individuals think that mega doses of vitamin C will help dodge the sickness bullet. But the body's cells can't absorb more than about 100mg per day and concentrations of vitamin C in the blood begin to level off at 200mg per day, according to a landmark study by the National Institutes of Health.

Although the Reference Values for nutrition labeling currently recommends at least 75mg of vitamin C per day, the Institute of Medicine recognized that this amount doesn't fill everyone's needs and changed the amount to:

- 75mg for females, 90mg for males,
- an additional 35mg for smokers (i.e., 110mg for female smokers and 125mg for male smokers),
- 80-85mg for pregnant women,
- 115-120mg for breastfeeding women.

Great sources of vitamin C are citrus fruits, tomatoes, berries, broccoli, spinach, sweet potatoes, and peppers.

Calcium

Humans are one of the few mammals whose bodies cannot manufacture calcium; it has to be ingested. It's the most plentiful mineral in our bodies, working with other minerals like magnesium and vitamins D3 and K2 to help promote strong healthy bones and teeth. In fact, vitamin K2 is largely responsible for putting calcium into our bones and out of our arteries. Magnesium transports calcium to our cells and vitamins D3 and K2 help our bodies absorb it. Incidentally, exercise helps our

Magnesium and vitamins D3 and K2 help our bodies transport and absorb calcium.

bodies use these minerals to strengthen our bones. Calcium is also needed for proper muscle contraction and relaxation, helps our blood to clot, transmits nerve impulses, and, in conjunction with magnesium and vitamin D3 and K2, helps prevent osteoporosis.

According to Harvard University Health Services, most Americans don't meet their RDA for calcium with diet alone. Although the government suggests 1,000mg (1 gram) of calcium daily, the recommended amount varies depending on age.

- Children need the most because their bodies demand calcium when their bones and teeth are developing,
- Adolescents between 9 and 18 are encouraged to consume 1,300mg (130%DV),
- Both males and females from 19- to 50-years-old should have 1,000mg daily,
- Adults over age 50 are advised to have 1,200mg (120%DV),
- Pregnant/breastfeeding women under the age of 18 require 1,300mg (130%DV),
- Pregnant/breastfeeding women over 18-years-old only need 1,000mg,
- Post-menopausal women should have 1,200mg of calcium per day to help stave off osteoporosis.

Remember our "Quick Guide" to nutrients? Anything with 5%DV or less is low in the nutrient, while 20%DV or more offers high amounts of the nutrient in the particular food item.

While there haven't been reports of anyone overdosing on calcium, the National Academy of Sciences (NAS) has set a limit of 2,500mg per day. An excessive amount of calcium may increase the risk of kidney stones and interfere with your body's absorption of minerals like iron and zinc. But consuming too much calcium seems to be much less of a concern than consuming too little. When our bodies don't get the calcium we require, we draw it from stored calcium in bones which may lead to problems like osteoporosis. When calcium is depleted from our bones they become thinner and weaker, making them more susceptible to breaking and fracturing.

One of the best sources of calcium is dairy products. However, some people lack lactase, the enzyme our bodies use to break down lactose, the natural sugar found in milk. For these individuals it may be difficult to fulfill the daily recommendation of 1,000mg of calcium per day unless they take calcium supplements. Remember, calcium will not absorb without magnesium and vitamins D3 and K2. If you decide to take calcium supplements, check with your physician first and then only go with the supplements with the USP (Unites States Pharmacopoeia) symbol. Some calcium supplements like dolomite and bone meal may contain toxic metals. If you're trying to cut back on fat, know that fat-free and reduced-fat milk products generally contain the same amount of calcium, without all the fat. Other foods high in calcium include sardines with bones, almonds, kidney beans, broccoli, oranges, and dark green leafy veggies like kale and spinach.

Iron

A trace mineral (we only need a small amount). The most important function of iron is to generate hemoglobin to carry oxygen through our blood to cells where it's used to produce energy. Low levels of oxygen in the hemoglobin of our red blood cells result in low levels of energy. A few other responsibilities of iron include boosting our immune system to fight infections, and changing beta-carotene into vitamin A. As I mentioned above, beta-carotene needs to be converted to vitamin A in our bodies, and iron helps make this change happen. Iron also helps produce collagen to hold the tissues of our bodies together and helps make amino acids which are proteins. Iron is also needed for neurotransmitters to function properly – a neurotransmitter is a chemical that helps nerve cells communicate with each other.

> Athletes need one-third more iron than non-athletes.

The recommended amount of iron is different according to your age and gender. For example, according to the Harvard University Health Services: For example, according to the Harvard University Health Services:

- Males over the age of 19 are advised to take 8mg per day,
- Women between the ages 19 and 50 should take 18mg,
- Women over 50 should cut back to 8mg per day,
- Pregnant women should increase their iron to 27mg per day.

Athletes need more iron because intense exercise, creating a greater turnover of red blood cells, causes iron elimination. Therefore, athletes are advised to take an additional one-third, or 11mg, more than non-athletes. Vegans are also encouraged to take in more iron than the suggested amount because they get most of their iron from plants sources, which don't get absorbed into the body very efficiently.

There are two types of iron – heme iron and non-heme iron. Heme iron is derived from meat, poultry, and fish. And although heme iron is absorbed by the body quickly, only about ¼ of consumed heme iron ends up absorbed, with the rest being excreted through feces. Non-heme iron, on the other hand, doesn't absorb into our bodies as easily because inhibitors reduce its absorption. Only 2-20% from food sources is absorbed. Calcium, tea, coffee, bran, and oxalic acid (in spinach) are some iron inhibitors. Consuming meats, poultry, fish, and foods with vitamin C, however, will increase the absorption of non-heme iron. A chicken spinach salad, for instance, will enable your body to absorb more heme iron than eating a spinach salad with only vegetables. Another factor to consider is that Nutritional Facts Labels only list the total amount of iron in the food item, not the amount of iron your body will absorb. Also, Nutritional Facts Labels don't segregate heme iron and non-heme iron.

Although our bodies require only a small amount (less than a teaspoon per day) of iron, iron deficiency is a major problem around the world. Without enough iron, the body can develop anemia. This occurs when the body doesn't get enough oxygen because of a deficiency of hemoglobin – iron's responsibility. Symptoms like fatigue, a weakening of the immune system, a pale appearance, loss of appetite, shortness of breath, difficulty concentrating, and irritability are signs that you should have your physician check your blood for iron deficiency. Sometimes iron supplements are required, but before you self-medicate, check with your doctor. Iron supplements can be dangerous, especially for people with hemochromatosis. In this condition, iron accumulates causing tissue and organ damage and other serious health issues like diabetes and heart disease.

Excellent sources of heme iron come from beef, lamb, poultry, and fish, including shellfish like oysters, clams, and shrimp. Non-heme iron is obtainable from nuts, fruits, vegetables, grains, and seeds.

Vitamin D

The vital player for the absorption of calcium and phosphorus for healthy teeth and bones. Vitamin D also regulates levels of calcium and phosphorus in our blood. The milk fortification program was established in the United States during the 1930s to combat rickets, a major problem for children at that time. Rickets is a disease caused by vitamin D deficiency and involves softening and weakening of bones, causing defective bone growth and problems like bowed legs and deformed skulls. Since the implementation of the milk fortification program, rickets has been made relatively rare in the United States.

As we age, we require larger amounts of vitamin D from outside sources

As we age, we require more vitamin D from outside sources because our bodies become less efficient at producing it.

because our bodies become less efficient at producing this vitamin. We get vitamin D from some foods, but mostly from sunlight. The ultraviolet (UV) rays from sunlight activate vitamin D synthesis in our skin. Sun exposure on the skin produces a vitamin D which is useless until enzymes in our liver and kidneys generate a chemical conversion which alters it to another form that our bodies can use to absorb calcium and phosphorus. According to the Mayo Clinic in Rochester, Minnesota, 10-15 minutes of sun exposure without sunscreen twice a week to the face, arms, hands, or back is usually enough. Beyond 15 minutes, a sunblock is recommended to protect the skin.

Also, people with darker skin, like African-Americans and Hispanics, may want to boost their dietary intake of vitamin D because their skin inhibits UV rays from getting to the lower part of the skin where vitamin D is generated. However, as always, consult with your doctor on what amount would be beneficial given your specific needs. Just as too little of this vitamin can cause problems, too much may result in weakness, vomiting, and nausea.

Not only do we get vitamin D from sunlight exposure, but we can also get it from foods like salmon, sardines, fortified vitamin D milk (whole, reduced-fat, and skim), fortified orange juice, fortified breakfast cereals (Grape-Nuts, Raisin Bran, and Total) and dark-green leafy veggies (mustard greens and kale).

Researchers are currently studying the effects vitamin D has on protecting against certain cancers like prostate, colon, and breast.

Potassium

A mineral electrolyte that carries an electrical charge found in all living animal and plant cells. As one of the most important electrolytes in our bodies, potassium's role is vital in keeping acidic and alkaline balance, delivering nutrients into cells, sending nerve impulses, regulating water balance in cells and tissues, assisting in building and repairing muscles, making muscles contract (including our heartbeat), and controlling blood

Potassium helps the body maintain a healthy acidic and alkaline balance.

pressure by expelling sodium out of cells. Individuals with high blood pressure usually have a lower potassium level compared to sodium levels.

The 2010 Dietary Guidelines agrees with the Institute of Medicine and also recommends 4,700mg per day. It's estimated that most American diets supply between 2,000 and 6,000mg each day, which suggests that potassium deficiency doesn't seem to be a problem in the United States. However, individuals who are bulimic or taking non-potassium sparing diuretics or laxatives may experience low levels of potassium due to loss of the mineral in their urine and feces. Bulimics lose potassium because they induce vomiting to control their weight and vomiting results in an increased loss of potassium in the urine. People with low levels of potassium (hypokalemia) may feel weakness and fatigue, dry skin, depression, slow reflexes, slowed heart rate, and even congestive heart failure, according to the American Heart Association.

It's highly unlikely that you'll consume too much potassium, even if you take potassium supplements (with your physician's advice, of course). However, large amounts of potassium injections may lead to potassium intoxication, which can cause muscular or respiratory paralysis, irregular heartbeat, and cardiac arrest. Without potassium injections, the extra potassium in your system is eliminated normally in urine, but taking in too much potassium through supplements means your body will find another way to eliminate the excess, typically through vomiting.

When people get muscle cramps during workouts, trainers will often suggest they increase their potassium by eating bananas. Contrary to popular belief, a banana contains only a moderate amount of potassium. Much better sources include foods like baked sweet potatoes, pinto beans, lentils, kidney beans, lima beans, split peas, tomato juice, prune juice, papaya, cantaloupe, avocados, spinach, and yogurt. If you're concerned about your potassium level, consult your family practitioner.

Contrary to popular belief, bananas contain only a moderate amount of potassium.

Magnesium

Another mineral that helps in the production of healthy teeth and bones. Over 300 biochemical reactions in the human body require magnesium.

Magnesium helps manage blood-sugar levels and supports several important enzymes. It's vital in the production process for energy. When certain enzymes split and transfer phosphate groups from the foods we eat to ADP (Adenosine Diphosphate – a key player in the body's energy metabolism), a substance called ATP (Adenine Triphosphate) is created to help produce energy. This process is what makes our muscles, including our heart and other organs, function.

According to a study sponsored by the National Institutes of Health, 68% of Americans are magnesium deficient. Other experts suspect that 80% might be a more realistic number. Even if you're reading nutrition labels specifically for magnesium intake, you could be in trouble because our bodies only absorb about one-third to one-half of the magnesium from foods we eat. Again, nutrition labels list the total amount of magnesium in the food and not the amount of magnesium our bodies will absorb.

Some symptoms associated with a magnesium deficiency include confusion, muscle contractions, muscle weakness, twitching, tiredness, and irregular pulse. People who take diuretics or consume too much caffeine will lose magnesium through their urine, which might be a reason to consult a doctor about magnesium supplements. There's a multitude of magnesium deficiency reports, but not enough evidence to establish any effects from high amounts of magnesium. Currently, the only known symptom of taking too much magnesium is diarrhea.

According to the Institute of Medicine:
- Men between the ages of 19-30 are advised to consume 400mg per day,
- Males 31 and over should increase to 420mg daily,
- Women (including breastfeeding women) ages 19-30 should take 310mg,
- Females 31 and older should increase to 320,
- Pregnant women should increase the recommended magnesium by 40mg.

Some great sources of magnesium are spinach, almonds, pumpkin seeds,100% bran, wheat germ, legumes (beans and peas), and halibut.

Looking at the amount of each nutrient our bodies require on a daily basis, it doesn't seem like we need many calories to accommodate these requirements. And I know people are trying to be more health conscious about the types of foods they order when they go out. People talk about ordering chopped salads, chicken Teriyaki sandwiches, or pastas with chicken and broccoli because those menu items sound healthier. But are they? The way foods are prepared at restaurants is crucial. When it comes to dining out, even the experts have a hard time trying to decide which food item is healthy.

Here are a few tips to remember when going out to dinner:

1. Steer clear of fried foods. Instead look for entrées that are broiled, roasted, baked, or steamed.
2. Ask for salad dressings, butter, sauces, and gravies to be served on the side so that you are in control of the amount that goes on your food.
3. Ask for a container and immediately put half your entrée away to take home for lunch the next day. American restaurants almost always give you double servings of food. Once the extra food is out of sight, you're less likely to reopen the container to eat it.
4. Order only one dessert per couple. Get just enough sweets to settle your cravings, but not enough to sabotage your weight management efforts.
5. Whenever possible, ask your waiter if the restaurant offers nutritional information for the foods on their menu. You might be amazed to see how much sodium and saturated fat is in restaurant food.

Think you can beat the experts?...

Trying to guess the calorie content of meals at restaurants and fast food joints is like trying to guess winning lottery numbers. "Healthy" meals are almost never as healthy as they appear on restaurant menus. Restaurant foods are so overloaded with hidden ingredients that even nutritionists are often confused as to the true amount of calories in each meal. After all, the chef's main agenda is to make food taste great, which in most cases means additional fat and sodium.

1. Cosi Tuna Melt or Cosi Bacon Turkey Cheddar Melt?

2. Boston Market's Turkey Carver Sandwich or Boston Market's Chopped Salad with Turkey?

3. Ruby Tuesday's Fresh Chicken and Broccoli Pasta or Ruby Tuesday's Bacon Cheeseburger?

4. Starbuck's Oat Bran Blueberry Coffee Cake or Starbuck's Chocolate Fudge Brownie?

5. Subway's Footlong Sweet Onion Chicken Teriyaki or Subway's Footlong Roast Beef?

6. McDonald's Caesar Salad with Grilled Chicken or McDonald's Quarter Pounder?

(Answers on page 47)

Answers to food comparisons:

1. Winner: Cosi' Bacon Turkey Cheddar Melt
        Calories: 682, Total Fat: 25g,
        Cholesterol: 98mg, Sodium: 1,780mg
   Loser: Cosi' Tuna Melt
        Calories: 1,012, Total Fat: 60g,
        Cholesterol: 122mg, Sodium: 1,948mg

2. Winner: Boston Market's Turkey Carver Sandwich
        Calories: 530, Total Fat: 17g,
        Cholesterol: 80mg, Sodium: 1,050mg
   Loser: Boston Market's Chopped Salad with Turkey
        Calories: 720, Total Fat: 54g,
        Cholesterol: 35mg, Sodium: 2,360mg
3. Winner: Ruby Tuesday's Bacon Cheeseburger
        Calories: 1,193, Total Fat: 85g
   Loser: Ruby Tuesday's Fresh Chicken and Broccoli Pasta
        Calories: 2,061, Total Fat: 128g
4. Winner: Starbuck's Chocolate Fudge Brownie
        Calories: 280, Total Fat: 16g,
        Cholesterol: 80mg, Sodium: 140mg
   Loser: Starbuck's Oat Bran Blueberry Coffee Cake
        Calories: 490, Total Fat: 26g,
        Cholesterol: 0mg, Sodium: 200mg
5. Winner: Subway's Footlong Roast Beef
        Calories: 580, Total Fat: 10g,
        Cholesterol: 40mg, Sodium: 1,800mg
   Loser: Subway's Footlong Sweet Onion Chicken Teriyaki
        Calories: 750, Total Fat: 10g,
        Cholesterol: 100mg, Sodium: 2,400mg
6. Winner: McDonald's Quarter Pounder
        Calories: 410, Total Fat: 19g,
        Cholesterol: 65mg, Sodium: 730mg
   Loser: McDonald's Caesar Grilled Chicken Salad
        Calories: 410, Total Fat: 24g,
        Cholesterol: 95mg, Sodium: 1,390mg

As you can see in the answers on page 47, there is much more fat, cholesterol, and sodium content in restaurant foods than you might suspect. I hope this sheds some light on why some people can't seem to lose weight when they dine out rather than prepare their food at home. One can't always know just what's being put in these foods to make them taste as good as they do.

Now that we know how to break down a Food Label and a little bit about the nutrients of the foods we're eating, let's find out how many calories your specific body and lifestyle require.

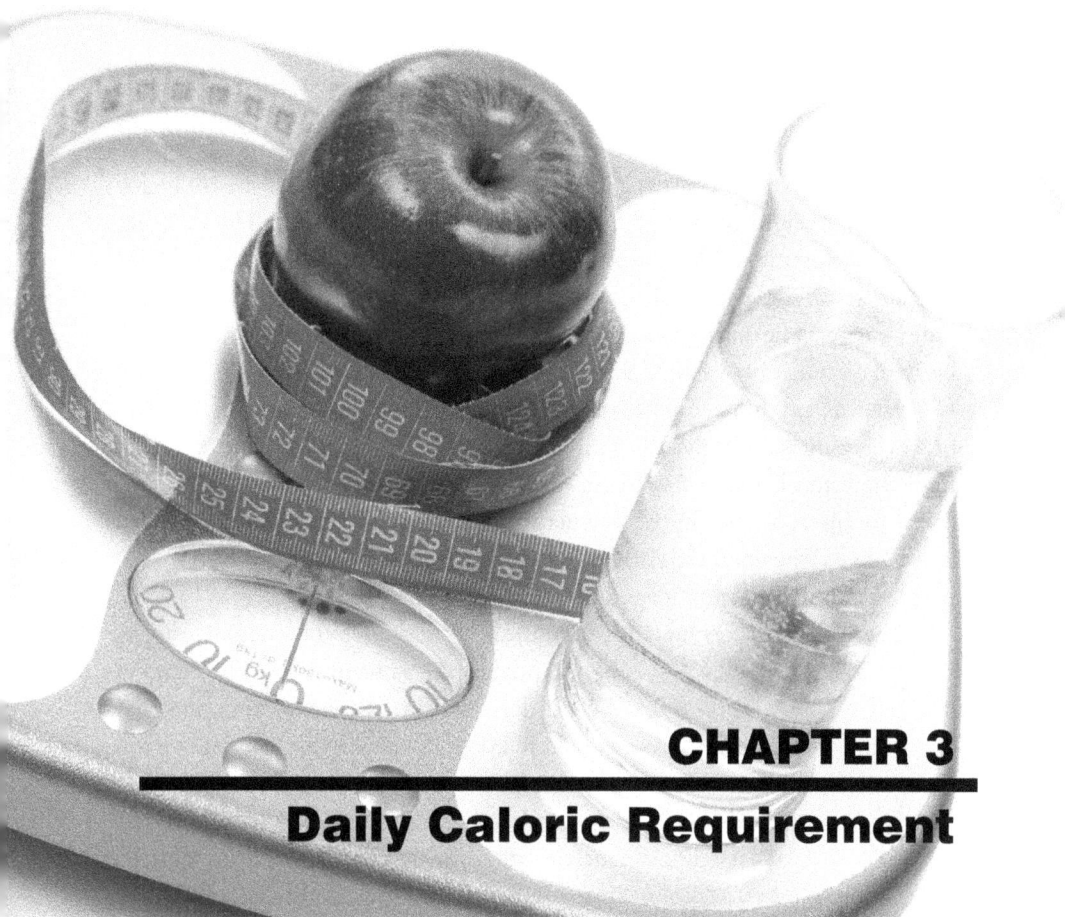

CHAPTER 3
Daily Caloric Requirement

In Chapter 1, we discussed the paramount strategies for achieving a *Transforming Your Lifestyle* physique. Now the question becomes: "How do I know how many calories I should consume to be at a healthier, happier weight?"

First, we need a basic understanding of the Body Mass Index (BMI). BMI is a measurement correlating height and weight to calculate total body fat. It's a term that's been recently popularized in mainstream America, but there are flaws with this calculation because no two bodies are alike. A BMI measurement can't distinguish muscle from fat, for example. Nor can it take into account factors such as pregnancy or body frame. Also, people younger than 18 are usually still growing, which means that their weight tends to fluctuate, making a BMI measurement less precise. Despite these weaknesses, the body mass index is still the measurement utilized by many physicians and obesity researchers.

Body Mass Index (BMI)

The BMI weight chart is a scientific estimate of where you should be for a "healthy" weight for your height, according to the National Heart, Lung and Blood Institute. There are three general categories defined by the BMI – healthy weight, overweight, and obesity. Each category has a body mass index range. The healthy weight BMI category ranges from 19 to 24.9. A body mass index between 25 and 29.9 is considered overweight, and obesity is defined as anything equal to or greater than 30. As BMI increases, the risk of developing serious health problems like type 2 diabetes, hypertension, high cholesterol, and heart disease also increases. Keep in mind, though, that there are discrepancies in this calculation, and an individual who has a lot of muscle mass (the good weight) may be categorized as overweight (even obese) because muscle adds poundage to bodies.

There are a few formulas to determine body mass index but they all result in approximately the same number. The formula I use is derived from calculating your personal weight in kilograms and dividing by the square of your height in meters. It takes a few steps to calculate because most of us don't use the metric system so we have to convert pounds into kilograms and inches into meters. If this seems complicated, you can visit my website, www.fitbodiesbysasha.com. Simply input your personal height and weight and my *BMI Calculator* will do the rest.

The BMI calculator at www.fitbodiesbysasha.com will compute your BMI after you input your personal height and weight.

For example, I'm 6'2" and weigh 215 pounds. Doing the BMI calculation, I find that my BMI is 27.69. Now, according to the BMI chart, I'm classified as "overweight." Yet in my defense, I have only 11% body fat – a little less than 24 pounds body fat and 191 pounds lean body mass. Because muscle is nearly 5 times denser than fat, my muscle mass means that I have more weight on me. So I'm still at a healthy weight.

Waist Circumference

To get a much better picture of an individual's health, we can use another gauge in combination with the BMI – the Waist Circumference (WC) measurement. It turns out that the type of fat – visceral fat or subcutaneous fat – can help predict diseases like type 2 diabetes. As we'll see in Chapter 6, visceral fat is located around the organs of the abdomen area, which is

BMI CHART

BMI (kg/m2)	19	20	21	22	23	24	25	26	27	28	29	30	35
Height (inches)	BODY WEIGHT (pounds)												
58	91	96	100	105	110	115	119	124	129	134	138	143	167
59	94	99	104	109	114	119	124	128	133	138	143	148	173
60	97	102	107	112	118	123	128	133	138	143	148	153	179
61	100	106	111	116	122	127	132	137	143	148	153	158	185
62	104	109	115	120	126	131	136	142	147	153	158	164	191
63	107	113	118	124	130	135	141	146	152	158	163	169	197
64	110	116	122	128	134	140	145	151	157	163	169	174	204
65	114	120	126	132	138	144	150	156	162	168	174	180	210
66	118	124	130	136	142	148	155	161	167	173	179	186	216
67	121	127	134	140	146	153	159	166	172	178	185	191	223
68	125	131	138	144	151	158	164	171	177	184	190	197	230
69	128	135	142	149	155	162	169	176	182	189	196	203	236
70	132	139	146	153	160	167	174	181	188	195	202	209	243
71	136	143	150	157	165	172	179	186	193	200	208	215	250
72	140	147	154	162	169	177	184	191	199	206	213	221	258
73	144	151	159	166	174	182	189	197	204	212	219	227	265
74	148	155	163	171	179	186	194	202	210	218	225	233	272
75	152	160	168	176	184	192	200	208	216	224	232	240	279
76	156	164	172	180	189	197	205	213	221	230	238	246	287

Source: National Heart, Lung, and Blood Institute

why it's sometimes called abdominal fat. And this is the type of fat which has been identified as a marker for chronic illnesses. According to the National Institutes of Health, a high Waist Circumference (WC) along with a BMI of 25 and above may be associated with an increased risk for type 2 diabetes, dyslipidemia, hypertension (high blood pressure), and cardiovascular disease.

The risk of health problems increases for a man when his waist is over 40 inches and for a woman when her waist is over 35 inches. You can easily determine your waist measurement by using a cloth measuring tape and placing it directly above your hipbone. Be sure the tape is horizontal all the way around your waist; most times the measuring tape will run across your naval. The measuring tape should be taut but not so tight that it creates a skin fold.

Caution! Levi jeans try to make you feel better about your waist size – they label their jeans two inches less than your actual waist measurement.

christopherSASHA

BMI	Obesity Class	Waist *less than* or equal to 40 in. (men) or 35 in. (women)	Waist *greater than* 40 in. (men) or 35 in. (women)
18.5 or less	Underweight	N/A	N/A
18.5 - 24.9	Normal	N/A	N/A
25.0 - 29.9	Overweight	Increased Risk	High Risk
30.0 - 34.9	Obesity I	High Risk	Very High Risk
35.0 - 39.9	Obesity II	Very High Risk	Very High Risk
40 or greater	Obesity III	Extremely High Risk	Extremely High Risk

Source: National Heart, Lung, and Blood Institute

I ask my clients to shoot for 19-24 on the BMI. Most clients then reply, "Fine. I'll only eat once a day and I'll reach that weight within a month." Wrong answer! As we'll discuss, your metabolism will come to a screeching halt if forced to survive after a drastic reduction in calories. And when you resume eating like before, you'll quickly gain back all your weight. Worse, statistics indicate that you'll most likely gain even *more* weight because you've lost more muscle, which is another culprit slowing your metabolism. Your metabolism will still be at a standstill until you learn how to rev it up.

The easiest way to use the BMI chart (page 51) is to find your current height and weight and follow that column to the top to find your current BMI. If you're either overweight or obese, make your first short-term goal to reduce your weight (through proper diet and exercise) to the preceding weight category which will be one point lower (to the left) on the BMI chart. When you reach this point, reward yourself and take pride! You just did a remarkable thing for your heart, blood pressure, and cholesterol level.

Continue this process until you reach your ultimate weight goal. Don't worry about falling off the wagon every once in a while as long as you get right back on and keep at it. Once you achieve your ideal weight, you will have learned how many calories you need to maintain your "healthy" weight.

This brings us to the next point of learning how many calories you need on a daily basis.

Metabolism

The amount of calories your body burns daily depends on your individual metabolism. The metabolism is very complex and it is not my intent to have us delve too deeply into this complicated biochemical process. Instead, let's discuss the basics on what the metabolism is all about and how your metabolism relates to a healthy weight for you.

First of all, your metabolism is the amount of calories in the food you eat that are converted into the energy your body needs to perform every function you do, from producing blood to exercising. Your metabolism won't be the same as mine, just as my metabolism won't be the same as a professional bodybuilder's. Everybody's metabolism is unique. Some metabolisms are higher and some are lower due to a host of factors like genetics and body composition.

There are three elements that make up your metabolism – your basal metabolic rate (BMR), your activity level, and your thermic effect of food (TEF). Each part burns a certain amount of calories during the day, which, when calculated together, comprise your metabolism, the amount of calories you expend on a daily basis. Our bodies burn calories every second of every day, even when we sleep.

You might ask, "Why do some people burn more calories than others?" One reason is that some people are genetically blessed with a high metabolism. Does that mean you're doomed from ever achieving a *Transforming Your Lifestyle* physique? Absolutely not! We can all learn how to kick-start our metabolism to attain the healthiest bodies we've ever had, both inside and out. All it takes is a little knowledge and determination. I'll provide the knowledge…it's up to you to do the rest. Remember, like anything in life, you get out of it what you put into it. It all comes down to one question, and the answer comes from deep within you: how badly do you want to reduce your risks of a myriad of chronic illnesses that the standard American diet (SAD) and lack of exercise lead to?

> Your basal metabolic rate (BMR), your activity level, and your thermic effect of food (TEF) make up your individual metabolism.

christopherSASHA

Basal Metabolic Rate (BMR)

We breathe every second of every day. Our hearts perpetually pump blood, our bodies maintain constant body temperature, and many other involuntary functions are performed 24 hours a day. These functions require calories to be expended, producing the energy our bodies need to survive.

The basal metabolic rate (BMR) is the minimum amount of calories necessary to survive in our most restful state. Put another way, the BMR is the minimum amount of calories needed for a person to remain asleep all day. It accounts for 60-75% of total calories on a daily basis. Every individual's BMR is different because no two people have exactly the same genetic blueprint, are the same age, height or weight, have the same daily activity level, have the same body composition, or are the same gender. These personal factors help determine your individual BMR, and therefore help determine the amount of calories required to lose, maintain, or even gain weight.

Fasting and crazy fad diets that require drastic calorie reductions lower your BMR and is likely to put your body in starvation mode.

Some determinants lower your basal metabolic rate while others raise it. Unfortunately, we lose muscle mass as we age, which lowers our BMR because muscle demands more calories than fat to maintain itself. This is why resistance training is important to maintaining a healthy weight as we age. Also, fasting and crazy diets that require drastic calorie reductions lower your BMR because your body is likely to go into starvation mode and cannibalize itself when it doesn't receive the necessary calories from the foods you consume. That's right – the body will eat its own muscle tissue to get the calories it needs to perform its required functions. *A gradual reduction of calories and an increase in exercise is the only proven method to properly lose weight and keep it off.*

Through exercise, we can redistribute our body composition which will increase our basal metabolic rate. By decreasing body fat and increasing lean muscle mass, our BMR will increase because muscle tissue requires more energy to maintain. Thus more calories will be burned, even when we're not doing anything!

There are a few factors we have no control over that affect our BMR. We can't change the fact that we're either male or female, for instance. Generally, males have higher basal metabolic rates because they have more muscle mass and a lower percentage of body fat. Sorry, ladies, but in general, it's true.

Also, tall, thin individuals tend to have a higher BMR compared to their shorter counterparts of equal weight. Finally, good old genetics plays a role in whether you'll have a faster or slower metabolism.

The first step to designing your personal daily caloric intake is to determine your individual basal metabolic rate. We'll calculate the specific amount of calories your body requires just to maintain your current weight at complete rest, without any movement. The best formula I've found is the Harris-Benedict Formula. With the exception of body composition (lean body mass versus body fat), this formula takes every factor into account to give a very close calculation of calories needed to maintain your current weight. Because body composition is not part of the equation, note that if you're either obese, or very muscular, you may not get as accurate a calculation as individuals who have an average amount of body fat (11-17% for men and 15-23% for women).

For your individual daily caloric intake, visit www.fitbodiesbysasha.com.

Harris-Benedict Formula

- Females: $655 + (9.6 \times W) + (1.7 \times H) - (4.7 \times A)$
- Males: $66 + (13.7 \times W) + (5 \times H) - (6.8 \times A)$

Note: **W** = bodyweight in kilograms (pounds / 2.2)

    H = height in centimeters (inches x 2.54)

    A = your current age

EXAMPLE 1:

A 36-year-old female who is 5'3" (160cm) and weighs 119 pounds (54kg) would have a BMR of 1,276 calories.

$655 + (518.4) + (272) - (169.2) =$ ***1,276 calories***

EXAMPLE 2:

A 36-year-old male who is 5'3" (160cm) and weighs 119 pounds (54kg) would have a BMR of 1,361 calories.

$66 + (739.8) + (800) - (244.8) =$ ***1,361 calories***

In these examples, both the male and female are the same age, height, and weight but the male requires a few more calories because, generally speaking, he has more muscle mass and less body fat. Again, these are the minimum amounts of calories these particular individuals need while at complete rest to maintain their current weight.

ACTIVITY LEVEL

The BMR represents between 60-75% of total calories required on a daily basis. Our *activity level* makes up the second part of our metabolism and accounts for 20-30% of our calories. When we speak of activity level, we mean every movement we make, from getting out of bed and showering to strenuous endeavors like glacier climbing and running marathons.

Some people have sedentary lifestyles. They walk to their cars to drive to work, walk to their desks where they sit all day, then walk back to their cars to drive home and watch television. Then they go to bed and get up the next morning and start the same cycle anew. Others might have a moderately active lifestyle. They might ride a bicycle to work a couple times during the workweek and work out three times a week. Still others are *very* active, having laborious jobs like construction and exercising several times each week.

Our activity level makes up the second part of our metabolism. It accounts for 20-30% of our calories.

The amount of activity you perform on a daily basis might be similar to one of these examples, or anywhere in between, or beyond. The main point is that the more movement and exercise you do, the more calories you burn, therefore the more weight you lose. Just as there are many definitions as to what constitutes a sedentary lifestyle, a moderately-active lifestyle and so forth, there are just as many multipliers attached to these distinct activity levels. One researcher might affix a certain multiplier to a certain activity level while another researcher might slap on a higher or lower multiplier to the same activity level. Remember, these formulas are just estimates as to how many calories we need to consume and how many calories are expended according to the type of lifestyle you may lead. Personally, I like to be as specific as possible to get the most accurate result. For this reason, I continue to use the Harris-Benedict Formula which utilizes an activity multiplier with five activity-level categories, where others formulas use only three.

According to the Harris-Benedict Formula, the BMR is multiplied by the activity level that best describes your specific current lifestyle. The five activity levels are:

Sedentary	Little or no exercise, desk job	BMR x 1.2
Lightly Active	Light exercise, sports 1-3 days/week	BMR x 1.375
Moderately Active	Moderate exercise, sports 3-5 days/wk	BMR x 1.55
Very Active	Hard exercise, sports 6-7 days/wk	BMR x 1.725
Extremely Active	Daily exercise, sports and physical job or 2X day training, i.e. marathon, etc.	BMR x 1.9

Continuing our example with the 36-year-old female who is 5'3" and weighs 119 pounds:
- Her BMR is 1,276 calories per day, just to survive and remain asleep the entire day,
- She has a *sedentary* lifestyle because she has a desk job and doesn't exercise, making her activity level multiplier 1.2,
- So the amount of calories her body requires to function properly and maintain her current weight is (1,276 x 1.2) = *1,531 calories per day.*

Now, let's make our 36-year-old female friend a little more active by working out on Tuesdays and Thursdays:
- Now she's *lightly active*, bumping her activity level multiplier to 1.375.
- The amount of calories she now needs to maintain her current weight rises to *1,755 calories per day* (1,276 x 1.375).

But what happens if she wants to compete in a fitness competition, which demands an *extremely active* lifestyle, requiring, let's say, cardio exercises at least twice a day along with resistance training each day?
- Now her activity level multiplier jumps to 1.9 and,
- The amount of calories her body will demand jacks up to *2,424 calories per day* (1,276 x 1.9).

There is NO cookie-cutter caloric intake for everyone.

As you can see, the more active you are, the more calories your body will demand just to maintain your current weight. However, if our avid fitness competitor wants to lean out and get ripped, she's going to have to lose some body fat by reducing her caloric intake. Otherwise, she'll remain at her current weight. To preserve as much muscle and burn as much body fat as possible, she'll want to lose one to two pounds of weight per week. We already know that a pound of body fat is approximately 3,500 calories, so if she cuts back 500 calories per day (500 calories x 7 days = 3,500 calories), she will theoretically lose about one pound a week. Instead of consuming 2,424 calories per day, she will want to decrease her caloric intake to 1,924 per day.

Is it now clear that there is no cookie-cutter caloric intake for everyone? Some diet books claim if you were to cut your caloric intake to 1,625 calories per day, you'll lose weight. Sure, you'll lose weight if you've been consuming 3,000 calories and drop your caloric intake by half. But is this the healthy way to lose weight? These diet books don't take into account that everyone is a different weight, height, gender, or age, and each has a different muscle mass and activity level. If our particular 36-year-old female were to scale down to 1,625 calories, she'd cut back too many calories at once and she'd risk losing muscle, thereby decreasing her metabolism and increasing the possibility of storing body fat. Her body needs a larger amount of calories and, if it doesn't get them, her body will start eating its own muscle tissue to get the calories it needs.

And this is just with our example of a female weighing 119 pounds. What about a male who weighs 220 pounds with a large percentage of muscle mass? The results would be much, much worse if he were to follow a 1,625 calorie diet.

The formulas used to help determine the amount of calories your specific body requires are not exact. There's no possible way to get the precise amount of calories that you, as an individual, require without doing specific, costly tests. However, the Harris-Benedict Formula calculation results are very close to the results these tests would provide. The numbers you come up with after you put your personal information into the formula provide an excellent starting point. To find your personal daily caloric intake, go to www.fitbodiesbysasha.com.

From here, you'll have to monitor your own progress by checking your weight, feeling how your clothes fit, and if possible, getting your body fat percentage checked periodically. Calipers are fine if the person taking the measurements knows how to use this piece of equipment. Otherwise, a better method to measure body fat is underwater immersion (hydrostatic testing). Many hospitals offer this service, though for a hefty price.

THERMIC EFFECT OF FOOD (TEF)

The final part that makes up your metabolism (your body's daily total expenditure of energy) is the thermic effect of food (TEF). This is the notion that your body has to burn calories to digest food. Theoretically, every time you eat you burn calories. Your body has to convert carbohydrates into simple sugars, proteins into amino acids, and fats into fatty acids – all to be utilized as energy. Food needs to be digested, absorbed into the bloodstream, and transported to be used as energy, stored as fat in the adipose tissue for future use, or disposed of as waste. The amount of calories burned depends on the type of food and how much of it you eat.

Protein is the hardest macronutrient for the body to digest. It requires more water and burns more calories to digest, consuming approximately 25% of the calories derived from the protein in your meal. Carbohydrates are easier to digest for the body to use as energy and it's estimated that somewhere between 10-15% of the calories originating from the carbs are burned in the process. Then there's fat which is very easily converted into fatty acids. All the calories used to digest, absorb, and carry the nutrients in the foods we eat into the bloodstream to be used for energy or stored for future use account for approximately 10% of total calorie expenditure.

> The thermic effect of food (TEF) makes up the final part of your metabolism.

I'm big on eating 5 or 6 mini meals (every 2-3 hours) per day because I believe it's the healthy way to fuel the body. When you have a headache and you take aspirin, you don't take a whole bottle all at once, do you? Only one or two aspirins every few hours will do the job. Anything beyond that is going to be wasted and will create more problems in the long run. The same is true with our diets. If you eat one or two meals a day, you're probably gorging over 1,000 calories at one time and your body doesn't need that many calories all at once. You wouldn't put 50 gallons of gas in your car tank when it only holds 20 gallons, right? The body will manage the calories it needs and store the excess as fat or dispose of it as waste. The best approach is to eat smaller meals throughout the day so your body can burn the calories as needed and get refueled when it runs low on glycogen.

Besides diminishing possible binges, hunger pangs, and lack of energy, one of the other benefits of eating smaller meals frequently throughout the day is that you burn more calories because your body will work to digest the food, which will raise your metabolism. Also, you won't enter starvation mode which inevitably thwarts your efforts at losing weight. Most of what you eat while in starvation mode, even healthy food, will likely be stored as body fat because your body will revert to doing what it was designed to do: it will prepare itself for famine. This is the most perplexing concept concerning diets for many of my clients.

Complaints

The major complaints I get from most clients when they first begin to increase the frequency of their smaller meals are nausea and initial weight gain. But these are both short-term side effects because your body is discombobulated. You're introducing a new eating regime to your body, and it will take a few weeks for your body to adapt to the change. If you experience either of these reactions, I would suggest making sure your meals are less than 500 calories each because you may be consuming more than you think. And keep in mind that your body might be a little sensitive to digesting food all the time.

In any event, these waves will subside after a while, so don't freak out. I promise the nausea will go away and the pounds will come off. Less fat will be stored when you consistently eat more frequent, smaller meals throughout the day. You can get through this short phase. For me, the first few months I moderated my eating, I would get sick when I ate breakfast. It took some time for my body to get used to having food in its system first thing in the morning but I did get over it and my body did adapt to the change. So will yours.

...our bodies burn more calories from the foods we eat after exercise.

Finally, let's not forget how the thermic effect of food (TEF) is drastically increased when a small variable like exercise becomes a part of our daily lifestyle. Numerous studies have indicated that our bodies burn more calories from the foods we eat *after* exercise. A study at the University of Nevada showed that the TEF of individuals who ate a high-carbohydrate 660 calorie meal after their resistance training session was *73% higher* than the TEF of participants who didn't work out! The researchers suggested that carbohydrates play an important role because the carbohydrates need to be converted to glycogen to replace the depletion of glycogen storages that were used for energy to perform the workouts. As the obesity epidemic continues to rise in the United States, more and more research is showing why exercise is a must to maintain a healthy weight.

From Obese to a Healthy Weight

Let's follow the metamorphosis of one American who begins in the 34.3% obese group (slightly more than one in three Americans) and who ends as a happier, healthier *transforming your lifestyle* individual.

As we know, the key to achieving and maintaining a healthy weight is to reduce calories slowly and increase exercise. And although this concept has been proven by research for years, people still seem baffled by it. Can it really be as simple as this? Yes. It can, and it is. Keep it simple and you *will* succeed.

26% of American adults report NO daily physical activity.

Starting from obese…

Our subject is a 35-year-old male named Waldo, who is 5′10″, weighs 250 pounds, and has a sedentary lifestyle. Waldo is an accountant in a Fortune 500 company who works a 55-70 hour week and claims he simply has no time to exercise. He continually consumes fast food and vending machine products, washing everything down with soda. Waldo doesn't eat breakfast, but by 11:00 a.m. he schleps to the Starbucks in his office building's cafeteria to devour a Cinnamon Chip Scone and a Grande Frappuccino blended crème-whip.

Waldo starts to feel hungry again by 3:30 and walks a block to the nearest McDonald's where he orders the value meal – a Double Quarter Pounder with Cheese, large fries and a large Coke. Waldo ends his day at the office at 6:30 p.m., picking up dinner at Kentucky Fried Chicken on his way home. After dinner, he usually snacks on a half pint of Haagen-Dazs ice cream as he watches whatever sport is playing on television, followed by the news. Then he goes to bed at 11:00 p.m. This is his basic ritual during the week.

Waldo had his annual physical and the doctor urged him – once again – to lose weight because his blood pressure and cholesterol levels were continuing to rise. Dr. Feelgood warned Waldo that he's a prime candidate for a heart attack or stroke with all the extra weight he's carrying around. Being human, and a creature of habit, Waldo disregarded the doctor's advice because he believes he's too young for a heart attack or stroke. He left the doctor's office, making a pit stop at Burger King before returning to work. He ordered a Double Whopper with Cheese, large fries, and a Coke.

A few weeks later, Waldo received a telephone call from his frantic sister-in-law, who told him that his younger brother was rushed to the hospital due to a heart attack. It happens that Waldo's 32-year-old brother had a weight problem similar to Waldo's even though he played basketball once a week with a few of his old college buddies. After witnessing his baby brother go through bypass surgery, Waldo began to realize that maybe heart attacks and strokes aren't diseases that are biased just towards the elderly anymore. That very day, Waldo decided he wasn't going to succumb to any preventable illnesses. He decided that a healthy lifestyle would help increase his chances for a longer, happier life.

The next day, after consulting with Dr. Feelgood about an exercise program, Waldo joined his local fitness club and hired a personal trainer to get him started on a workout routine. The personal trainer suggested that Waldo do resistance training three times per week in addition to some form of cardio (biking, walking, elliptical, etc.) at least twice per week. Remembering Dr. Feelgood's advice to diet and exercise to get rid of his unwanted weight, Waldo found a nutritionist to help him with his diet. The nutritionist, Ms. Powerfoods, asked Waldo to keep a food diary for two weeks. She showed him how to graph his diary, making nine columns for the time he ate, the food he ate, calories, total fat, saturated fat, carbs, protein, sugar, and fiber. After learning Waldo had issues with high blood pressure and cholesterol levels, she also asked that he record the amount of sodium and cholesterol in each food, making a total of eleven columns.

FOOD DIARY

Food diaries are your best plan of attack when trying to lose weight. A food diary is a detailed account of everything you eat and drink throughout the day. When you write on paper what you eat and drink every day, it's much easier to locate the extra, forgotten calories. If you're consuming too many calories, this simple journal makes it easy to find a few calories to eliminate here and there to help reduce your daily caloric intake.

For example, one of my clients would drink soda during her workday and a couple of glasses of wine with dinner a few nights per week. When she added these drinks to her food journal, she found she was drinking an additional 4,800 calories a week just from these beverages alone. Another client would sneak a piece of chocolate from the candy dish at the receptionist's desk at work every time he passed by. He calculated over 400 calories a day, on average, from these seemingly innocent bites of chocolate. These are the "forgotten" calories that you don't realize you're consuming. And they add up quickly.

The August 2008 edition of the *American Journal of Preventative Medicine* published a study about the effectiveness of food diaries in helping people lose weight. The study included 1,685 individuals with an average age of 55. They were asked to keep a food diary, eat a healthier diet, and exercise three hours per week. There was a strong correlation between how frequently these individuals kept detailed diaries and the amount of weight they lost during the study. The individuals keeping a detailed food diary more frequently lost more weight.

I'm a huge advocate of these little detailed food accounts. It's not necessarily an easy task, but you need to sit down and write a food diary for at least two weeks to get a realistic idea as to what you're consuming on a daily basis. Go to www.fitbodiesbysasha.com to find my Electronic Food Journal calculator. It will automatically calculate your daily caloric intake. Initially, all of my clients are required to perform this chore, and I still do it periodically myself.

The food diary has to be completely honest, otherwise there's no point in keeping it. The clients that I have to hound for their diaries are the ones who are in denial. They're afraid to really see the kind of foods they're eating and the amount of calories, fat, and sugar they're devouring on a daily basis. You may be able to fool others, but you can never fool yourself. I've had several clients lie in their food diaries because they were embarrassed about what they were eating and drinking. But once they truly opened up about their diet, I was able to help them help themselves.

If done properly, your food journal should be by your side all day for at least a week, and preferably two. This way you can record everything you eat and drink right away so you don't forget the little pieces of chocolate or the sips of soda that might be adding unwanted pounds. If you wait until the end of the day to log your foods, you will likely forget most of your food intake for the day. Most people are astounded by the amount of calories they ingest without even recognizing they ate or drank something.

TIME	FOOD ITEM	CALORIES	TOTAL FAT	SAT. FAT	CARBS.	PROTEIN	SUGAR	FIBER	SODIUM	CHOLESTEROL
11:00 a.m.	Frappuccino Blended Crème - Whip	610	19g	12g	92g	15g	79g	0g	420mg	60mg
11:00 a.m.	Cinnamon Chip Scone	620	25g	11g	92g	7g	53g	1g	440mg	30mg
1st Meal Total:		1,230	44g (33%)	23g	184g (60%)	22g (7%)	132g	1g	860mg	90mg
3:30 p.m.	Double Quarter Pounder w/ Cheese	740	42g	19g	40g	48g	9g	3g	1,380mg	155mg
3:30 p.m.	French Fries (large)	570	30g	6g	70g	6g	0g	7g	330mg	0mg
3:30 p.m.	Coca-Cola Classic (large-32 fl. Oz.)	300	0g	0g	80g	0g	80g	0g	20mg	0mg
2nd Meal Total:		1,610	72g (40%)	25g	190g (47%)	54g (13%)	89g	10g	1,730mg	155mg
8:00 p.m.	2 Chicken Breasts (original recipe)	720	42g	10g	14g	74g	0g	0g	2,040mg	230mg
8:00 p.m.	Mashed Potatoes (with gravy)	140	5g	1g	20g	2g	1g	1g	560mg	0mg
8:00 p.m.	Cole Slaw	180	10g	1.5g	22g	1g	18g	3g	270mg	5mg
3rd Meal Total:		1,040	57g (49%)	12.5g	56g (21%)	77g (30%)	19g	4g	2,870mg	235mg
9:30 p.m.	1/2 Pint Haagen-Dazs (Butter Pecan)	620	46g	22g	42g	10g	36g	0g	220mg	220mg
Daily Total:		4,500	219g (44%)	82.5g	472g (42%)	163g (14%)	276g	15g	5,660mg	700mg

Example of Waldo's Food Diary for Monday

Creating a food diary showed Waldo that when he did eat, he ate a plethora of high-calorie, high-fat, high-sugar, high-sodium, and high-cholesterol foods. With his food journal, Waldo can clearly see why he is obese, has pre-diabetes symptoms, and has concerns with his sodium and cholesterol levels. He now realizes his body has become a ticking time-bomb over the years, ready to explode with any number of deadly illnesses. But he also realizes that it's not too late to change his beliefs and behavior modifications to his diet and lifestyle.

After calculating each category in Waldo's food diary, we find that he consumes approximately 4,500 calories per day. What's more, the calories are mostly derived from "bad" carbs and "bad" fats. According to his Body Mass Index (BMI), Waldo, like 34.3% of adult Americans, comes in at over 30 and is therefore categorized as obese.

Using the Harris-Benedict Formula, Waldo requires 2,729 calories to maintain his current obese weight. Waldo's Basal Metabolic Rate (BMR) is:

$$66 + (13.7 \times W) + (5 \times H) - (6.8 \times A)$$

$$66 + (1,557) + (889) - (238) = \textbf{\textit{2,274 calories per day}}$$

Note: **W** = 250 pounds or 113.64 kilograms

H = 5'10" or 177.8 centimeters

A = 35-years-old

His current activity level is *sedentary* which indicates his basal metabolic rate (BMR) should be multiplied by 1.2 making his approximate daily caloric intake equal 2,729 calories. Remember, this is the amount of calories needed just to maintain his current weight at 250 pounds with little or no exercise in his daily routine. Waldo is currently consuming 1,771 calories more than his body's requirement, which means that he will continue to gain more and more weight as time passes.

Waldo's Calorie Adjustments

Now we have a benchmark. From here, I would personally recommend Waldo lose one to two pounds per week. We know that a slow reduction in calories combined with an increase in daily physical activity has been scientifically proven to properly lose weight *and keep it off.* Waldo realizes that he didn't gain all his extra weight overnight, so he won't be able to lose all his extra weight overnight. Plus, he doesn't want to drastically reduce calories and slow his metabolism. He understands that this would put his body in a defense starvation mode and his body would likely store the calories eaten as fat thinking a famine is about to strike.

Your body will store more body fat and slow down its metabolism.

Ms. Powerfoods has helped Waldo create a healthy diet with less refined carbs, fat, sodium, cholesterol, and sugar. She has replaced these foods with high-quality protein, more complex carbohydrates, and more fiber. Also, she made the meals lower in calories and had Waldo eat three main meals with a snack between each so he eats every 2-3 hours.

I would recommend reducing Waldo's caloric intake by 250 calories, so that he would now be consuming 4,250 instead of 4,500 calories per day. Notice that we don't want to drop Waldo's consumption to 2,729 calories and risk slowing his metabolism.

Waldo's Exercise Adjustments

For Waldo, I would also include some type of physical activity (weight lifting, cardio) to burn an additional 250 calories per day. The reduction of 250 calories from his diet, coupled with expending 250 calories through exercise, will create a total deficit of 500 calories per day, or 3,500 calories per week. Since one pound of body fat is approximately 3,500 calories, Waldo will theoretically lose one pound per week.

Ideally, I would have Waldo lift weights for one hour on Mondays, Wednesdays, and Fridays while doing 45-60 minutes of cardio on Tuesdays, Thursdays, and Saturdays. And I'd recommend that he change his routine frequently to keep it interesting. The most important part of exercise is to have fun. Otherwise it becomes a chore and the odds are that Waldo will eventually quit. When you begin your exercise regimen, remember to change things up. If kickboxing gets you all fired-up, do it. If listening to your favorite jams while climbing the StairClimber relaxes you, do that. The point is to find many different cardio activities you enjoy and keep changing the type of cardio exercises to stay motivated.

Some cardio machines calculate the amount of calories that get burned while doing a specific exercise. Don't believe it. At best, the calculations are extremely rough estimates. The problem is that these machines don't take into account all the factors (gender, height, weight, age, body mass, etc.) that would need to be considered to help determine a more accurate estimate of calories burned. My experience tells me that the estimates from these machines are typically off from 30-67%, based on the more accurate calorie-counting heart rate monitor watch that I use, which accounts for my age, gender, height, and weight.

Cardio exercises are excellent for your cardiovascular system (heart and lungs) and for burning calories to lead to weight loss. But as you lose weight, you'll also lose muscle. And as we already know, less muscle means a slower metabolism and more stored fat. We simply must include weight training to keep our muscles working hard and strong while increasing our metabolism. I typically break the body parts into antagonistic muscle groups exercises. For example, chest and back on Mondays, legs and shoulders on Wednesdays, and biceps and triceps on Fridays. Then I continually change the routines with a method called periodization, which you'll find explained in Chapter 9. I'll do 15 repetitions of each exercise for a couple of weeks, then negatives (pages 206-208) for each exercise for a couple of weeks, then low repetitions/high weight for a couple of weeks, etc.

An increase in muscle will increase your metabolism with less calories stored as fat.

Not only do I change the number of repetitions for each exercise, I also change the exercises for each body part every week. This way I target different angles of my muscles to keep my body strong while protecting my joints from each angle, making my body perform more functionally. One week I might do leg presses, barbell forward lunges, and lying leg curls. The next week I might do squats, dumbbell forward-backward lunges, and deadlifts. If you continue to change your routines, you'll be less likely to become bored and more likely to create a habit of exercising every day for a happier, healthier you.

Checking Back in with Waldo

It's been 2 months since Waldo changed his diet and started working out. He's lost 8 pounds in 10 weeks and has more energy than he's had in a long time. He's also noticed his clothes are looser and he's had to tighten his belt by 2 notches. But wait a minute. Didn't I say that if you were to reduce 3,500 calories per week, you'd lose 1 pound of body fat per week? Waldo should have lost *10 pounds* in the past 10 weeks, right?

The reason Waldo only lost 8 pounds is probably due to lifting weights. Waldo has had a sedentary lifestyle for quite some time so any lifting of weights is going to cause the muscle to overexert, forcing the muscle to grow. Muscle is almost 5 times heavier and about 4 times more dense than fat. This explains why Waldo's clothes are looser and yet he only lost 8 pounds of bodyweight. The scale can't distinguish between muscle and fat. More than likely, he gained 2 pounds of muscle weight, which is awesome! The extra muscle will increase his metabolism with less calories stored as fat and that is exactly our goal. Congratulations, Waldo!

If you're losing weight like Waldo, reward yourself with a weekend getaway or buy a new suit, or do something you enjoy. I recommend that you reward yourself after achieving each short-term goal. Of course I wouldn't recommend using food or alcohol as the reward. The extra calories will thwart your efforts for your ultimate goal – a healthy weight. Also, if you get into the habit of associating food as a reward, food will probably become a comfort for you, leading you back to being overweight, or worse – obese.

HITTING A PLATEAU

Oh no! Waldo has hit a plateau after being on his new diet and exercise regime for 14 weeks. He can't get his weight below 238 pounds. Many dieters give up on their weight loss program when they hit a plateau. They think they've lost all the weight they can lose, and they get frustrated. Please – don't give up and quit. This is just a time to revise your diet and exercise programs.

Waldo decided to cut his breakfast and afternoon snack out of his diet to drastically reduce his daily caloric intake in order to get below his stagnant weight. His strategy worked for a couple of weeks, then he saw the numbers go slowly back up on his weigh-ins. Apparently, Waldo cut back too many calories and his metabolism began to slow down, making his body store more calories as fat. Not a wise move, Waldo.

What he should have done was create another food diary for a week or two to see if he's taking in more calories without noticing that he's doing so. Maybe he's been slacking off with his workouts and yet is still consuming the same amount of calories. The calories then wouldn't be burning off but would become stored as fat instead. It's amazing how many calories are utilized during and after physical activity. Personally, I burn a little over 800 calories during my workouts, which are about 1 hour and 15 minutes; plus another 300 calories during the first hour after my workout. Fewer calories are needed on days you don't work out. Since I know I burn approximately 1,100 calories on the days I work out, I know that I should cut back somewhere around 800 calories on the days I don't work out.

During Waldo's plateau, he learned that he still needs to eat every 2-3 hours, but that he should cut a few calories here and there on those days he doesn't work out. After making a few adjustments with his diet and exercise routine, Waldo was back on track and losing weight again. It's been 12 months since Waldo embarked on his healthy lifestyle and he's feeling like he's in his twenties again. His lower back isn't sore all the time, his blood pressure and cholesterol levels have dropped, and people are complimenting him on his noticeable weight loss.

> Eventually, you will come to a point where caloric intake will equal caloric expenditure.

This is a huge milestone for Waldo because he reached his short-term goal of escaping from the "obese" category and lowering his risk for many chronic illnesses. At 200 pounds, Waldo is still overweight but continues to strive toward his ultimate goal, 170 pounds. He's lost 50 pounds with another 30 to go. Again, he rewards himself by buying the new set of golf clubs he's been wanting.

Seven months later, Waldo hit another plateau. He's been stuck at 175 pounds for a month. This time he's recorded a food diary to see if he's been straying from his daily caloric intake. After viewing his diet on paper, he knows he's been true to his diet (3,100 calories) and he's been working out 6 days per week. So what could be keeping Waldo from continuing his weight loss progress?

Eventually, one comes to a point where caloric intake equals caloric expenditure. That's the point Waldo has hit and will continue to remain at unless he either slightly decreases his daily calories, or increases his physical activities. At 175 pounds, Waldo works out 6 days each week which demands approximately 3,100 calories per day, according to the Harris-Benedict Formula. Waldo's Basal Metabolic Rate (BMR) is:

$$66 + (13.7 \times W) + (5 \times H) - (6.8 \times A)$$
$$66 + (1,090) + (889) - (245) = \textit{1,800 calories per day}$$

Note: **W** = 175 pounds or 79.55 kilograms

H = 5'10" or 177.8 centimeters

A = 36-years-old

Waldo now has a "very active" lifestyle, which means his BMR (1,800 calories) should be multiplied by 1.725 making his daily caloric intake about 3,105 calories. In order for Waldo to continue his weight loss, he needs to either slightly decrease his daily calories again or increase his physical activities. Waldo decided to cut back another 100 calories from his diet. Also, he remembered that his personal trainer once told him that walking

15 minutes a day will take off approximately one pound of bodyweight in a month. So, instead of taking the elevator, he now walks up and down 10 flights of stairs to get to and from his office twice a day.

ACHIEVING A HEALTHY WEIGHT

Almost 2 years later, Waldo has reached his ultimate goal of being at a healthy weight for his height – 170 pounds. *Waldo decided against fad diets and took the road that has been proven by scientists for years to get his extra weight off and keep it off.* During this time he learned how to eat properly with portion control and has embedded new eating behaviors that will last him a lifetime.

Waldo now knows that he needs to keep tabs on his diet and look for signs, like his clothes becoming tighter and the numbers on the scale creeping back up, in order to maintain a healthy weight. He also knows that this isn't a fad diet, but rather a lifestyle that needs to continue for him to remain healthy. After all, the side effects Waldo has experienced with this new lifestyle are more energy, no more constant back and knee pains, lower blood pressure and cholesterol levels, less work for his heart, being able to move around without running out of breath, and having more self-esteem and confidence. And these are just some of the side effects *you'll* experience after losing weight and keeping it off. Isn't being a healthy weight worth feeling and looking great?

Your weight will fluctuate from time to time (even day to day) for many reasons, such as having undigested food in your digestive system, a high-sodium meal that causes water retention, or adding muscle from weight training. Another reason might be eating a few more calories than you should have the night before, which could become a peril to your weight loss or weight management program if not recognized. Remember to weigh yourself once a day, always at the same time and on the same scale. It's best to weigh in first thing in the morning, naked, after going to the bathroom because there will be no undigested food or water in your digestive system thus making your reading a true weight.

It's all about how accurate you want to be, thereby leading to your best results. If you find you're gaining weight, your clothes are getting tighter, or your body fat percentage is creeping up, it's time to reevaluate your diet and exercise program. This is where your food diary becomes your best ally. This little daily record will show where you can cut calories and make little tweaks that could result in huge changes in your physique. You only have one body in this one life. Allow me to be your coach and let's keep it at top performance!

CHAPTER 4

Learn How to Eat at Fast Food Restaurants

There are times when you have no other choice but to stop at a fast food joint. As much as I try to stay away from these high-calorie, sodium-infested establishments, it seems as though, about once a week, I find myself in a drive-thru. Still, not too bad when you consider *one quarter of Americans eat fast food every single day.* The problem I have with this type of food is not only the amount of fat and dietary cholesterol, but the extreme amount of sodium in most menu items. The Double Whopper with Cheese Sandwich from Burger King, as just one example, has 1,500 milligrams (1500mg) of sodium, which, according to the 2010 Dietary Guidelines, is a full day's worth. The problem with too much dietary sodium is that it puts you at risk for hypertension and eventually strains the heart, leading to a possible heart attack, stroke, or a plethora of other diseases. According to a report by the non-profit Center for Science in the Public Interest (CSPI), 150,000 Americans die

> One quarter of Americans eat fast food every single day.

> 150,000 Americans die prematurely of high blood pressure each year.

prematurely of high blood pressure each year.

Even with the bad rap fast food restaurants take, I'm still convinced that it's not the food itself that ruins a diet, but rather the choices we make when ordering. I believe the U.S. Dietary Guidelines place too much emphasis on carbohydrates and not enough on protein and fat. First, life is protein. Our bodies' biochemical processes and behaviors are made possible because of protein. Second, fat is my preferred source of energy. Properly losing unwanted weight is essentially losing body fat. Remember, we want to metabolize the fat but preserve the muscle because muscle revs up our metabolism. When our bodies have an overabundance of carbs, they'll use glucose (carbs) as the main energy source and not burn as much fat. With time, fat accumulates and you gain weight. However, when carbs are reduced, our bodies will have to tap into our stored fat to produce energy. Studies have shown an active person's diet with food proportions consisting of total fat around 30%, protein 30% and carbs 40% help lose body fat and keep it off.

So, in this chapter, we'll analyze the big three fast food establishments – McDonald's, Wendy's, and Burger King – and we'll look at the percentage breakdown of the three macronutrients (fat, carbohydrates, and protein) of their foods to help you understand why people gain weight consuming these foods when they could actually *lose* weight.

Too much food, too much of the wrong foods, and lack of exercise collectively represent only a part of the problem with our obesity epidemic. We also have a lack of *nutrition education*. Currently, a few states have enacted menu labeling legislation, forcing restaurant chains to post the nutrition information of their foods so as to help consumers make better food choices. Many other states have legislative proposals to offer information like calories, fat content, carbohydrates, protein, and sodium for each menu item for health conscious Americans. But until every state mandates that all restaurants offer nutrition information for each menu item, we need to learn which foods we should consume only sparingly. This chapter will give you the knowledge you need to make better decisions when ordering from these fast food chains.

McDonald's

Best Overall Breakfast Sandwich

The Egg McMuffin takes the lead as the most balanced nutritional breakfast item with 290 calories, 11 grams (11g) total fat, 4.5g saturated fat, 30g carbohydrates, and 17g protein. To make it lower in carbs and calories, I don't eat the top half of the English muffin. Which brings me to the second leading breakfast item: the English muffin. The English muffin is low in fat, but it's also low in protein and a bit high in refined carbohydrates.

Worst Overall Breakfast Sandwich

The Big Breakfast is a Big Disappointment with a caloric value that could feed a small village (730 calories, 46g total fat, 14g saturated fat, 53g carbohydrates, and 27g protein). Fifty-six percent of its calories come from fat. What's more, about half the fat consists of our enemies – saturated and trans fats. Although there are 27g of protein in this monster meal, the protein is only 15% of the meal. Also, if we're changing out eating habits so that we're eating

Breakfast is the MOST important meal of the day.

5 or 6 times a day, we can only eat half of the Big Breakfast in any one sitting. Most of this breakfast is likely to be stored as fat because it's too many calories for the average body to utilize at one time.

I would also run from the Hotcakes because of their high calories, high carbohydrates, and low protein. In fact, even though they would take me all of about 5 minutes to eat, I would have to run with my thunder thighs at 5.2 mph for *60 minutes* to burn off the calories in these Hotcakes. And while I'm running, I'd jump through hoops to get away from any of the trans fat-infested biscuit breakfast sandwiches. All the biscuit items are mostly saturated and trans fats, baked fresh to clog your arteries.

All of these items are mostly fat and therefore high in calories. Breakfast is the most important meal of the day. Try to focus more on protein, a little on carbohydrates, and some fat to get the day off to a great start. Believe me, you'll feel better and not so weighed down.

Pound for pound, the McDonald's Hash Browns (a processed food) contain more fat and calories than the notorious Big Mac.

FOOD	CALORIES	TOTAL FAT	SAT. FAT	TRANS FAT	CARBS	PROTEIN
Egg McMuffin	290	11	4.5	0	30	17
		34%			42%	24%
Sausage McMuffin	370	21	9	0.5	31	14
		51%			34%	15%
Sausage McMuffin with Egg	450	26	10	0.5	31	20
		54%			28%	18%
English Muffin (with butter or margarine)	150	2	1	0	27	5
		12%			74%	14%
Bacon, Egg and Cheese Biscuit	440	24	8	5	36	19
		50%			33%	17%
Sausage Biscuit	410	26	8	5	34	10
		57%			33%	10%
Sausage Biscuit with Egg	500	32	10	5	36	18
		57%			29%	14%
Bacon, Egg and Cheese McGriddle	450	21	7	1.5	46	20
		42%			40%	18%
Sausage, Egg and Cheese McGriddle	560	32	11	1.5	48	21
		51%			34%	15%
Sausage McGriddle	420	22	7	1.5	44	11
		47%			42%	11%
Hash Browns	140	8	1.5	2	15	1
		53%			44%	3%
Hotcakes (margarine 2 pats & syrup)	600	17	4	4	102	9
		26%			68%	6%
Big Breakfast	730	46	14	7	53	27
		56%			29%	15%

Best Overall Dry Salad

It might be the best for you, but it's also the most boring – the Side Salad (15 calories, 0g total fat, 0g saturated fat, 3g carbohydrates, and 1g protein). Thank goodness the next best salad has some substance – the Caesar Salad with Grilled Chicken (200 calories, 6g total fat, 3g saturated fat, 10g carbohydrates, and 28g protein). For all the other nutrition in this salad, I'll sacrifice a few calories for some flavor.

Worst Overall Dry Salad

The California Cobb Salad with Crispy Chicken takes the lead as being the worst salad McDonald's has to offer. It weighs in with 360 calories, 18g total fat, 6g saturated fat, 22g carbohydrates, and 29g protein. An extremely close runner-up is the Bacon Ranch Salad with Crispy Chicken (340 calories, 16g total fat, 5g saturated fat, 23g carbohydrates, and 27g protein).

FOOD	CALORIES	TOTAL FAT	SAT. FAT	TRANS FAT	CARBS	PROTEIN
California Cobb Salad w/ Grilled Chicken	260	11	5	0	10	32
		37%			15%	48%
Caesar Salad w/ Grilled Chicken	200	6	3	0	10	28
		26%			20%	54%
Bacon Ranch Salad w/ Grilled Chicken	240	9	4	0	11	31
		33%			17%	50%
California Cobb Salad w/ Crispy Chicken	360	18	6	1.5	22	29
		44%			24%	32%
Caesar Salad w/ Crispy Chicken	300	14	4.5	1.5	22	24
		41%			28%	31%
Bacon Ranch Salad w/ Crispy Chicken	340	16	5	1.5	23	27
		42%			27%	31%
Side Salad	15	0	0	0	3	1
		0%			75%	25%
Fruit and Walnut Salad	310	13	2	0	44	5
		37%			57%	6%

A salad can't be eaten without some type of dressing, so let's see what other kind of damage we can do ...

Best Overall Dressing

The Low-Fat Balsamic Dressing offers low calories with high flavor (40 calories, 3g total fat, 0g saturated fat, 4g carbohydrates) but it drops the ball by offering no protein. I'm big on protein being in every meal I eat because it helps slow the release of insulin. Low-Fat Family Recipe Italian Dressing is also very good.

Worst Overall Dressing

This comes as no shock. Creamy Caesar Dressing ranks as the worst dressing with 190 calories, 18g total fat, 3.5g saturated fat, 4g carbohydrates, and 2g protein. However, the Ranch Dressing comes close by offering 170 calories, 15g total fat, 2.5 saturated fat, 9g carbohydrates, and 1g protein. Creamy, cheese-based dressings are some of the worst diet offenders.

> Creamy, cheese-based dressings are some of the worst diet offenders.

FOOD	CALORIES	TOTAL FAT	SAT. FAT	TRANS FAT	CARBS	PROTEIN
Low - Fat Balsamic Dressing	40	3	0	0	4	0
		63%			37%	0%
Low - Fat Family Recipe Italian Dressing	50	2.5	0.5	0	7	1
		42%			51%	7%
Cobb Salad Dressing	120	9	1.5	0	9	1
		67%			30%	3%
Creamy Caesar Dressing	190	18	3.5	0	4	2
		87%			9%	4%
Ranch Dressing	170	15	2.5	0	9	1
		77%			21%	2%

Let's put it all together …

Best Overall Salad with Dressing

I know it ruins the whole concept of a Caesar Salad, but you get the most nutrition for your buck with the Caesar Salad with Grilled Chicken topped with Low-Fat Family Recipe Italian Dressing (260 calories, 8.5g total fat, 3.5g saturated fat, 17g carbohydrates, and 29g protein). Based on a 1,500 calorie per day diet, you're allowed 300 calories per meal/snack, five times a day. Therefore, based on calories, this makes a perfect meal or snack.

> If you don't like salads, chances are you're not going to order this. I face the same dilemma with flaxseed oil. Intellectually I know it's good for the body, but I can't stomach the side effects it gives me. So I pass on flax and substitute something else.

Try to choose from any of the salads with *grilled* chicken and use any of the "low fat" dressings. When in doubt, order a non-cream based or non-creamy vinegar-based selection.

Worst Overall Salad with Dressing

Beware of the innocent Side Salad with any of the creamy salad dressings because the fat content ranges from 59%-80%. You might be thinking that you've made a healthy choice by getting the Side Salad, but (along with any of the creamy salad dressings) it offers especially low protein and extremely high fat. The Side Salad with Creamy Caesar Dressing is the worst (205 calories, 18g total fat, 3.5g saturated fat, 7g carbohydrates, and 3g protein). Translation: 80% fat, 14% carbohydrates, and 6% protein. Remember, we're trying to keep our fat intake around 30%, carbohydrates 40%, and protein 30%.

I would run from any of the salads with *crispy* chicken. And I would also steer clear of the Creamy Caesar and Ranch dressings. Besides those recommendations, if you're trying to make healthier food choices and have no other choice but to order from McDonald's, you're going to have to deal with a few extra fat calories with the choices offered by their salads. Remember, it's always better to eat a little something than nothing at all. Do what you can here, then try to eat a little less fat and carbohydrates, and a little more protein, in your next meal.

Best Overall Sandwich

By far, the best sandwich McDonald's has to offer is the Chicken McGrill, which has 400 calories, 16g total fat, 3g saturated fat, 38g carbohydrates, and 27g protein. It fits close to our guidelines with 36% fat, 38% carbohydrates, and 27% protein. The second best sandwich McDonald's has to offer is the Chicken McGrill without mayonnaise. Some might argue this is the most nutritious sandwich at McDonald's, but I think the fat content is a little too low, and, more importantly, the refined carbohydrates are a little too high. We want to keep our insulin rising and ebbing as slowly as possible – no spikes and no plummets. The refined carbs are going to automatically jack our insulin level up, so let's have fewer refined carbs. Besides, the fat will slow down the insulin spike.

In defense of McDonald's, they're getting better with this section of their menu.

Worst Overall Sandwich

If you want high calories and high fat, the Double Quarter Pounder with Cheese is your sandwich. Less than 3 of these behemoths will fulfill the daily caloric intake for a typical person, not to mention filling their arteries. It boasts 730 calories, 40g total fat, 19g saturated fat, 46g carbohydrates, and 47g protein. I would refrain from ordering any of the sandwiches with cheese so I could cut back on the extra calories and saturated fat. If you stay away from the cheese, you'll be on the right track.

FOOD	CALORIES	TOTAL FAT	SAT. FAT	TRANS FAT	CARBS	PROTEIN
Hamburger	260	9	3.5	0.5	33	13
		31%			51%	20%
Cheeseburger	310	12	6	1	35	15
		35%			45%	19%
Double Cheeseburger	460	23	11	1.5	37	25
		45%			32%	22%
Quarter Pounder w/ Cheese	510	25	12	1.5	43	29
		44%			34%	23%
Double Quarter Pounder w/ Cheese	730	40	19	3	46	47
		49%			25%	26%
Big Mac	560	30	10	1.5	46	25
		48%			33%	18%
Big 'N' Tasty	520	29	9	1.5	41	24
		50%			31%	19%
Big 'N' Tasty w/o Mayonnaise	420	18	7.5	1.5	41	24
		38%			39%	23%
Big 'N' Tasty w/ Cheese	570	33	11	1.5	43	27
		52%			30%	19%
Big 'N' Tasty w/ Cheese w/o Mayonnaise	470	22	9.5	1.5	43	27
		42%			36%	23%
Filet - O - Fish	400	18	4	1	42	14
		41%			42%	14%
Chicken McGrill	400	16	3	0	38	27
		36%			38%	27%
Chicken McGrill w/o Mayonnaise	300	5	1.5	0	38	27
		15%			50%	35%
Crispy Chicken	500	23	4	1.5	50	24
		41%			40%	19%
Crispy Chicken w/o Mayonnaise	400	12	2.5	1.5	50	24
		26%			50%	24%
McChicken	420	22	4.5	1	41	15
		47%			39%	14%
McChicken w/o Mayonnaise	320	11	3	1	41	15
		31%			51%	19%

christopherSASHA

French Fries, Chicken McNuggets and Chicken Selects Premium Breast Strips

The only thing McDonald's French Fries have to offer nutritionally is a whole lot of fats (especially our enemy – trans fat) along with needless calories. The same holds true for the Chicken McNuggets. By the way, what *are* these things made of? The Chicken Selects Premium Breast Strips are advertised as being made with breast meat but I don't think the 66g of fat (12g saturated fat and another 9g trans fat) can justify 77g of protein. Besides, the body can't utilize that amount of calories at one time. If you're not burning calories right after consuming these monsters, most of the calories will turn to fat or be excreted from your body. The 92g of carbohydrates will mostly convert to fat. And the 66g of fat doesn't need to go through much transformation to also be stored in your body as fat.

FOOD	CALORIES	TOTAL FAT	SAT. FAT	TRANS FAT	CARBS	PROTEIN
Small French Fries	230	11	2	2.5	30	2
		43%			52%	5%
Medium French Fries	350	16	3	4	47	4
		41%			54%	5%
Large French Fries	520	25	5	6	70	6
		43%			53%	4%
Chicken McNuggets - 4 pc	170	10	2	1	10	10
		52%			24%	24%
Chicken McNuggets - 6 pc	250	15	3	1.5	15	15
		54%			23%	23%
Chicken McNuggets - 10 pc	420	24	5	2.5	26	25
		51%			25%	24%
Chicken Selects - 3 pc	380	20	3.5	2.5	28	23
		47%			29%	24%
Chicken Selects - 5 pc	630	33	6	4.5	46	39
		47%			29%	24%
Chicken Selects - 10 pc	1270	66	12	9	92	77
		47%			29%	24%

christopherSASHA

FOOD	CALORIES	TOTAL FAT	SAT. FAT	TRANS FAT	CARBS	PROTEIN
1% Low - Fat Milk Jug (8 fl. Oz.)	100	2.5	1.5	0	12	8
		22%			47%	31%
1% Low - Fat Chocolate Milk Jug (8 fl. Oz.)	170	3	1.5	0	26	9
		16%			62%	22%
Minute Maid Apple Juice Box (6.75 fl. Oz.)	90	0	0	0	23	0
		0%			100%	0%
Orange Juice (12 fl. Oz.)	140	0	0	0	33	2
		0%			94%	6%
Coca - Cola Classic (child size - 12 fl. Oz.)	110	0	0	0	29	0
		0%			100%	0%
Coca - Cola Classic (small - 16 fl. Oz.)	150	0	0	0	40	0
		0%			100%	0%
Coca - Cola Classic (medium - 21 fl. Oz.)	210	0	0	0	58	0
		0%			100%	0%
Coca - Cola Classic (large - 32 fl. Oz.)	310	0	0	0	86	0
		0%			100%	0%

Beverages

It should go without saying that bottled water is the best beverage choice but the 1% Low-Fat Milk Jug has a well-balanced nutritional distribution with 22% total fat, 47% carbohydrates, and 31% protein. If you have a sweet tooth, the 1% Low-Fat Chocolate Milk Jug comes pretty close to fulfilling our nutritional ratio. The Minute Maid Apple Juice Box and Orange Juice are high in sugar and should be consumed in small amounts. If you like apples and oranges, try eating a whole apple or orange. The benefit is that you'll get all the flavor, plus the fiber from the apple skin and the pulp from the orange will slow the spike in your blood sugar, reducing your risk for weight gain and giving you a sense of satiety.

Water is the best choice of beverages.

christopher SASHA

As for Coca-Cola Classic ... it's just a bad idea. First of all, according to researchers at the Harvard School of Public Health, just *one* soft drink per day is associated with weight gain and type 2 diabetes. Secondly, it's *loaded* with 29g of sugar per 12 fluid ounces. The number one ingredient is High Fructose Corn Syrup. Translation: SUGAR. We'll discuss the health dangers of High Fructose Corn Syrup in Chapter 5. Every 4g of sugar is equal to 1 teaspoon of table sugar. So our 32 ounce Large Coca-Cola Classic soda converts to approximately 22 teaspoons of sugar! It's no wonder that, according to an article in the May, 2006 issue of the *American Chronicle*, women who increased their daily intake of regular soda from one or fewer per week to one or more per day gained, on average, a little more than 10 pounds over a 4-year period. Also, their risk of diabetes rose by 85% compared with women who consumed less than one soda per month. It's a better idea to drink 32 ounces (one quarter of a gallon) of water than soda. Your dentist may never forgive you, but your body and teeth will thank you for it.

> Just ONE soft drink per day is associated with weight gain and type 2 diabetes.

Desserts

As we discussed earlier, a snack should contain about 300 calories, which totally eliminates the McFlurries and Triple Thick Shakes. When it comes to desserts, *practice portion control.* Because avoiding foods you love can be counter-productive, I would recommend having them only once or twice per week. Be smart about your choices, and if you can't stay away from that cheesecake, try two bites ... and that's it. If you can't control yourself, "out of sight, out of mind" might be a good motto until you learn portion control.

The Fruit 'N Yogurt Parfait, with or without granola, isn't too bad. The Fruit 'N Yogurt Parfait (without granola) is a little lower in carbohydrates, which means fewer calories. However, they still weigh in with almost double the calories and less fiber than a piece of whole fruit like an apple or orange. Another option is the Vanilla Reduced Fat Ice Cream Cone. Try ordering it in a dish rather than the cone to lower the sugars and therefore the calories.

From a nutritional standpoint, McDonald's has a menu that makes it difficult to find a somewhat healthy meal. However, the corporation is beginning to join the new American health craze. The Cleveland Clinic, one of the nation's top heart hospitals, where patients struggle daily with coronary artery disease, served McDonald's hamburgers and fries in their food court, to which eyebrows were raised from patients and doctors alike. The concerns spawned the Fruit and Walnut Salad, a staple that McDonald's is now offering throughout the nation. Veggie burgers and carrot sticks have also recently made it onto the menu at the Cleveland Clinic. Hopefully those items will soon be available nationwide, too, so you can look forward to new healthy fare at a McDonald's near you.

FOOD	CALORIES	TOTAL FAT	SAT. FAT	TRANS FAT	CARBS	PROTEIN
Fruit 'N Yogurt Parfait	160	2	1	0	31	4
		11%			79%	10%
Fruit 'N Yogurt Parfait (w/o Granola)	130	2	1	0	25	4
		13%			75%	12%
Apple Dippers (1 package)	35	0	0	0	8	0
		0%			100%	0%
Low - Fat Caramel Dip (1 package)	70	1	0.5	0	14	0
		14%			86%	0%
Vanilla Reduced Fat Ice Cream Cone	150	3.5	2	0	24	4
		22%			67%	11%
Strawberry Sundae	280	6	3.5	0	51	6
		19%			72%	9%
Hot Caramel Sundae	340	7	4.5	0	62	7
		19%			73%	8%
Hot Fudge Sundae	330	9	6	0	55	8
		24%			66%	10%
Baked Apple Pie	250	11	3	4.5	34	2
		41%			56%	3%
M&M's Candies McFlurry (12 fl. Oz. cup)	620	20	12	1	96	14
		29%			62%	9%
Oreo McFlurry (12 fl. Oz. cup)	560	16	9	2	88	14
		26%			64%	10%
Chocolate Triple Thick Shake (16 fl. Oz.)	580	14	8	1	102	13
		22%			69%	9%
Strawberry Triple Thick Shake (16 fl. Oz.)	560	13	8	1	97	13
		21%			70%	9%
Vanilla Triple Thick Shake (16 fl. Oz.)	550	13	8	1	96	13
		21%			70%	9%

Wendy's

Wendy's has a cool concept based on having everything individualized so you can customize your meal. All the condiments come in separate packages, so you can choose the toppings and add the dressing you like. If you prefer a sandwich bun instead of a kaiser roll, you can substitute and make a meal that fits your health goals – providing you know what you're looking for.

Salads

The only salads that I would order as is would be the Side Salad (dry and b-b-boring) and the Fresh Fruit Bowl with Low-Fat Strawberry Yogurt. All the other salads are way too high in calories with 41%-72% total fat. As we've discussed, our portion sizes have gotten out of control. But by making a few changes to the salads, we can reduce the fats and calories. For example, the Chicken BLT Salad comes with 680 calories, 47g total fat, 13g saturated fat, 30g carbohydrates, and 38g protein. By excluding the home-style garlic croutons and exchanging the honey mustard dressing with the low-fat version, we're able to slash 26g, or 55% of the total fat, thereby reducing total calories. At the same time, our protein value goes from 22% to 31%. Two simple changes make the Chicken BLT Salad much healthier. It's not the healthiest, but it's still healthier.

FOOD	CALORIES	TOTAL FAT	SAT. FAT	TRANS FAT	CARBS	PROTEIN
Chicken BLT Salad (as-is)	680	47	13	0	30	38
Percentages		61%			17%	22%

Get rid of the home-style garlic croutons and use the low-fat honey mustard dressing instead…

FOOD	CALORIES	TOTAL FAT	SAT. FAT	TRANS FAT	CARBS	PROTEIN
Chicken BLT Salad (fixed)	440	21	9	0	31	35
Percentages		42%			27%	31%

FOOD	CALORIES	TOTAL FAT	SAT. FAT	TRANS FAT	CARBS	PROTEIN
Mandarin Chicken Salad	550	26	3	0.5	52	30
		42%			37%	21%
Spring Mix Salad	500	42	10.5	0	24	13
		72%			18%	10%
Chicken BLT Salad	680	47	13	0	30	38
		61%			17%	22%
Taco Supremo Salad	680	31	14	3	68	32
		41%			40%	19%
Homestyle Chicken Strips Salad	670	45	12	2.5	38	30
		60%			22%	18%
Caesar Side Salad	290	23.5	4.5	0	13	9
		71%			17%	12%
Side Salad	35	0	0	0	7	2
		0%			78%	22%
Fresh Fruit Bowl w/ Low-Fat Strawberry Yogurt	220	1	0	0	49	6
		4%			86%	10%
Mandarin Orange Cup	80	0	0	0	20	1
		0%			95%	5%
Fresh Fruit Cup	60	0	0	0	16	1
		0%			94%	6%
Oriental Sesame Dressing	190	11	1.5	0	21	1
		53%			45%	2%
House Vinaigrette Dressing	190	18	2.5	0	8	0
		84%			16%	0%
Honey Mustard Dressing	280	26	4	0	11	1
		83%			16%	1%
Creamy Ranch Dressing	230	23	4	0	5	1
		89%			9%	2%
Fat Free French Style	80	0	0	0	19	0
		0%			100%	0%
Reduced Fat Creamy Ranch	100	8	1.5	0	6	1
		72%			24%	4%
Low Fat Honey Mustard	110	3	0	0	21	0
		24%			76%	0%

FOOD	CALORIES	TOTAL FAT	SAT. FAT	TRANS FAT	CARBS	PROTEIN
Spring Mix Salad (as - is)	500	42	10.5	0	24	13
Percentages		72%			18%	10%

Lose the honey roasted pecans and exchange the house vinaigrette dressing with fat free French dressing...

FOOD	CALORIES	TOTAL FAT	SAT. FAT	TRANS FAT	CARBS	PROTEIN
Spring Mix Salad (fixed)	260	11	6	0	30	11
Percentages		37%			46%	17%

By eliminating the honey roasted pecans and substituting the house vinaigrette dressing with fat-free French dressing, we can cut in half the calories, as well as the total percentage of fat, in the Spring Mix Salad. Again, by making these trivial changes, we can turn the original Spring Mix Salad with 500 calories and 72% fat into a leaner salad of 260 calories and 37% fat. If you want nuts in your salad, I would opt for the almonds because they're higher in protein and lower in fat. Almonds have fat, but it's predominantly monounsaturated fat, which is the "good" fat that helps prevent heart disease. (More on monounsaturated fat in Chapter 6.) If you want to lower calories and lower total fat, only add half the packet of almonds and you'll have the best of both worlds. ***Remember, moderation is the key.***

Remember, "Low-Fat," "Reduced Fat", and "Fat Free" dressings are lower in fat, but the caloric distribution changes from fats to carbohydrates. It's paramount to pay attention to the *type* of fat that's in the dressings. If the majority of the fat in regular dressing is "hydrogenated," "partially hydrogenated", or "modified," go with the low fat, reduced fat, or fat free to avoid any trans fat. However, if the majority of the fat comes from heart healthy monounsaturated fat (like olive oil dressings), reconsider according to the amount of calories you want to consume for the day. Also, know that most of the calories in fat free dressings are in the form of sugars to make up for lost flavor. The result: you might save on fat – but not calories – and you won't lose weight.

FOOD	CALORIES	TOTAL FAT	SAT. FAT	TRANS FAT	CARBS	PROTEIN
Junior Hamburger	280	9	3.5	0.5	34	15
		29%			49%	22%
Junior Cheeseburger	320	13	6	0.5	34	17
		37%			42%	21%
Junior Cheeseburger Deluxe	360	16	6	0.5	37	18
		40%			41%	19%
Junior Bacon Cheeseburger	380	18	7	0.5	34	20
		43%			36%	21%
Hamburger, Kids' Meal	270	9	3.5	0.5	33	15
		30%			48%	22%
Cheeseburger, Kids' Meal	320	13	6	0.5	34	17
		37%			42%	21%
Classic Single with Everything	430	20	7	1	37	25
		42%			35%	23%
Big Bacon Classic	580	29	12	1.5	46	35
		45%			31%	24%
Ultimate Chicken Grill Sandwich	360	7	1.5	0	44	31
		17%			49%	34%
Spicy Chicken Fillet Sandwich	510	19	3.5	1.5	57	29
		33%			44%	23%
Homestyle Chicken Fillet Sandwich	540	22	4	1.5	57	29
		37%			42%	21%

Best Overall Sandwich

If there were ever a perfect sandwich in the fast food industry, the Wendy's Ultimate Chicken Grill Sandwich would be it. Ordering it the way it's originally prepared delivers 360 calories, of which only 17% is total fat, 49% carbohydrates, and a respectable 34% protein. When I go to Wendy's, this is the puppy I order. It has both flavor and nutrition. The downside is that the bun is refined carbs, which increase blood sugar fairly quickly. Our bodies take the refined carbs in the bun and convert them into glucose (blood sugar) for fuel, and we either burn it as energy or store it as fat.

The Junior Hamburger isn't too bad, either. The protein is a little low and the carbs are a little high, but, overall, its nutritional ratio is acceptable.

Worst Overall Sandwich

The Big Bacon Classic is the worst sandwich offered at Wendy's (580 calories, 29g total fat, 12g saturated fat, 46g carbohydrates, and 35g protein). Here is where *portion size* takes on meaning. First of all, avoid anything with the words "Big", "Biggie", or "Great Biggie" in the name because they'll eventually mean "Big Problems" for your health! The Big Bacon Classic starts off as the reasonably healthy Junior Hamburger mentioned above. But then they add another 2 ounce patty of beef (110 calories, of which 63% is fat), a slice of American cheese (70 calories, 64% fat), bacon (20 calories, 68% fat), mayonnaise (30 calories, 90% fat), and a kaiser roll instead of a sandwich bun (40 calories, 11% fat). By adding these extra components, the calorie count gets jacked up by 270, of which 57% is FAT. A few calories here and there eventually add on many unwanted, unhealthy calories.

Do you understand now why portion size is paramount in the "battle of the bulge?"

French Fries, Homestyle Chicken Strips and Nuggets

The French fries contain the most trans fat, the fat that will clog your arteries the quickest. I can devour the medium sized French fries in less than 5 minutes. But then I have to pay the hefty price of a 6-mile brisk walk, which will take about an hour and 15 minutes just to burn off the calories I picked up in 5!

Try to limit anything that's fried by ordering the smallest size, and just take a few bites to appease your craving. After that, throw the rest away.

FOOD	CALORIES	TOTAL FAT	SAT. FAT	TRANS FAT	CARBS	PROTEIN
French Fries, Kids' Meal	280	14	2.5	3.5	37	3
		44%			52%	4%
French Fries, Medium	440	21	3.5	5	58	5
		43%			53%	4%
French Fries, Biggie	490	24	4	6	65	5
		44%			52%	4%
French Fries, Great Biggie	590	29	5	7	77	6
		44%			52%	4%
Homestyle Chicken Strips w/ Deli Honey Mustard Sauce	580	34	6	3	39	29
		53%			27%	20%
Homestyle Chicken Strips w/ Spicy Southwest Chipotle Sauce	550	31	5.5	3	37	28
		52%			27%	21%
Homestyle Chicken Strips w/ Heartland Ranch Sauce	610	39	7	3	34	28
		58%			23%	19%
4 Piece Kids' Meal Nuggets w/ Barbecue Sauce	220	11	2.5	1.5	21	9
		45%			39%	16%
4 Piece Kids' Meal Nuggets w/ Sweet & Sour Sauce	225	11	2.5	1.5	22	8
		45%			40%	15%
4 Piece Kids' Meal Nuggets w/ Honey Mustard Nugget Sauce	310	23	4.5	1.5	16	8
		68%			21%	11%
5 Piece Nuggets w/ Barbecue Sauce	260	14	3	1.5	24	11
		47%			36%	17%
5 Piece Nuggets w/ Sweet & Sour Sauce	265	14	3	1.5	25	10
		47%			38%	15%
5 Piece Nuggets w/ Honey Mustard Nugget Sauce	350	26	5	1.5	19	10
		67%			22%	11%

christopherSASHA

Baked Potatoes and Chili

Surprisingly, none of the baked potatoes, with the exception of the Bacon and Cheese with Country Crock Spread, are bad choices, though they're a little higher in carbs and lower in protein than our desired ratio. My main concern is that white potatoes are high on the *glycemic index*, which means they'll convert into sugar in your system fairly quickly, and, if not burned as energy, will likely turn to body fat. I would choose the Sour Cream and Chives and the Broccoli and Cheese Baked Potatoes over the Plain Baked Potato because the fat in the sour cream and the fiber in the broccoli will slow down the digestive process, thereby lessening the spike in your blood sugar level. The downfall is that the calorie count will be higher, but in this case, I'd sacrifice a few calories for flavor.

Glycemic Index is the measure of how foods affect blood-sugar levels.

The Small Chili with Crackers and Cheese is a sound choice because the nutritional ratio fits within our goals, carrying 35% total fat, 38% carbohydrates, and 27% protein. The Large Chili with Crackers and Cheese is a little higher in calories but fits into our nutritional ratio as well.

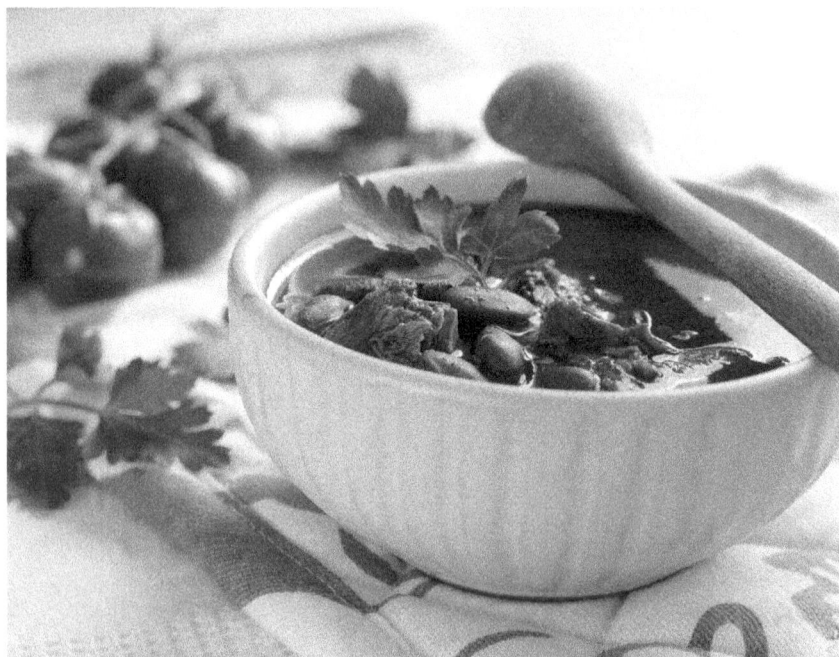

FOOD	CALORIES	TOTAL FAT	SAT. FAT	TRANS FAT	CARBS	PROTEIN
Plain Baked Potato w/ Spread	330	7	1.5	0.5	61	7
		19%			73%	8%
Sour Cream and Chives w/ Spread	400	13	5	0.5	62	8
		30%			62%	8%
Broccoli & Cheese w/ Spread	440	15	3	0.5	69	10
		30%			61%	9%
Bacon & Cheese w/ Spread	560	25	7	0.5	69	16
		40%			49%	11%
Small Chili	220	6	2.5	0	23	17
		25%			43%	32%
Small Chili w/ Crackers and Cheese	320	12.5	6	0.5	31	22
		35%			38%	27%
Large Chili	330	9	3.5	0.5	35	25
		25%			44%	31%
Large Chili w/ Crackers and Cheese	430	15.5	7	0.5	43	30
		32%			40%	28%

christopherSASHA

Beverages and Frosty

Tea is the best beverage at Wendy's because it packs antioxidants that help prevent heart disease and some types of cancers. The coffee is okay to order too but watch out for too much caffeine. Caffeine stimulates our pancreas to produce insulin and depletes calcium from our bones, causing them to become porous and susceptible to osteoporosis. Caffeine also depletes our bodies of magnesium, a mineral involved in more than 300 metabolic reactions.

With the exception of the 2% reduced fat milk, I wouldn't recommend the other beverages. The cola and lemon lime drinks are all sugar. And colas add phosphoric acid, which interferes with the body's absorption of calcium, the mineral that helps strengthen our bones and teeth. Researchers at Tufts University believe colas may seriously weaken a woman's bones.

Be aware of names. Marketers use words that seem minute in our minds when we quickly read them. Wendy's uses the words "junior", "small", and "medium", which implies "a little". But the "little" Frosties are crammed with high calories and a lot of fat and sugars.

Most Americans can barely squeeze 8 glasses of water into their bodies throughout the day, but for some reason they're able to guzzle 16 ounces (two glasses) of a 430 calorie Frosty during a single half-hour lunch break!

FOOD	CALORIES	TOTAL FAT	SAT. FAT	TRANS FAT	CARBS	PROTEIN
Coffee	4	0	0	0	1	0
		0%			100%	0%
Tea	0	0	0	0	0	0
		0%			0%	0%
2% Reduced Fat Milk	120	4.5	3	0	13	8
		33%			41%	26%
1% Low - Fat Chocolate Milk	170	2.5	1.5	0	28	8
		14%			67%	19%
Diet Cola, Medium (20 oz.)	0	0	0	0	0	0
		0%			0%	0%
Lemon Lime Drink, Medium (20 oz.)	120	0	0	0	31	0
		0%			100%	0%
Cola, Medium (20 oz.)	120	0	0	0	34	0
		0%			100%	0%
Junior Frosty (6 oz.)	160	4	2.5	0	28	4
		22%			68%	10%
Small Frosty (12 oz.)	330	8	5	0	56	8
		22%			68%	10%
Medium Frosty (20 oz.)	430	11	7	0	74	10
		23%			68%	9%

Burger King

Breakfast

All of Burger King's breakfast sandwiches are high in calories and fat, and low in protein. The Croissan'wich with Sausage, Egg and Cheese is a nightmare with 520 calories, of which 67% is fat. What's more, 149 calories are saturated and trans fats. Limit your consumption of any sandwich with sausage because it jacks up the calories and almost doubles the saturated fat.

If I had to choose one of the breakfast sandwiches, I would go with the Sourdough Breakfast Sandwich with Ham, Egg and Cheese. The ham consists of 73% protein, only 27% fat, and 0 carbs. To make a case in point, by exchanging the ham with sausage, its cousin sandwich (the Croissan'wich with Sausage, Egg and Cheese) increases its calories by 160 and doubles both total fat and saturated fat. The lactic and propionic acids in the sourdough bread will slow stomach emptying and thereby slow digestion, which slows the increase and decrease in blood sugar and lessens the amount of excess calories to be stored as body fat. Blood sugar levels increase while the food we eat is digesting and decrease after digestion. I wouldn't even consider the French Toast Sticks or Hash Brown Rounds because they're loaded with saturated and trans fats.

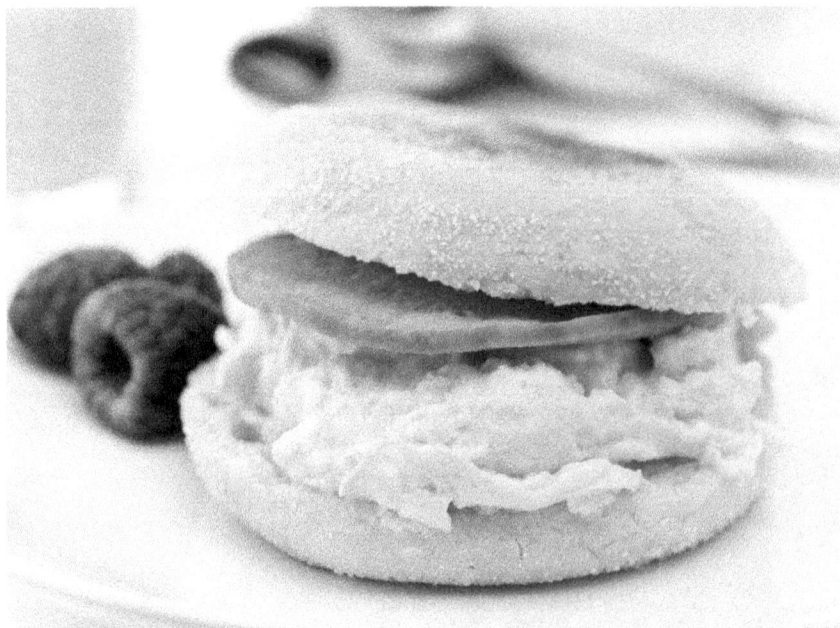

FOOD	CALORIES	TOTAL FAT	SAT. FAT	TRANS FAT	CARBS	PROTEIN
Croissan'wich, with Sausage, Egg and Cheese	520	39	14	2.5	24	19
		67%			18%	15%
Croissan'wich with Sausage and Cheese	420	31	11	2.4	23	14
		65%			22%	13%
Croissan'wich with Egg and Cheese	320	19	7	1.9	24	12
		54%			31%	15%
Sourdough Breakfast Sandwich with Sausage, Egg and Cheese	540	39	13	0.9	30	20
		64%			22%	14%
Sourdough Breakfast Sandwich with Bacon, Egg and Cheese	380	22	8	0.3	30	16
		52%			31%	17%
Sourdough Breakfast Sandwich with Ham, Egg and Cheese	380	20	7	0.3	30	19
		48%			32%	20%
French Toast Sticks (5)	390	20	4.5	4.5	46	6
		46%			48%	6%
Hash Brown Rounds, Small	230	15	4	4.9	23	2
		58%			39%	3%
Hash Brown Rounds, Large	390	25	7	8.4	38	3
		58%			39%	3%

Sandwiches

Three of Burger King's sandwiches, Chicken Whopper Junior (with mayonnaise), Chicken Whopper Junior (no mayonnaise), and Chicken Whopper (no mayonnaise), fit close to our nutritional guidelines. Unfortunately, most of the carbohydrates are refined and will convert to sugar quickly, but this is a necessary sacrifice when consuming fast foods. If you don't like chicken and crave a burger, the Whopper Junior (no mayonnaise) is fairly close to our nutritional ratios.

The BK Veggie Burger items are a little low in protein and a little high in carbohydrates. As for the remaining sandwiches offered by Burger King, their total fat ranges from 40%-59% and they're low in protein, ranging from 14%-27%. The worst sandwich is the Double Whopper with Cheese (with mayonnaise). It has a whopping 1,070 calories, 70g of total fat, 27g of saturated fat, 53g of carbohydrates, and 57g of protein. You might think that 57g of protein and 53g of carbohydrates would balance out the fat, but remember that fat grams are worth 9 calories each, while carbohydrates and protein grams are only 4 calories each. So when you do the math, the Double Whopper with Cheese (with mayonnaise) consists of 59% total fat, only 20% carbs and barely 21% protein. Yikes … call the cardiologist!

FOOD	CALORIES	TOTAL FAT	SAT. FAT	TRANS FAT	CARBS	PROTEIN
Hamburger	310	13	5	0.5	31	17
		38%			40%	22%
Double Hamburger	450	24	10	0.9	31	28
		48%			27%	25%
Cheeseburger	360	17	8	0.7	31	19
		43%			35%	22%
Double Cheeseburger	540	31	15	1.3	32	32
		52%			24%	24%
Bacon Cheeseburger	400	20	9	0.6	32	22
		46%			32%	22%
Bacon Double Cheeseburger	580	34	17	1.3	32	35
		53%			22%	25%
King Supreme Sandwich	550	34	14	1.2	32	30
		55%			23%	22%

Whopper Sandwich (with mayonnaise)	710	43	13	1	52	31
		54%			29%	17%
Whopper Sandwich (no mayonnaise)	550	25	10	0.9	52	31
		41%			37%	22%
Whopper with Cheese (with mayonnaise)	800	50	18	1.4	53	36
		56%			26%	18%
Whopper with Cheese (no mayonnaise)	640	33	16	1.3	53	35
		46%			33%	21%
Double Whopper (with mayonnaise)	980	62	22	1.9	52	52
		57%			22%	21%
Double Whopper (no mayonnaise)	820	45	19	1.8	52	52
		49%			26%	25%
Double Whopper with Cheese (with Mayonnaise)	1070	70	27	2.1	53	57
		59%			20%	21%
Double Whopper with Cheese (no mayonnaise)	910	52	25	2.1	53	57
		52%			23%	25%
Whopper Junior (with mayonnaise)	390	22	7	0.5	32	17
		50%			33%	17%
Whopper Junior (no mayonnaise)	310	13	5	0.5	31	17
		38%			40%	22%
Whopper Junior with Cheese (with mayonnaise)	440	26	9	0.7	32	19
		54%			29%	17%
Whopper Junior with Cheese (no mayonnaise)	360	17	8	0.6	32	19
		43%			36%	21%

Chicken Whopper (with mayonnaise)	580	26	5	0.5	48	39
		40%			33%	27%
Chicken Whopper (no mayonnaise)	420	9	2.5	0.4	47	38
		19%			45%	36%
Chicken Whopper Junior (with mayonnaise)	350	14	2.5	0.3	30	26
		36%			34%	30%
Chicken Whopper Junior (no mayonnaise)	270	6	1.5	0.2	30	25
		20%			44%	36%
Chicken Specialty Sandwich (with Mayonnaise)	560	28	6	2.2	52	25
		45%			37%	18%
Chicken Specialty Sandwich (no mayonnaise)	460	17	4.5	2.2	52	25
		33%			45%	22%
BK Veggie Burger (with mayonnaise)	390	16	2.5	0.1	46	15
		37%			47%	16%
BK Veggie Burger (reduced fat mayonnaise)	330	10	1.5	0.1	45	14
		28%			55%	17%
BK Veggie Burger (no reduced fat mayonnaise)	290	7	1	0.1	44	14
		21%			60%	19%
BK Fish Filet	520	30	8	0.4	44	18
		52%			34%	14%

French Fries, Onion Rings, Chicken Tenders, Baked Potato and Chili

The French fries and onion rings are basically half fat and half carbohydrates. Let's look at the ingredients used to deep fry these products to impart their irresistible flavor. Yum… they're loaded with saturated and trans fats! The main ingredient is "partially hydrogenated oil," a trans fat. The trans fat starts as soybean oil (a relatively healthy oil with a fair amount of Omega-3s). But then hydrogen atoms are added and pressurized in the oil, hence the name "hydrogenated" oil. Modified potato starch is the next ingredient in Burger King's French Fries. It's a starch (carbohydrate) made from corn, wheat, potato, or rice that has been treated physically or chemically to modify one or more of its physical or chemical properties, and it usually contains less than .5% (.005) protein. The function of modified potato starch is to help batters and coatings adhere to poultry and fish products.

Next, potato dextrin is added, which is another carbohydrate. Potato dextrin is derived from potatoes by the application of heat. It also forms a strong adhesive paste. Potato dextrin isn't nutritionally harmful, but do you really want to eat something that is used widely in adhesives like postage stamps, envelopes, and wallpaper? The last ingredient I want to mention is dextrose, a sugar to make the food taste better, but addicting so you crave more. Dextrose (also called corn sugar) is glucose sugar refined from corn starch and used as a sweetener, a source of rapidly absorbed energy that, if not used, will likely convert to body fat. Dextrose spikes the insulin level, which results in carbs being stored as fat.

> The higher the glycemic index, the higher the spike of insulin your pancreas creates.

In order to delay the absorption of food molecules and further slow the insulin spike, try eating some protein first. When I crave French fries or onion rings, I always order the smallest size offered, eat half and give the other half away. I also order something with a lot of protein (usually chicken) to counterbalance the fat and carbohydrates. I end up with more calories but it slows the insulin level rollercoaster.

The Chicken Tenders have more fat than the French fries or onion rings. On the bright side, they also have a little more protein. As with the French fries and onion rings, the Chicken Tenders have the monster trans fats provided by hydrogenated oils and other unhealthy refined carbs and sugars. Try to consume these bad boys sparingly. The Baked Potato sounds healthy, but as mentioned before, it's very high on the glycemic index. The glycemic index is a measure of how foods affect blood-sugar levels. The higher the glycemic index, the higher the spike of insulin your pancreas creates leading to a higher chance these calories will be stored as body fat. Try ordering the potato with sour cream, which will increase the calories but will slow the digestive process. The Chili isn't a horrible choice and is better than any of the fried foods, but be aware that the beef used in this concoction isn't very lean.

I know it sounds like an impossible challenge trying to be healthy in an unhealthy world, but it gets easier as you practice. I promise!

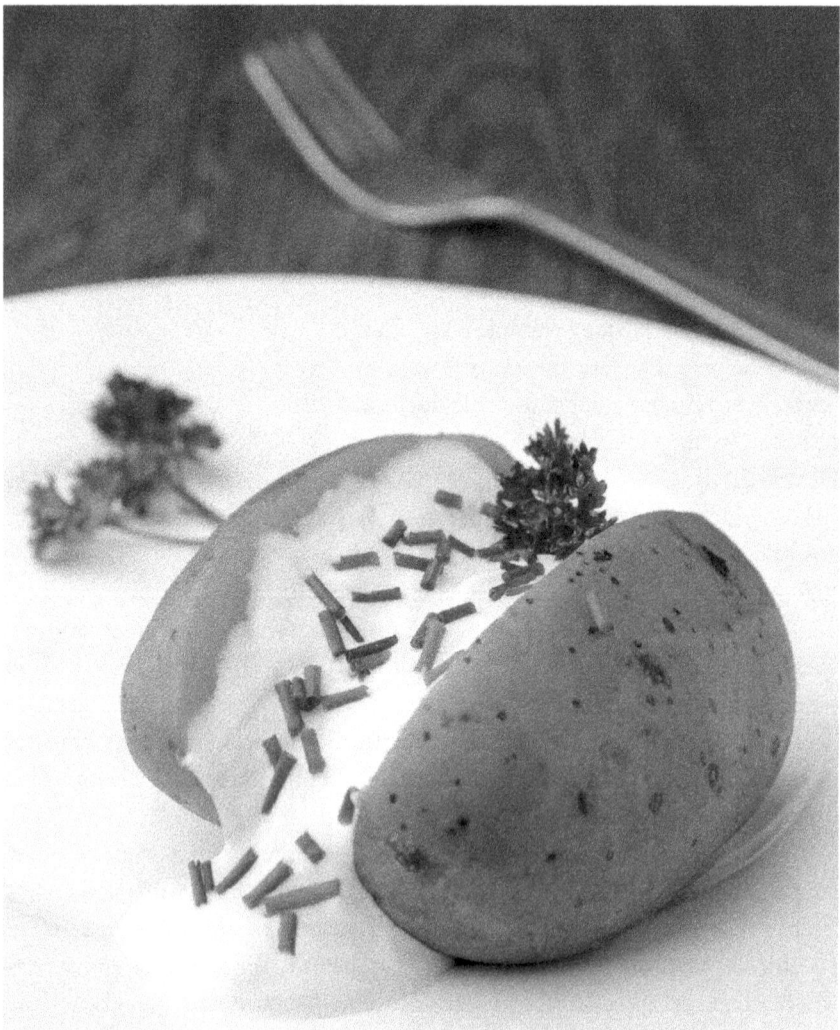

FOOD	CALORIES	TOTAL FAT	SAT. FAT	TRANS FAT	CARBS	PROTEIN
French Fries, Small	230	11	3	3	29	3
		44%			51%	5%
French Fries, Value	340	17	4.5	4.4	43	4
		45%			50%	5%
French Fries, Medium	360	18	5	4.7	46	4
		45%			51%	4%
French Fries, Large	500	25	7	6.4	63	6
		45%			50%	5%
French Fries, King	600	30	8	7.8	76	7
		45%			50%	5%
Chicken Tenders, 4 Pieces	170	9	2.5	2	10	11
		49%			24%	27%
Chicken Tenders, 5 Pieces	210	12	3.5	2.3	13	14
		50%			24%	26%
Chicken Tenders, 6 Pieces	250	14	4	2.7	15	16
		50%			24%	26%
Chicken Tenders, 8 Pieces	340	19	5	3.6	20	22
		50%			24%	26%
Onion Rings, Small	180	9	2	2	22	2
		46%			50%	4%
Onion Rings, Value	280	13	3.5	3.1	35	4
		43%			51%	6%
Onion Rings, Medium	320	16	4	3.6	40	4
		45%			50%	5%
Onion Rings, Large	480	23	6	5.4	60	7
		44%			50%	6%
Onion Rings, King	550	27	7	6	70	8
		44%			50%	6%
Baked Potato with Chives	260	0	0	0	61	6
		0%			91%	9%
Chili	190	8	3	0.3	17	13
		38%			35%	27%

Dipping Sauces...

The only Dipping Sauces I would consider would be the Barbecue Dipping Sauce and the Sweet & Sour Dipping Sauce. With all the fats and carbohydrates in the Onion Rings and Chicken Tenders, there's no need to add more. At least these two sauces are low in calories and carbs. All the other sauces are loaded with fats and sugars. Remember that just because an item correlates with another item on the menu, it doesn't mean that you have to order them together. For example, the Zesty Onion Ring Dipping Sauce doesn't have to be ordered with the Onion Rings. Instead, try the Barbecue Dipping Sauce, if you really want sauce. Or better yet, have the onion rings by themselves and save yourself the extra calories, fats, and sugars.

FOOD	CALORIES	TOTAL FAT	SAT. FAT	TRANS FAT	CARBS	PROTEIN
Barbecue Dipping Sauce	35	0	0	N/A	9	0
		0%			100%	0%
Honey Flavored Dipping Sauce	90	0	0	N/A	23	0
		0%			100%	0%
Honey Mustard Dipping Sauce	90	6	1	N/A	9	0
		60%			40%	0%
Sweet & Sour Dipping Sauce	40	0	0	N/A	10	0
		0%			100%	0%
Ranch Dipping Sauce	140	15	2.5	N/A	1	1
		94%			3%	3%
Zesty Onion Ring Dipping Sauce	150	15	2.5	N/A	3	0
		92%			8%	0%

Salads and Dressings...

Either of the Chicken Caesar Salads (with no dressing) will give you a nutritious snack or meal. It's when you add dressing that the questions of too much fat and not enough protein come into play. Light Done Right Light Italian Dressing isn't done so right. It has 72% fat in it. Who are they kidding? This is why it's so important to read and understand Nutritional Facts Labels and Ingredient Lists, as we learned in Chapter 2.

Any of the salads with Kraft Fat Free Ranch Dressing are going to be your best bets at Burger King. Personally, I prefer the Chicken Caesar Salad with Croutons with the Kraft Fat Free Ranch Dressing because it has a sufficient

FOOD	CALORIES	TOTAL FAT	SAT. FAT	TRANS FAT	CARBS	PROTEIN
Chicken Caesar Salad (no Dressing or Croutons)	160	6	3	0	5	25
		31%			12%	57%
Chicken Caesar Salad with Croutons (no Dressing)	250	9	3	N/A	19	27
		30%			29%	41%
Side Garden Salad (no Dressing)	180	16	2.5	N/A	10	0
		0%			83%	17%
Kraft Catalina Dressing	180	16	2.5	N/A	10	0
		78%			22%	0%
Kraft Ranch Dressing	220	23	3.5	N/A	2	0
		96%			4%	0%
Kraft Thousand Island Dressing	110	9	1.5	N/A	7	1
		72%			25%	3%
Signature Creamy Caesar Dressing	140	13	2	N/A	4	1
		85%			12%	3%
Light Done Right Light Italian Dressing	50	4.5	0.5	N/A	4	0
		72%			28%	0%
Kraft Fat Free Ranch Dressing	60	0	0	N/A	6	0
		0%			100%	0%

amount of calories to hold me over for a few hours. The carbohydrate ratio is a little low, but that allows me to have a few more carbs in other foods I consume throughout the day.

Remember that it's okay to have a few more fats or carbohydrates in one meal as long as you try to lower them in the other foods you eat throughout the day.

FOOD	CALORIES	TOTAL FAT	SAT. FAT	TRANS FAT	CARBS	PROTEIN
Chicken Caesar Salad with Croutons (no Dressing)	250	9	3	N/A	19	27
Kraft Fat Free Ranch Dressing	60	0	0	N/A	6	0
Calories	310	9	3		25	27
Percentages		28%			35%	37%

I would stay away from the other dressings Burger King offers because they have too much fat and sugars. The Kraft Catalina Dressing has 10g of sugar – over 2 teaspoons of sugar in 1 serving. Kraft Thousand Island Dressing isn't far behind with 7g of sugar.

Beverages...

The only beverage with any nutritional value at Burger King is the 1% Milk cup. Everything else is packed with carbohydrates (i.e., sugar). The Minute Maid Orange Juice has fructose, which is a sugar and should be consumed in moderation. Sugar has not only been associated with obesity but also cancer, type 2 diabetes, osteoporosis, and tooth decay because it depletes your bones and teeth of calcium. Your bones and teeth need calcium to continue to be strong and healthy.

The Coca-Cola Company has become such a behemoth in our world that 94% of the world's population can identify the Coca-Cola trademark. It's the most widely recognized English word after "okay". What's more, people drink nearly 10,450 soft drinks from the Coca-Cola Company *every second of every day*. Talk about crazy.

FOOD	CALORIES	TOTAL FAT	SAT. FAT	TRANS FAT	CARBS	PROTEIN
Coca Cola Classic, Kids and Value	120	0	0	0	31	0
		0%			100%	0%
Coca Cola Classic, Small	160	0	0	0	41	0
		0%			100%	0%
Coca Cola Classic, Medium	230	0	0	0	56	0
		0%			100%	0%
Coca Cola Classic, Large	330	0	0	0	82	0
		0%			100%	0%
Coca Cola Classic, King	430	0	0	0	108	0
		0%			100%	0%
Diet Coke, all sizes	0	0	0	0	0	0
		0%			0%	0%
Sprite, Kids	120	0	0	0	30	0
		0%			100%	0%
Sprite, Small	160	0	0	0	40	0
		0%			100%	0%
Sprite, Medium	220	0	0	0	55	0
		0%			100%	0%
Sprite, Large	320	0	0	0	80	0
		0%			100%	0%
Sprite, King	420	0	0	0	105	0
		0%			100%	0%
Dr. Pepper, Kids	120	0	0	0	30	0
		0%			100%	0%
Dr. Pepper, Small	160	0	0	0	39	0
		0%			100%	0%
Dr. Pepper, Medium	220	0	0	0	54	0
		0%			100%	0%
Dr. Pepper, Large	320	0	0	0	79	0
		0%			100%	0%
Dr. Pepper, King	410	0	0	0	104	0
		0%			100%	0%
1% Milk (8 oz.)	110	2.5	1.5	N/A	12	8
		22%			47%	31%
Minute Maid Orange Juice	140	0	0	0	33	0
		0%			100%	0%
Frozen Coca Cola Classic, Medium	370	0	0	0	92	0
		0%			100%	0%
Frozen Coca Cola Classic, Large	460	0	0	0	116	0
		0%			100%	0%
Frozen Minute Maid Cherry, Medium	370	0	0	0	92	0
		0%			100%	0%
Frozen Minute Maid Cherry, Large	450	0	0	0	113	0
		0%			100%	0%

Shakes and Desserts...

Again, the interesting thing is why the marketing team chose to use the words "small" and "medium" to describe the size of their shakes. Like Wendy's Frosties, there's nothing "small" or "medium" about Burger King's shakes. Undoubtedly they're betting on the fact that consumers associate these puny adjectives with calorie-conscious items. After all, you're ordering from a menu with no nutritional facts. When I see the word "small" on a menu, I think low calories. The hard fact is that these shakes harbor between 410 and 790 calories, of which, 46%-52% come from fat. Surprisingly, the vanilla flavor has the highest fat content of all the shakes.

The Dutch Apple Pie is fried, which means it contains trans fat just like the fries, chicken tenders, and onion rings, so I would stay away. The Hershey's Sundae Pie is half fat and half sugar which is likely to store as fat if not burned off by some type of activity. If you can control temptation, try having just one Nestle Toll House Freshly Baked Chocolate Chip Cookie. It will satisfy your sweet tooth and deliver only 220 calories instead of the total 440 calories if both cookies are eaten. Remember, we don't want to deprive ourselves from any of the foods we love, but we must practice ***portion control.***

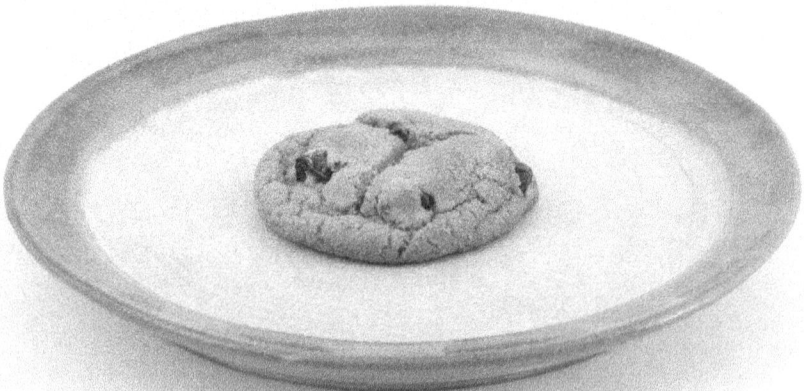

FOOD	CALORIES	TOTAL FAT	SAT. FAT	TRANS FAT	CARBS	PROTEIN
Vanilla Shake, Value	410	24	15	1.1	42	8
		52%			40%	8%
Vanilla Shake, Small	560	32	21	2	56	11
		52%			40%	8%
Vanilla Shake, Medium	720	41	27	2	73	15
		51%			41%	8%
Chocolate Shake (syrup added), Small	620	32	21	2	72	12
		46%			46%	8%
Chocolate Shake (syrup added), Medium	790	42	27	2	89	15
		48%			45%	7%
Strawberry Shake (syrup added), Small	620	32	21	2	71	11
		47%			46%	7%
Strawberry Shake (syrup added), Medium	780	41	27	2	88	15
		47%			45%	8%
Dutch Apple Pie	340	14	3	3	52	2
		37%			61%	2%
Hershey's Sundae Pie	300	18	10	1.5	31	3
		54%			42%	4%
Nestle Toll House Freshly Baked Chocolate Chip Cookies (2)	440	16	5	0.4	68	5
		33%			62%	5%

Fast food doesn't need to be totally eliminated from your diet, but it certainly needs to be watched carefully. I know it might be hard to order healthy food from these fast food joints at first, but think about how just a few calories here and there can add up to real pounds and heart disease. Then reconsider the fried foods, soft drinks, extra biggie sizes, cheeses, and creamy dressings and substitute with salads, grilled chicken, smaller sizes, fruits, and low-fat dressings. You don't have to gain weight in a fast food restaurant – you can actually lose weight, but only if you choose to learn how to order the right foods.

christopherSASHA

We've covered a lot so far. But you'll get the best results for *transforming your lifestyle* from understanding the functions of the foods we put in our bodies – specifically, about both the nutrients our bodies need, as well as the stuff we can do without. When you understand this, you'll easily make healthier food choices.

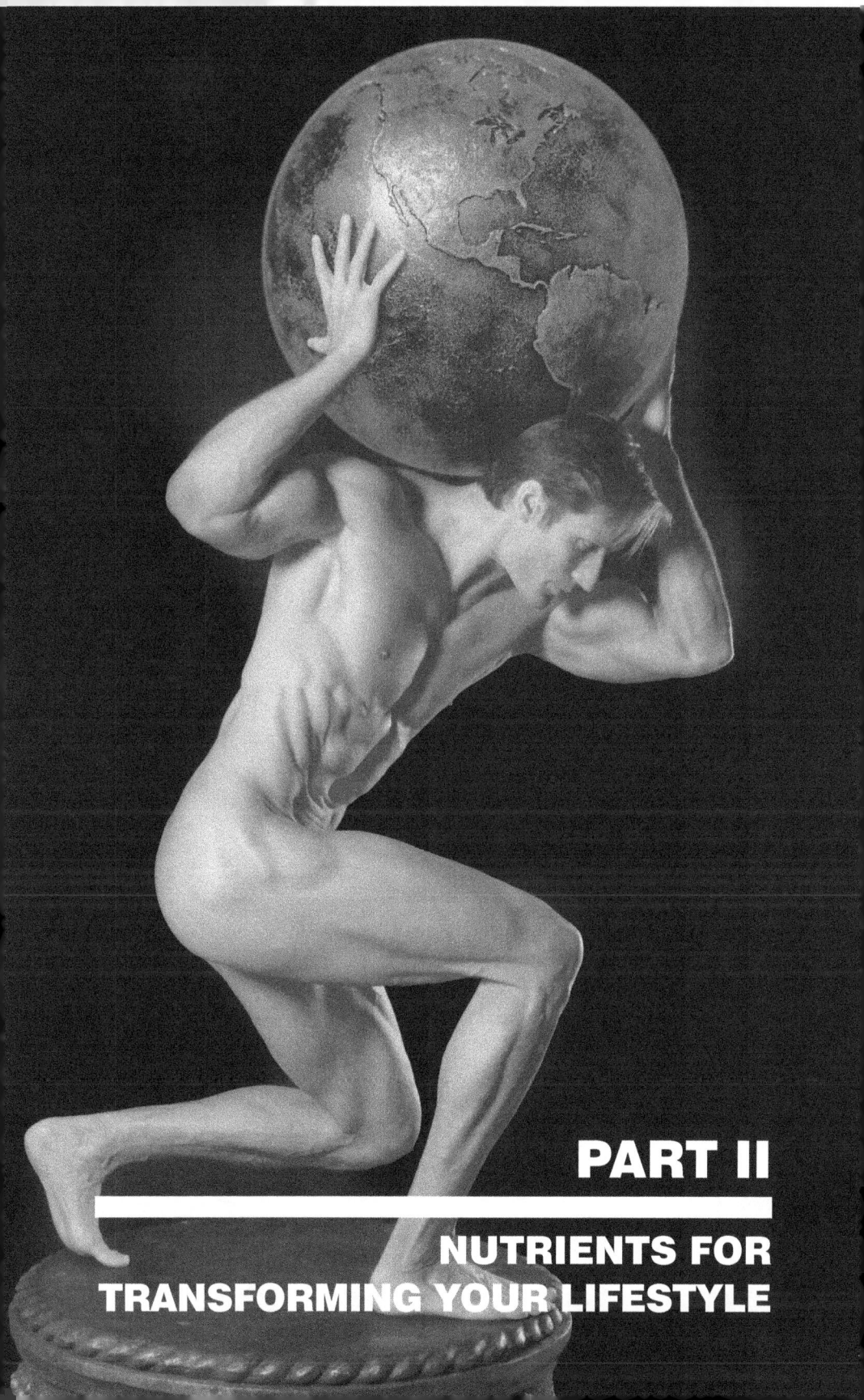

PART II

NUTRIENTS FOR TRANSFORMING YOUR LIFESTYLE

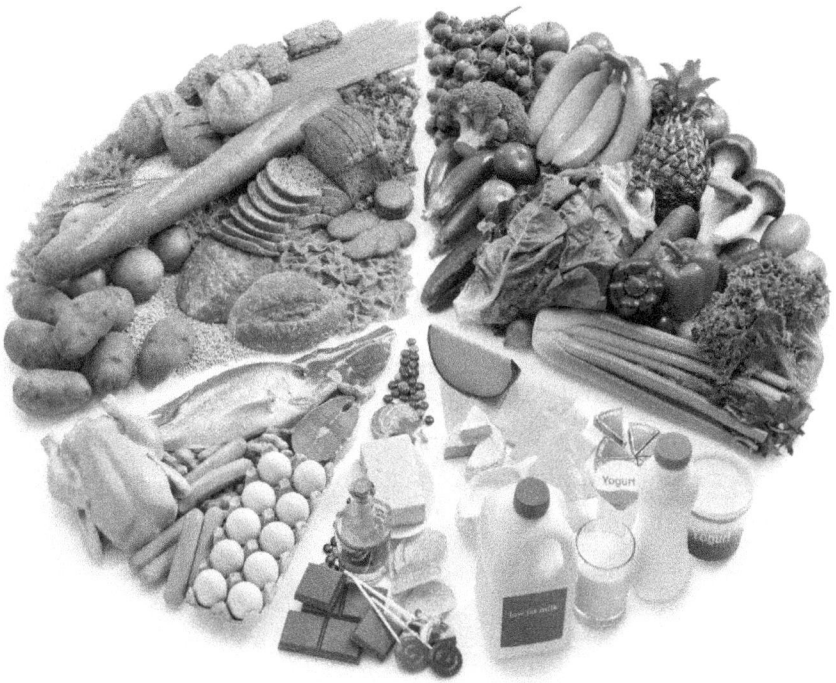

CHAPTER 5
Carbohydrates

Carbohydrates are a major source of energy for our bodies, whether for breathing, reading, or exercising. Carbs supply *all* the cells in the body with the energy they need. To build muscle mass, carbs are a necessity because they fuel the body for exercise, help transport protein to muscles for growth, and help prevent the muscle you already have from breaking down. Sugars, fibers, and starches are the most common forms of carbohydrates and, despite the word on the street about their dangers, "good" carbohydrates are an important part of a healthy diet. On the other hand, too many "bad" carbs (highly processed foods) can actually increase your risk for type 2 diabetes and coronary heart disease. The best sources for carbohydrates are vegetables, fruits, and whole grains, which yield fiber and various vitamins and minerals.

Carbohydrates, excluding fiber, are broken down in the intestine into their simplest form, sugar (glucose), which then enters the blood. As the blood sugar level rises, it triggers the pancreas to produce insulin. The function of insulin is to drive the glucose into cells where it's either used as energy, stored in our muscle tissue and liver as glycogen, or stored as body fat. The words "sugar" and "storage" together concern me because if the sugar isn't used, the two combined equal body fat. Liver glycogen maintains a normal blood sugar level to fuel the brain, while muscle glycogen is fuel for muscles. Glycogen is a good thing because if your blood sugar (glucose) level drops, glycogen can be converted back to glucose to be used for energy.

Dr. Atkins based much of his famous diet on the belief that carbohydrates are not a necessary macronutrient. And – technically – he was right because carbs aren't necessary since proteins can go through a biochemical process called gluconeogenesis to be converted to glucose if needed. The problem, however, with a no-carbohydrate diet is with the long term effects: reduced athletic performance and possible brain damage. The brain can only utilize glucose for energy, and the glucose that's converted from protein may not be enough.

Here's a no-brainer…

Your brain needs a constant amount of glucose (a form of energy derived primarily from the carbohydrates consumed) in order to function properly. When glucose (blood sugar) levels are low, you may begin to feel faint, dizzy, shaky and/or irritable because your brain cells aren't getting enough blood sugar, or energy. Your brain also needs carbohydrates, along with an amino acid (protein) called tryptophan to produce serotonin, a brain neurotransmitter that helps you feel less stress, less pain, and signals your body that you're full.

I was dieting for a photo shoot. I had 3 weeks to get ready. I had to fine-tune my six-pack midsection and I was about 10 pounds overweight. Although I was skeptical of the Atkins Diet, I decided to give it the old college try. I bought nothing but meat from the grocery store so that I could be heavily armed with all the protein and fat my body would need to build the perfect physique. I ate Porterhouse steaks for breakfast, went to buffets to load up on all the roast beef I could eat for lunch, consumed 24 egg-white omelets and a pound of bacon for dinner – and let's not forget whey protein shakes 3 times a day. For the week before the shoot, I forced myself to wake up 2 times in the middle of each night to cram another 30 grams of protein into my system.

In just those 3 weeks, I lost 10 pounds and my body fat dwindled to a mere 3.9%. It was a phenomenal shoot and I was extremely happy with the results I'd gotten with this crazy diet. But the inside of me was a horribly different story. I had the physique of a Ferrari but the performance of a Yugo. I got sick easily. I was exhausted from the time I woke up in the morning until the time I went to bed. I couldn't focus on anything for very long. Most importantly, my cholesterol level noticeably increased. That's when I realized that the Atkins Diet may work for the short term, but in no way would I be able to sustain this diet for the rest of my life. This confirmed for me once again that **diets don't work long-term**.

Complex Carbohydrates

There are 2 basic types of carbohydrates: complex and simple. Complex carbohydrates, also called "good" carbs, are not sweet. They're in all plant-based foods and they usually take longer for the body to digest. Simple carbohydrates are in fruits and refined, processed foods that digest rather quickly. Complex carbs are commonly found in multi-grain bread, wholemeal pasta, brown rice, and vegetables.

Complex carbs can be further divided into two groups: high fiber and low fiber. High-fiber complex carbs are not digestible by humans because we lack the enzyme to break them down. But don't think there aren't any health benefits. Though we lack the enzyme to break fiber down, it's crucial for cleaning our digestive system by assisting waste matter to pass more thoroughly, which will help reduce the risk of developing colon cancer. Fiber also gives a sense of satiety because it slows the digestion process so blood sugar levels don't skyrocket then plummet shortly afterwards, resulting in feeling hungry shortly after eating. High-fiber vegetables, like lettuce and broccoli, are healthy and are linked with lowering incidences of heart disease, cancer, hypertension, arthritis, and type 2 diabetes. A high-fiber diet may also lower your risk of other disorders like irritable bowel syndrome and hemorrhoids. Some low-fiber complex carbohydrates include squash, potatoes, rice, and all cereals and grains.

Whole grains, also known as cereals, are good sources of fiber, vitamins and minerals, and are low in fat. Whole grains consist of three elements: bran, germ, and endosperm. All three contain valuable nutrients. The bran coats the outer layer of the cereal grain. The germ is the part capable of germination, and the endosperm makes up most of the seed plant.

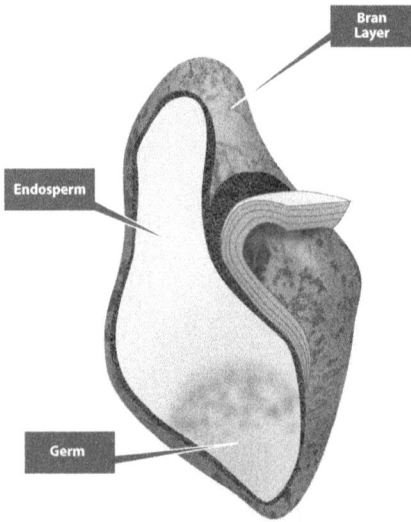

Whole grains haven't had their bran or their germ removed by milling, which makes them a better source of fiber. In contrast, refined grains (white flour or white rice) have both the bran and the germ removed from the grain. Although some vitamins and minerals are added back into the refined grains after the milling process, they still don't contain as many nutrients as whole grains.

The average American consumes less than one serving of whole grains a day and 85% of the grains we do eat are refined.

Instant rice might save cooking time, but will likely add inches to your waistline.

The purpose of refined grains is to promote a much longer shelf life and to reduce cooking time. For instance, whole grain rice takes about 45 minutes to cook while Uncle Ben's Instant Rice (enriched long grain rice) takes 5 minutes. Because we live in an instant gratification society, we naturally grab the Uncle Ben's Instant Rice, falsely thinking that we made a healthy decision. Quite the contrary. That instant rice might save you 40 minutes of cooking time, but will eventually add inches to your waistline. Instant rice turns to sugar quickly in your system, therefore leading to stored body fat if not utilized as energy. Try to choose whole grains rather than refined grains.

Here's a list of some excellent sources of complex carbohydrates:

1. Starches – Sourdough rye bread, brown rice, oats, barley, legumes and vegetables
2. Fiber (insoluble) – Whole-wheat breads and cereals, wheat bran, carrots, cauliflower, and apple skin
3. Fiber (soluble) – Oat bran, legumes, barley, rice bran, and apple pulp

EXAMPLES OF WHOLE GRAINS	EXAMPLES OF REFINED GRAINS
Wild Rice	White Bread
Brown Rice	White Rice
Oatmeal	Corn Flakes
Whole-wheat Breads & Pastas	"Enriched" Breads & Pastas
Popcorn	Pretzels

Fiber

Let's discuss fiber for a moment. Fiber is a part of plant food (whole grains, fruits, vegetables, nuts, seeds) that the body can't digest, which means that it doesn't provide calories. Fiber is important for the health of the digestive system, helps reduce the risk from some chronic diseases like cardiovascular disease, type 2 diabetes and obesity, and is linked to preventing some types of cancer, especially colon cancer. Some other benefits include the prevention of constipation, hemorrhoids, diverticulosis (an intestinal disorder), as well as the lowering of cholesterol and blood sugar. There are two types of fiber: soluble and insoluble. Neither type is digestible by the human body. Therefore fiber isn't absorbed into the bloodstream and used for energy. Rather it passes through the intestines. Both types of fiber have their own important benefits and functions.

Soluble Fiber

Soluble fiber has been shown to help lower low-density lipoprotein (LDL), the "bad" cholesterol, thus reducing the risk of heart disease. It also regulates blood sugar, which helps prevent diabetes. It binds with fatty acids and prolongs the time it takes the stomach to empty so that sugar is released and absorbed into the bloodstream at a slower pace. Oats have the highest proportion of soluble fiber of any grain; however, other good sources include kidney beans, lima beans, soy beans, lentils, chick peas, barley, rice bran, flax seed, fruits (apple pulp, strawberries, and oranges) and vegetables (carrots and corn).

Insoluble Fiber

Insoluble fiber aids in regular bowel movements, preventing constipation and speeding the removal of toxic waste through the colon. It also controls and balances the pH (acidity/alkalinity) in the intestines to help prevent colon cancer. Foods high in insoluble fiber include whole-wheat breads, wheat cereals, wheat bran, rye, brown rice, fruit skins (apple skins), and vegetables (cauliflower, Brussels sprouts, and cabbage). Remember the old saying, "Eat your cabbage to clean yourself out"? How many times did I hear that from my grandmother?!

Consume at least 25 grams of fiber each day.

Most American adults don't consume nearly enough dietary fiber on a daily basis. Every gram of fiber is 4% of the Daily Recommended Allowance, therefore 25 grams of fiber is our goal. The American Heart Association suggests eating a variety of fiber sources. Don't torture yourself by trying to choose one specific type of fiber over the other. *Eating enough fiber is the important thing.*

Breads

Be careful when choosing "healthy" breads. Even though the package may say "100% Whole-Wheat", "7 Grain", "12 Grain", etc., that doesn't always mean that these breads really are whole-grain breads. By using fancy wording and by placing flakes of grains and seeds on the surface of their breads, food companies make it problematic for the health-conscious person to recognize a whole-grain food. Mindful that consumers are interested in whole-grain products, companies make foods sound like they're whole-grain and healthy when they actually aren't.

That's misleading and a form of false advertising that ought to be illegal.

Food manufacturers make foods 'sound like' they're healthy when actually they aren't. Protect yourself by reading Nutrition Facts Labels and Ingredient Lists discussed in Chapter 2.

But somehow the food manufacturers get away with it. So, read Food Labels and Ingredient Lists carefully, as explained in Chapter 2. Whole-grain products will list the main ingredient as whole wheat, whole oats, stone ground whole wheat, or some other whole grain cereal. If the label says "made with wheat flour" it may be a marketing ploy because *even highly processed cookies are made with wheat flour.*

When it comes to breads and other foods, we first need to understand what "enriched" means. Essentially, manufacturers strip most

christopher SASHA

of the nutrients out of grains during processing to make the flour. Then, to improve the nutritional value of the food, they add back a few nutrients. So when the Ingredient List on the back of bread specifies "enriched flour," *it is not a whole-grain product.*

Enriched flour is the first ingredient listed in 5 of the 8 breads I randomly selected from grocery store shelves. Each of these breads added back the nutrients niacin, iron, riboflavin, and folic acid. Please don't fall into the trap marketers have created, adding flakes of grain or seeds on the top of their bread. Many times these breads aren't healthy but the flakes of grain or seeds deceive the consumer into believing they are. Always check the Ingredient List. If it has the word "enriched" listed, it's processed and nutrients have been stripped away.

'Enriched flour' means it's not a whole-grain product.

Further, high fructose corn syrup ranks as one of the top ingredients in 5 of the 8 breads, meaning that most of the bread will be converted into sugar quickly when digested in the body. If you're not utilizing the calories for energy shortly after consuming these processed breads, chances are these calories will be stored as body fat.

BREAD	CALORIES	TOTAL FAT	SUGAR	DIETARY FIBER	CARBS	PROTEIN
Natural Ovens Bakery - Original	60	1.5 g	1 g	4 g	7 g	7 g
White Bread	130	2 g	3 g	2 g	23 g	4 g
Cracked Wheat Bread	90	1.5 g	1 g	1 g	16 g	3 g
Butternut - All Whole-Grain 100% Whole Wheat	60	0.5 g	2 g	2 g	12 g	3 g
Natural Harvest - 7 Grain	100	1.5 g	3 g	1 g	19 g	4 g
Sara Lee - Heart Healthy Plus - 100% Multi-Grain made with real Honey	100	1.5 g	4 g	2 g	19 g	5 g
Brownberry - Rye (seeded)	70	0.5 g	<1 g	2 g	14 g	2 g
Pepperidge Farm - Pumpernickel	80	1 g	<1 g	2 g	15 g	3 g

Sara Lee has a bread labeled Heart Healthy Plus – 100% Multi-Grain (made with real honey). This is a great example of marketers vying for your business. Even though the stone ground whole wheat flour is a good start, they taint the product by making the third, fourth, and fifth ingredients all sugar (honey, brown sugar, and high fructose corn syrup respectively). Remember, four grams of sugar equals one teaspoon. You might see a slice of bread, but your body recognizes it as a teaspoon of sugar. "Enriched white bread" is the most corrupted of all because it has nearly the same effect as pure sugar. It's even worse than ice cream! At least ice cream also packs in some nutrients like calcium and protein, along with the sugar.

4 grams of sugar equals 1 teaspoonful.

Natural Ovens Bakery makes a few types of bread that I like. The company was founded by a husband and wife team with backgrounds in biochemistry and nutrition. Their bread has twice the fiber and twice the protein of the average bread and less than half the carbohydrates, not taking net carbs (discussed on page 134) into account. It also contains 310 milligrams (310mg) of heart-healthy Omega-3s. All this nutrition is jam-packed into only 60 calories. When it comes to bread, the rule of thumb is the denser and heavier, the better. Because this bread doesn't have preservatives, refrigerate or freeze it. Otherwise, you'll quickly end up with a loaf of mold.

BREAKFAST CEREALS

The same cautions we use with breads we have to use with breakfast cereals. Be on guard against marketers' attempts to dupe us into purchasing calorie-laden cereals. Kellogg's Frosted Mini-Wheats audaciously calls itself "Lightly sweetened" when its top ingredients are "sugar" and "high fructose corn syrup." In fact, this cereal's calorie count is the highest in sugar of all the cereals listed in the graph – and 22% of its total calories are attributed to these two sweeteners.

Other cereals advertise in big print "Antioxidants" and "Soy Protein" to catch our attention. When vetting the list of ingredients, you'll notice that these ingredients are near the bottom of the list – which means there is very little of them in their cereal.

I once had a similar experience when I visited Thailand and bought a few cashmere suits. I thought I was getting a real bargain until my tailor at home told me there was no more than 1% cashmere in the suits, the rest of the material being cheaper wool. Apparently, if an item has only a minute amount of a particular substance in it, they can still over-emphasize it, a practice known as "puffing." Only you can refrain from being victimized. **Read the Ingredient List.**

All Bran, Special K, Oat Bran, Kellogg's Frosted Mini-Wheats, Life, Cheerios, Total, Rice Krispies, Cornflakes, Crispix, and Rice Chex all list sugar and/or high fructose corn syrup as top ingredients. It's no wonder Americans are getting fatter even when they try buying cereals that sound healthy. Food manufacturers know what they're doing when they include sugar, or a form of it, in the top ingredients. Sugar is one of the most psychologically addicting substances we know. We crave it. We can't get enough. By the time you wake up in the morning, your body has taken care of all the calories you ate for dinner the night before and your blood sugar level is low. When your blood sugar level is low, you get that hungry feeling and want a quick fix to satisfy the discomfort. The quickest fix we can get is from carbohydrates, which all contain some form of sugar. So you schlep to the kitchen for a bowl of cereal (loaded with sugar) and your hunger slowly dissipates.

Sugar is one of the most psychologically addicting substances we know.

You start associating the cereal with comfort and you get hooked – all part of the food manufacturers' plan! Then, the sugar leaves the stomach, is absorbed quickly into the bloodstream, and you start to feel hungry again. The vicious cycle continues and you consume more carbohydrates, or sugar. And if you're not moving and burning calories, most of these sugars are likely to be stored as body fat. The more refined carbohydrates you eat, the fatter you're likely to get.

In order to slow this unhealthy cycle, you need to include protein and fiber in your diet. Then the digestive system has to break through protein and fiber before it can utilize the sugar. This slows the digestive process and the absorption of the sugar into the bloodstream, giving the sugars less chance to be stored as fat. It also helps you feel full for longer. This is why I have Kashi - Go Lean cereal first thing in the morning. It has three times the fiber and three times the protein of the average breakfast cereal. I then have plenty of time to plan my next meal without my hunger driving me straight for the carbs.

BREAKFAST CEREALS	CALORIES	TOTAL FAT	SUGAR	DIETARY FIBER	CARBS	PROTEIN
Kashi - GO LEAN	140	1 g	6 g	10 g	30 g	13 g
Quaker Oatmeal (non instant)	150	3 g	1 g	4 g	27 g	5 g
Cream of Wheat (non instant)	120	0 g	0 g	1 g	24 g	4 g
All Bran (original)	80	1 g	6 g	10 g	23 g	4 g
Oat Bran	210	3 g	9 g	6 g	28 g	7 g
Total	100	0.5 g	5 g	3 g	23 g	2 g
Special K (original)	110	0 g	4 g	<1 g	22 g	7 g
Cheerios (original)	110	2 g	1 g	3 g	18 g	3 g
Cornflakes	100	0 g	2 g	1 g	24 g	2 g
Life (original)	120	1.5 g	6 g	2 g	25 g	3 g
Kellogg's Frosted Mini-Wheats	180	1 g	10 g	5 g	41 g	5 g
Wheat Puffs	50	0 g	0 g	1 g	11 g	2 g
Crispix	110	0 g	2 g	1 g	24 g	2 g
Rice Krispies	120	0 g	3 g	0 g	29 g	2 g
Rice Chex	120	0.5 g	2 g	<1 g	26 g	2 g

Simple Carbohydrates

In contrast to complex carbohydrates, simple carbohydrates are digested very easily. They are rapidly broken down and absorbed into the bloodstream, signaling the pancreas to quickly produce insulin. Eventually these sugars are converted to fat if not used as energy. The aftermath of consuming too many simple carbohydrates is a burst of energy followed by a swift drop in energy, leaving you feeling more tired than before. A classic example of the effects of simple carbohydrates is when you give kids a lot of candy to eat. They'll start out hyper for a short time, then fall fast asleep.

Simple carbs give a quick burst of energy followed by a swift drop in energy, leaving you feeling more tired than before.

Simple carbohydrates, also called simple sugars, come from fruits, milk and dairy products, processed foods, and anything with refined sugar added.

Refined processed foods (soft drinks, desserts, candy) contain almost no vitamins or minerals and are usually loaded with calories.

Consuming large amounts of refined carbohydrates over an extended amount of time can lead to type 2 diabetes and a host of other chronic illnesses. Once again, *moderation is the key to Transforming Your Lifestyle.*

Because simple carbohydrates digest easily, making you feel hungry again soon, it's better to eat whole fruits rather than fruit juices. Fruit juices offer just the sugar from the fruit, whereas whole fruits contain vitamins, nutrients, and fiber. Your body has to metabolize these substances before utilizing the sugars for energy. Therefore the digestive process is slowed, allowing proper absorption of the sugars, meaning less will have a chance to be stored as fat.

Types of Sugars

When sugar is first extracted from the juice of the beet or cane plant, it's molasses, a strong-tasting, thick, black liquid. To lessen the taste and crystallize the sugar, it goes through a refining process. After molasses, sugar becomes brown sugar which retains varying amounts of molasses. The product at the end of the refining process is refined white sugar.

There are many types of sugars that are all virtually empty calories. Sugars usually end with "-ose" – sucrose, lactose, maltose. Sugar alcohols (a type of carbohydrate that is not sugar or alcohol but has a similar chemical structure that partly resembles sugar and partly resembles alcohol) end with "-itol" – sorbitol, mannitol, xylitol. And then there are the artificial sweeteners. This knowledge will help you when reading the elaborate names on Nutrition Facts Labels.

According to the United States Department of Agriculture (USDA), total sugar consumption has risen in America from an estimated 114 pounds per person in 1975 to over 136 pounds in 2007. USDA figures indicate that the type of sweeteners consumed has changed mostly from refined sugar (sucrose) to predominantly high fructose corn syrup, which some studies suggest may play a role in weight gain by undermining appetite control.

> Sugar-sweetened beverages, including sports and energy drinks, may be the single largest driver of the obesity epidemic.

You may wonder why Americans would switch from refined sugars to corn sweeteners. Well, consumers didn't consciously decide to make the change. That decision was made by food manufacturers because corn sweeteners like high fructose corn syrup are cheaper, easier to use, and sweeter than refined sugar. So less is needed. Damn those food manufacturers. They know that sugars metabolize quickly, allowing the stomach to empty rapidly, and making you feel hungry again more quickly, encouraging you to eat more. The ultimate result, obviously, is weight gain. This is a vicious cycle that needs to be broken.

In 2004, the National Academy of Sciences suggested that added sugars *should not exceed 25% of daily calories, or 500 calories based on a 2,000 calorie diet.* In 2005, the World Health Organization (WHO) recommended limiting intake of added sugars to *no more than **10%** of daily calories, or 200 calories based on a 2,000 calorie diet.* This would help slow the worldwide rise in obesity that is fueling the growth of chronic diseases such as type 2 diabetes and cancer. In 2006, experts advocated a 15% decrease in added sugar consumption, which implies that sugar may be one of the pernicious foods causing obesity and chronic diseases. In fact, the *New England Journal of Medicine* had an article in the April 30, 2009 issue declaring that "sugar-sweetened beverages (soda sweetened with sugar, corn syrup, or other caloric sweeteners and other carbonated and non-carbonated drinks, such as sports and energy drinks) may be the single largest driver of the obesity epidemic."

> ...sugar may be one of the pernicious foods causing obesity and chronic diseases.

There seems to be a perpetual list of sweeteners manufacturers have created to make foods taste better, or sweeter, in hopes that the consumer would purchase more of their products. Let's describe the more common types of sugars to gain a better awareness of what we're putting into our bodies. I'm not by any means promoting a "no sugar" diet, because sugar is okay in moderation – *as long as you eat a healthy diet and balance the extra calories.*

Natural Sugars

Molasses

A thick, dark syrup derived from the juice that is boiled down from sugar cane. Used mainly for cooking.

Brown Sugar

A combination of white sugar and molasses.

Sucrose

Better known as table sugar, white sugar, or just sugar. It has about 16 empty calories per serving (4 grams), and has virtually no nutritional value. It occurs naturally in every fruit and vegetable as a result of photosynthesis (the process plants use to convert the sun's energy into food). Sucrose is a catalyst for tooth decay. Bacteria in the mouth convert sucrose to acids that break down tooth enamel. And, of course, that's in addition to the part it plays in obesity, type 2 diabetes, cancer, and other major chronic diseases.

Fructose

The sweetest "natural" sugar found in fruit and the major component of honey. New research shows that fructose has the ability to raise triglyceride levels considerably, which may lead to heart disease. It converts to fat more easily than any other type of sugar, one of the reasons Americans are getting fatter. Fructose doesn't metabolize the same as sugar (cane or beet) which alters the way metabolic-regulating hormones function. Fructose doesn't *increase* leptin, an appetite hormone that signals our brains when we're full, nor does it *suppress* ghrelin, the hormone that increases our feelings of hunger.

Fructose also forces the liver to jack up the levels of fat in the bloodstream in the form of triglycerides. But for me, the most compelling evidence to limit my fructose consumption is the recent studies indicating that fructose depletes adenosine triphosphate (ATP). ATP is the usable form of energy our bodies use to move and function. So what does this mean? When ATP is depleted, we lose our energy. And when we're sluggish, we tend to eat more

Fructose enables pancreatic cancer cells to proliferate.

christopherSASHA

to pick up our energy level, thus resulting in the consumption of more and more calories, leading to more and more stored body fat.

Today, most of the average 158 pounds of sugar consumed per individual per year is in the form of fructose. Approximately 25% of the average diet is sugar, mostly fructose. A recent UCLA study found that fructose enables pancreatic cancer cells to proliferate. I'm not suggesting that you throw fruit out or banish it from your diet. Some whole fruit is good for your body. It offers desperately needed fiber. What I am proposing is beverages like fruit juices and sodas sweetened with fructose should be limited. Even the Ingredient List on so-called health drinks need to be vetted because manufacturers add fructose to sweeten otherwise boring drinks. ***Warning:*** diabetics are encouraged to use fructose because it doesn't signal the pancreas to produce insulin.

Lactose

A type of sugar found in milk and milk products (cheese, butter, ice cream, etc.). Lactose is about 1/6th as sweet as sucrose. Lactose intolerance is the inability to digest lactose and it's genetic; about 70% of the world's population gets an upset stomach drinking milk or eating dairy products.

Maltose

Also called malt sugar. It's the worst sugar of all. Maltose is the primary sugar in beer, which can result in the appropriately named "beer belly", when too much is consumed.

High Fructose Corn Syrup

You probably don't think of sugar when you look out over a corn field, but that's where many sweeteners in processed foods originate. High fructose corn syrup was developed in the 1970s because it's much cheaper than sucrose and twice as sweet so less needs to be used. It's also easier to blend into beverages.

High fructose corn syrup is a liquid so it gets into the bloodstream quickly. And you know by now what happens next. Americans consumed *1,000%* more high fructose corn syrup in 1990 than what they consumed when it was introduced in the 1970s. Americans consumed almost 63 pounds of it in 2001, according to the USDA. It's the primary sweetener in soft drinks

> Americans consumed 1,000% more high fructose corn syrup in 1990 compared to the 1970s.

and can also be found in everything from breads to pastas to jellies to yogurts to baked goods and condiments like ketchup. It's also in many "health" foods like protein bars, energy drinks, and natural sodas.

Dextrose

Also called corn sugar or grape sugar. It's refined from corn and cheaper than sucrose for manufacturers to mix into beverages. Dextrose is 70%-75% as sweet as sucrose and is absorbed quickly.

Honey

Nature's original sweetener. A sweet fluid made by bees from the nectar of flowers, honey is significantly sweeter than sucrose. Recent studies suggest that honey helps in preventing fatigue and enhancing athletic performance. Supposedly, ancient Greek and Roman athletes used honey to increase their strength and stamina. Research has also shown that honey may assist in quicker muscle recovery following heavy exercise. So what are you waiting for? Try stirring a spoonful of honey into a glass of water after your daily workout.

Sugar Alcohols (Nutritive Sweeteners)

Sorbitol

A sugar alcohol (nutritive sweetener) that occurs naturally in some fruits (apples, cherries, plums, pears, prunes, peaches) and vegetables and also can be manufactured from corn syrup. It's a bulk sweetener the body metabolizes slowly, which results in fewer calories than regular sugar – about 2.5 calories per gram as opposed to 4 calories from sucrose, or sugar. Sorbitol doesn't cause tooth decay and has been safely used for over half a century. Since it's about 60% as sweet as sucrose, it's popular among diabetics and others trying to reduce their sugar intake but still craving something sweet. Sorbitol is in a myriad of dietetic food products like sugar free candies, gums, breath mints, sugar-free maple syrups, brownies, cookies, pancake and cake mixes, and sugar-free hot fudge toppings. It's even in products like toothpaste and mouthwash and some medicines.

Unfortunately, sorbitol is not a perfect sugar substitute. Since the body absorbs it slowly, the unabsorbed sugars may retain water in the intestines which can cause a range of gastrointestinal problems, including diarrhea, abdominal pain and bloating, especially in children who have lower body weight.

> I recently had a bout with this "safe" sugar substitute when I was watching a movie and innocently devoured a half bag of sugar-free gummy bears. About an hour later I felt abdominal pains and realized I suddenly had a major case of gas, gas and more gas. I couldn't make it stop. My stomach looked like I was five months pregnant! After lying in the fetal position all night, I finally felt back to normal in the morning.

This goes to prove that even those who read Food Labels and try to follow a healthy diet can still be sabotaged by marketers and nutritional labels. Luckily, there are petitions for the FDA to better inform the public of potential gastrointestinal symptoms in foods containing one or more grams per serving of sorbitol.

Mannitol

A sugar alcohol that comes from seaweed or the Manna plant. It can be manufactured for commercial and medical purposes. Mannitol is also found in pineapples, sweet potatoes, fresh mushrooms, and other fruits and vegetables. It's about 70% as sweet as sucrose and has been in use for over 60 years. The good news is that diabetics benefit from mannitol because it has approximately 1.6 calories per gram compared with 4 calories per gram of regular sugar. Like other sugar alcohols, mannitol metabolizes at a slow rate so it doesn't raise the blood sugar or insulin levels as much as sugar. The bad news, however, is that because it absorbs slowly from the intestines, excesses may produce laxative properties in some people.

You commonly see mannitol in the dust that blankets chewing gum. It keeps the gum from getting moist and sticking to the wrappers. Mannitol is also used as a bulking agent in powdered foods. It thickens and stabilizes processed foods, and is the sweetener in "breath-freshening" candies.

Xylitol

Finally, a sugar alcohol that may be an elixir in the sugar substitute industry! Xylitol is a natural substance produced in our bodies. It's also found in fruits (strawberries, plums, pears, raspberries) and vegetables (lettuce, mushrooms, carrots) and can be extracted from birch tree pulp, giving it the nickname "wood sugar." It's used as a sweetener in beverages, chewing gum, mints, hard candy, cough syrups, toothpaste, mouthwash, dietetic foods, and nasal spray (a clean nose reduces problems with allergies, asthma, and sinus infections).

First discovered by a German chemist in 1891, xylitol was rediscovered by a group of Finnish scientists during World War II when there was a dearth of sugar. According to these Finnish researchers, xylitol may boost calcium absorption, thus helping to prevent osteoporosis and bone weakening. Xylitol is used in dietetic foods because it's as sweet as sugar but is absorbed more slowly, which means there's less change in insulin levels. Study after study has concluded that the use of xylitol can diminish sugar cravings, which reduces insulin levels resulting in possible weight loss.

Xylitol may also help in the battle against tooth decay. It blocks cavity-causing bacteria from producing acids that can otherwise damage the teeth or gums. Trident Gum's assertion that, "Chewing Trident after eating cleans and protects teeth from cavities," was developed after they reformulated their gum to include xylitol. Xylitol also builds immunity, protects against chronic degenerative diseases, and provides anti-aging benefits. It's also as sweet as sucrose but has only 2.4 calories per gram.

So why, with all of these benefits, isn't xylitol more popular in the United States? Economics. Xylitol is more expensive than cane sugar and other sugar alcohols, so it doesn't help corporate America unless they jack up the prices of their products – and that wouldn't fare well in a competitive market.

Like most sugar alcohols, xylitol in high dosages can have a laxative effect. I'm not sure what's meant by "high dosages" because people have consumed as much as 400 grams (400g) on a daily basis for extended periods of time without any side effects. However, I wouldn't recommend testing its limits.

Maltitol

Maltitol is a substance hydrogenated (hydrogen atoms added and pressurized) from maltose that has a chemical structure similar to both sugars and alcohols, but, like all sugar alcohols, it is neither sugar nor alcohol. It's about 90% as sweet as sugar and has approximately 2.1 calories per gram.

Maltitol is used as a bulking agent in sugar-free, no-sugar-added, reduced calorie, and light foods. It can be found in yogurts, sauces, jellies, chocolates, breakfast cereals, fruit fillings, frozen desserts, and dietetic bars. Almost every sugar-free chewing gum contains maltitol. Like other sugar alcohols, about half remains undigested in the intestines and can cause gastrointestinal problems. Many individuals complain about its side effects (severe diarrhea and gas), yet it also seems to be a popular choice for manufacturers.

Isomalt

Discovered in the 1960s, isomalt became popular in the United States in 1990. This sweetener is only about 45%-65% as sweet as sucrose and carries only 2 calories per gram. It's used in beverages, baked products, fruit spreads, candy, toffee, chewing gum, chocolates, cough drops, nutritional supplements, jams, ice cream, and pharmaceuticals. Isomalt is an excellent sugar-free bulk sweetener and doesn't cause an increase in insulin levels, which makes it great for dietetic products. In large amounts, it can create intestinal havoc in some people because, like other sugar alcohols, it only partially digests in the intestines.

Artificial (Non-nutritive) Sweeteners

Saccharin

Discovered in 1879 and the oldest of all artificial sweeteners, saccharin was widely used during both World Wars to compensate for sugar shortages. It's between 200-500 times sweeter than sugar and goes undigested so there are no calories. Saccharin has no effect on blood insulin levels, which makes it an asset for diabetics. Commonly known as the table top sweetener (Sweet 'n Low), saccharin is also used in many other foods, cosmetic products, vitamins, and pharmaceuticals.

In 1977, a controversial study finding bladder cancer in rats that had been fed high dosages of saccharin became public and was amplified by the media. The FDA proposed banning saccharin but Congress instead required saccharin products to carry health warning labels until further studies could be conducted. At the time, there was no other sugar substitute on the market. What the initial study failed to disclose was that the "high dosages" the rats were fed added up to the equivalent of about *800* diet sodas per day.

Since then, more than 30 human studies have indicated that saccharin is safe for humans at *normal* levels of consumption. The average user of saccharin ingests less than one ounce per year. According to the American Diabetes Association, saccharin is safe for people with diabetes. In 2000, President Clinton signed a bill removing the warning label.

Aspartame

First discovered in 1965 by accident, aspartame is about 180-200 times sweeter than sugar, yet according to the American Dental Association, is safe and doesn't contribute to tooth decay. It's beneficial to diabetics and individuals dealing with weight management because it doesn't affect blood sugar levels and has no calories. Aspartame is a component in reduced-calorie and sugar-free products like diet soft drinks (Diet Coke, Diet Pepsi), chewing gum, yogurt, breakfast cereals, table top sweeteners (Equal, NutraSweet), frozen desserts, sugar-free cough drops, vitamins, and pharmaceuticals.

75% of all food additive-related complaints in the U.S. are about aspartame, **which is supposedly safe**.

Though discovered in 1965, aspartame didn't meet FDA approval for dry foods until 1981 and soft drinks until 1983. Aspartame has been the most scrutinized food ingredient in history, with over 200 scientific studies trying to confirm its safety. It went through rigorous studies and FDA review boards for many years due to misrepresentation and inconclusive studies. There have been allegations of more than 90 different symptoms caused by aspartame including headaches, nausea, anxiety attacks, brain tumors, Parkinson's, Alzheimer's, and even death. And there are concerns about its links to brain cancer and leukemia.

Two of the three components of aspartame are methanol and phenylalanine. Methanol, which is capable of causing blindness, liver damage, and death, is poisonous and flammable and used in the making of formaldehyde (that's right – embalming fluid!), paint stripper, and carburetor cleaners. Phenylalanine is an amino acid which is a health hazard for people with the rare genetic disease phenylketonuria (PKU). Phenylalanine cannot be metabolized by these individuals and is a toxin to their brain. Therefore, the FDA requires that aspartame products include a warning label stating that the sweetener contains phenylalanine.

Some studies show there are side effects. Others show there are no side effects. However, at least six FDA officials (including the FDA commissioner who approved aspartame to be a safe food additive) were given executive positions at G.D. Searle Company, or its affiliates, after the substance was approved. And G.D. Searle just happens to be the international pharmaceutical company that makes aspartame. Coincidentally, 75% of all food additive-related complaints in the United States are about *aspartame, which is supposedly safe.* That should make you think twice about using this substance!

There's enough drama in the history of aspartame's FDA approval to make a movie. What research are you going to believe?

Sucralose

Discovered in 1976, sucralose, now known popularly as Splenda, was first approved for use in Canada in 1991 but didn't get FDA approval in the United States until 1998. It is reported to be 600 times as sweet as sugar and, like other artificial sweeteners, it doesn't cause tooth decay and doesn't affect blood glucose or insulin levels. The manufacturer of sucralose claims the body cannot metabolize this artificial sweetener but the FDA's "Final Rule" report states that 11%-27% can be absorbed in humans – after all, sucralose is made with chlorine and real sugar.

Like aspartame, Sucralose, too, went through a long series of safety studies – more than 100 of them over 20 years. Although the studies were conducted on both animals and humans, the bulk of them were performed on animals by – you guessed it! – the manufacturer. There have not been any independently controlled human studies on this substance including any long-term studies on its possible side effects. *My question is, why would the FDA accept studies from the manufacturer?* Even more disturbing, the FDA reported many of the tests that were accepted came with "inconclusive" results.

There haven't been any independently controlled human studies on Sucralose.

Does it comfort you knowing that sucralose is in candy, ice cream, dietary supplements, medical foods, breakfast bars, soft drinks (Coke C2, Diet Coke with Splenda, Pepsi Edge, Pepsi ONE, Diet RC Cola), milk products, fruit juices, salad dressings, chewing gum, jams and jellies, coffees and teas, baked goods, etc.? This is why reading the Nutrition Facts Label is so important if you want to be healthy. You just don't know what food manufacturers are putting in the foods that you consume every day.

Stevia

A shrub that grows wild in South America. It's been used for centuries by the native Indians of Paraguay and Brazil for uses like making sweet herbal tea and treating heartburn, obesity, and hypertension. It's all-natural and between 250-300 times sweeter than sucrose. Stevia wasn't discovered commercially until 1918. Since then, other benefits have surfaced such as weight reduction and the prevention of tooth and gum decay. As usual, always consult your health care professional for medical advice about adding this or any sweetener to your diet.

Stevia has undergone approximately 900 studies, with numerous toxicological studies showing it to be safe for human use. It has been embraced in Japan for over 30 years with no complaints of adverse reactions. (Compare that to the 75% complaint-rate of Aspartame!) It's also approved and used in countries like China, South Korea, Taiwan, Thailand, Malaysia, and Israel where it is used in products like chewing gum, desserts, table top sweeteners, baked goods, soy sauce, fruit juices, tobacco products, candy, yogurts, and soft drinks. Japan has banned artificial sweeteners, which has caused the ***Coca-Cola Company to replace ASPARTAME with Stevia in all Diet Coke consumed in Japan. In fact, 40% of the Japanese sweetener market is Stevia.***

Yet as common as this sweetener is elsewhere, in the U.S., the FDA has denied three food additive petitions for Stevia. Although the FDA approved rebaudioside A (a highly purified form of the Stevia plant) as Generally Recognized As Safe (GRAS) for use in food in December, 2008, the FDA has not approved Stevia itself as being safe. There seems to be something very strange in this. Could it all be based on economics?

History shows that until 1984 health food stores in the U.S. were selling Stevia. Then the FDA received an "anonymous firm" complaint about the herb which ultimately resulted in the ban of all sales and import of the substance. At that time, the FDA performed unexpected raids on companies that were using Stevia in teas and they proceeded to confiscate the inventory as if it was some type of illegal hallucinogen. The FDA also ordered a distributor of Stevia supplements to destroy all literature he had on the subject. Allegedly, one FDA inspector told a health store company president they were trying to stop the consumption of Stevia *because NutraSweet (Aspartame) complained to the FDA.* In 1991, the FDA stamped Stevia as an unsafe food additive and put restrictions on its import. This was done at the request of an aspartame manufacturer. Apparently, at the time, Stevia was NutraSweet's main competitor in the U.S. According to national records, after Stevia's ban,

NutraSweet hired several FDA board members – at higher paying salaries. Hmmm!

Whey Low

The new kid on the block. Whey Low is all natural, tastes exactly like sucrose, and has been accepted by the FDA as safe for food use. It packs the same sweetness and functional properties as table sugar with only 4 calories per serving as opposed to 16 calories from ordinary sugar. There are three ingredients in Whey Low: sucrose (table sugar), fructose (fruit sugar), and lactose monohydrate (milk sugar). Whey Low is perfect for baking because, unlike artificial sweeteners, it can withstand high temperatures. More good news! I have yet to read of any side effects from this product.

Sugar Addiction

Basically, sugar is a natural nutrient that makes food taste sweet. Sugar has been extracted from sugar cane for over 2,000 years and from sugar beet since the 17th century. So why, all of the sudden, is there such an obesity and diabetes epidemic? Why has it only been recently that sugar has become so psychologically addicting?

Could it be that mere natural sugar is the culprit for the rise of diabetes to the third most frequent disease in America? Or could the recent obesity epidemic that currently victimizes 2/3rds of American adults be the result of natural – unrefined – sugar? Or could the real culprit of diabetes and obesity be processed foods using refined sugars that have been stripped of their nutrients – refined sugars like high fructose corn syrup? The fact is, sugar is still the cheapest preservative food manufacturers use to increase the shelf life of their processed foods. It's been around for a long time, but the preservative methods used now are only relatively recent developments.

> Sugar has been around for over 2,000 years. Why all of a sudden, is there such an obesity and diabetes epidemic?

You see, it's not only portion sizes that have made Americans fatter in the past 30 years – it's refined carbohydrates like white flour foods, white rice, crackers, noodles, cereal, and refined white sugar. In the early 1900s, the average American consumed about 5 pounds of sugar per year. Today, every year, the average American consumes his or her own *body weight* in sugar. Carbohydrates have sugar in them, but our bodies aren't designed to metabolize these massive amounts of refined sugars.

Sugar may be the greatest psychological addiction in the United States. Some researchers believe food addiction is similar to drug addiction – and that some people have overeating behaviors that parallel the compulsive drug-using behavior of drug addicts. In fact, a scanning technology showing activity in the living brain has found many similarities between drug addicts and food addicts. One study revealed that cocaine addicts who were shown syringes, white powder, and cash demonstrated many of the same brain responses as another study group that was shown ice cream.

Breaking an addiction to heroin, cocaine, or other addictive drug may actually be easier than breaking a sugar addiction because an individual may be able to avoid drugs completely. Sugar, on the other hand, can't be completely avoided because it's in almost every processed food.

Sugar has rightfully been given the nickname "white poison" because of its links with:

- heart disease
- type 2 diabetes
- cancer
- high blood pressure
- weight gain (leading to obesity)
- tooth decay.

> Some people have overeating behaviors that parallel the compulsive drug-using behavior of drug addicts.

More than 70 years ago, Dr. Otto Warburg won the Nobel Prize in medicine when he discovered that cancer cells require glucose (sugar) for growth. All cells have a requirement for glucose, but cancer cells consume as much as 4-5 times more glucose than normal, healthy cells. In fact, they're unable to multiply rapidly without it.

And sugar robs the body of vitamins and minerals and weakens the immune system. The human body simply wasn't designed to consume the large amounts of sugar we're currently consuming and it's little wonder why diabetes and obesity are at an all time high in the United States.

The only way we can repress "Fat America" is to decrease calories, especially calories from sugars, and increase our physical activity and nutrition literacy.

Net Carbohydrates

Net carb? Low carb? Net impact carb? Effective carb count? What do these phrases mean?

These are all marketing tools used by food manufacturers who boldly stamp them on any product that contains fiber, sugar alcohols, or glycerine. Since the Atkins Diet, companies have been reformulating food products with lower amounts of net carbohydrates. These catchy terms are just a tactic to give products more shelf appeal. *The FDA has not legally defined any of these phrases.* The catchy phrases were created by companies only to grab consumers' attention. Since most consumers don't have the time to calculate the "real" total carbohydrates in foods, thoughtful marketers try to do all the work for us.

Yeah, right.

As we discussed earlier in this chapter, fiber is basically a calorie-free carbohydrate that is not digestible by the human body, so it doesn't affect blood sugar. Strictly speaking, sugar alcohols are carbohydrates and a source of calories, but manufacturers argue that they have little effect on blood sugar. Glycerine is used as a lubricant for foods like protein bars to make them easier to digest. Food manufacturers argue fiber, sugar alcohols, and glycerine should not be tallied in the amount of total carbohydrates. To arrive at the "net carbohydrate value," we subtract the combined grams of fiber, sugar alcohols, and glycerine from the total grams of carbohydrates in that particular food.

But wait. Is the calculation that easy? Nothing is that easy in the food industry!

An American Dietetic Association publication recommends people with diabetes who are trying to manage their blood sugars should count *half* of the grams of sugar alcohol because approximately half of the sugar alcohol is digested. Remember, this is a general calculation and *is not an officially approved label.*

The net carbohydrate value calculation could be different from company to company or even from product to product within the same company. Until the FDA ensures that these terms are consistent with other nutrient content labeling claims, and because I know we don't have the enzyme to break down fiber and utilize it as energy, I only subtract the grams of *fiber* from the total grams of carbohydrates to determine a more accurate carbohydrate count.

Now that we understand that "good" carbs are a necessity for good health, let's challenge your beliefs about fats, and why they don't always deserve the bad rap they've gotten.

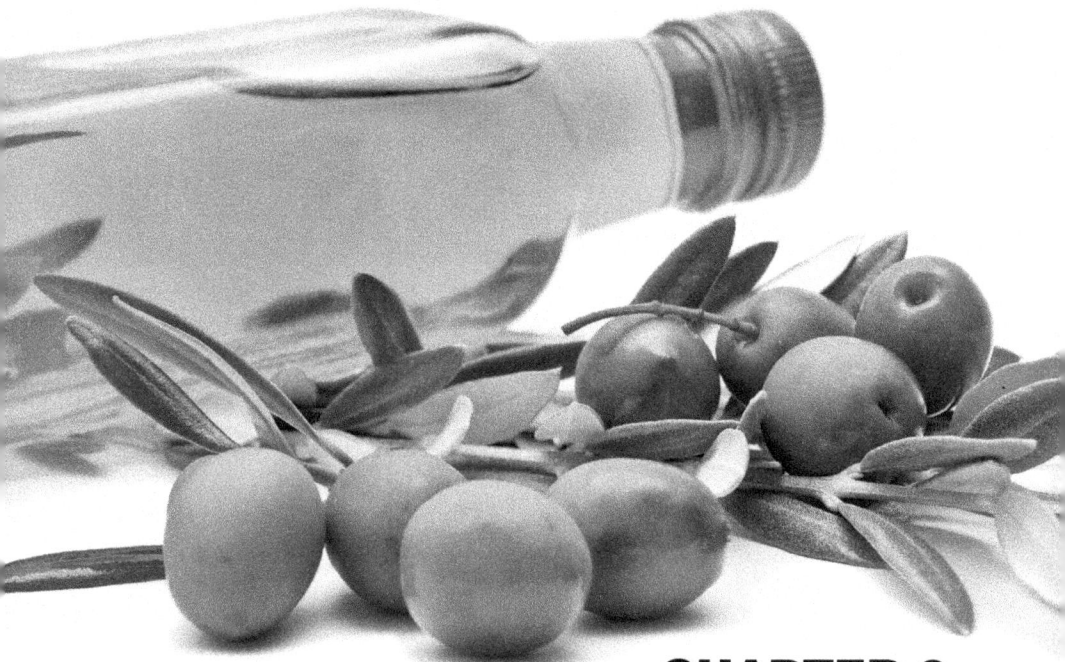

CHAPTER 6

Fats

You may not believe this, but our bodies need fat to survive.

As we discussed in Chapter 5, carbohydrates are a major source of energy. But fats are the other major source of energy that our bodies require for a myriad of bodily functions. Body fat cushions our organs, protects our bodies against cold, provides energy (approximately 9 calories per gram, as opposed to 4 calories per gram from carbohydrates or protein), aids in the absorption of vitamins A, K, D, and E, and is necessary for producing hormones such as estrogen. Women who don't produce enough estrogen are at higher risk for osteoporosis and heart disease. Fats give us a sense of satiety, a feeling of fullness, so we eat less. They slow the digestive process because our bodies have to break through fat before utilizing carbs. This cuts back on the rise of blood sugar levels, resulting in fewer calories to be stored as body fat.

Excess body fat is linked to cardiovascular disease, stroke, type 2 diabetes, hypertension, osteoporosis, respiratory disease, and certain types of cancer.

Fat is an essential component of all cells and is important for proper growth and development, and maintenance of good health. Our nervous system (spinal cord, brain, nerves, ganglia) requires fat to protect it and to transmit messages from our brain to our muscles. There are documented cases of clients who have been anorexic and bulimic for years who can't walk because they have degenerative neurological problems that some doctors attribute to very low fat.

The word fat has had a bum rap for quite some time, but now it's making a comeback.

So why in the world would somebody go on a fat-free diet? The word "fat" has had a bum rap for quite some time, but now it's making a comeback. What we're learning is that there are different types of fat – some good, some bad. Our bodies break down fat into fatty acids known as saturated, polyunsaturated, and monounsaturated. There's also a special type of man-made polyunsaturated fat called "trans fat".

Let's start with the bad fats – saturated and trans fats. These are the dark, evil fats that have been linked to obesity, high blood cholesterol, heart attack, stroke, and some types of cancer.

The Bad Fats

SATURATED FATS

Saturated fats are found in some animal foods such as red meat and the dark meat of poultry. They're also in whole-fat dairy products, butter, tropical oils, egg yolks (but not the egg whites, called albumen), seafood, and organ meats such as liver, brains, and kidneys. They signal your body to produce cholesterol, which may raise blood cholesterol levels.

There are two types of cholesterol: body-manufactured cholesterol and dietary cholesterol. Both come from two sources – your body and food.

There are 2 types of cholesterol: body-manufactured cholesterol and dietary cholesterol.

Cholesterol is naturally produced by your liver to make hormones and is essential for the body to function properly. Your body utilizes it to make bile that breaks down seeds, skins, and fats.

Cholesterol is a soft, waxy substance coated with a layer of protein which makes a *lipoprotein*. There are two types of lipoprotein. One is Low-

Density-Lipoprotein (LDL), which is the "bad" cholesterol. It's the major cholesterol carrier in the blood, and if there's a surplus of LDL, there's a possibility that the walls of the arteries feeding the heart and brain could become clogged with a hard plaque. In time, this plaque can block the blood flow to the heart causing a heart attack. Or it could possibly block the blood flow to the brain, leading to a stroke.

LDL is the "bad" cholesterol, while HDL is the "good."

High-Density-Lipoprotein (HDL) is the "good" cholesterol based on the belief that it removes cholesterol from arteries and sends it back to the liver where it is either recycled or excreted in bile and disposed from the body.

High cholesterol is usually the result of too much LDL cholesterol in your system. Having high cholesterol can be an inherited trait and one you may have no control over. But it can also be a condition caused by a diet high in saturated fat and/or lack of exercise. If the latter is the cause, you – *and only you* – have total control and you can correct the problem.

Remember, not *all* cholesterol is bad. Cholesterol is essential in forming cell membranes and for the production of sex hormones, vitamin D, and bile. But your body produces all the cholesterol it needs in your liver, so there's no need to consume it.

According to the National Cholesterol Education Program's (NCEP's) Expert Panel on Detection, Evaluation and Treatment of High Blood Cholesterol in Adults most recent guidelines, your total cholesterol level (both LDL plus HDL) should be lower than 200.

Less than 200: **Acceptable**
Between 200 and 239: **Borderline high**
Above 239: **Too high**

Ways to lower your cholesterol....

1. Lower Dietary Cholesterol – The American Heart Association recommends that you limit your average daily cholesterol intake to less than 300 milligrams (300mg). That's about one whole egg! That's right. One large egg has about 213mg of cholesterol. So if you have a total cholesterol level at or above 200, I would recommend saying good-bye to mom's homemade Sunday Brunch omelets.

Another no-brainer is to lower your saturated fat by using fat-free and low-fat dairy products rather than saturated foods. Try to exchange saturated fats with monounsaturated fats and polyunsaturated fats. For instance, replace butter with olive oil which is mostly monounsaturated fat. Also, try eating fish a couple times each week.

2. Stop Smoking - Not only for your lungs' sake, but for your cholesterol. Smoking lowers HDL levels, which is the cholesterol we want and need. It also increases the tendency for blood clots. According to the American Lung Association of Indiana Lung Center, after you stop smoking for 24 hours, your risk of heart disease diminishes. Furthermore, after one year of not smoking, your risk of coronary heart disease falls to half that of a continuing smoker.

3. Moderate Your Alcohol Consumption - One drink per day has been shown to increase HDL cholesterol levels and reduce the risk of blood clots. Anything more than one drink per day is inviting other health dangers, such as alcoholism, obesity, high blood pressure, stroke, cancer, and even suicide. Let's define ONE drink:

- Beer - 12 oz.
- Hard Liquor (whiskey, vodka, gin, etc) - 1/2 oz.
- Wine – 6.5 oz.

Many women I know seem to think no matter how big the wine glass is, it's still only one drink. So, in order to moderate your alcohol, don't bring out the 60 oz. margarita glass you got for your 21st birthday.

4. Above all... Exercise, Exercise, Exercise – Exercise has been proven to increase HDL cholesterol levels, helps control weight, and lowers the risk of diabetes and high blood pressure. It doesn't matter how you exercise… just do *something*. Tango through your neighborhood, do gardening or yard work, go dancing, or do housework. What about dancing while you're cleaning the house? It'll make it more enjoyable while helping you keep in shape!

Saturated fat is most likely to deposit plaque and cholesterol as it treks through our arteries, which is then likely to raise LDL. The old school of thought was that a total score of both LDL and HDL below 200 indicated that you were less likely to be at risk for cardiovascular diseases. Now, however, cardiologists are growing more concerned about the actual size of the LDL particles. The smaller they are, the more likely they are to contract beneath the blood vessel linings, narrowing the walls of the arteries and cutting off the blood flow to the heart and brain. The result? An unpleasant ride in an uncomfortable restraining bed in the back of an ambulance on a less-than-scenic trip to your local hospital. If you don't watch your saturated fat intake, you may well be subjecting yourself to either a heart attack or stroke.

> The average age at which American men die of heart disease is 73, yet James Near and Gordon Teter (Chairman and CEO of Wendy's respectively) died at the ages of 58 and 56. Burt Baskin, cofounder of Baskin Robbins, died with 31 flavors under his belt at the age of 54. Incidentally, it was Baskin's taste buds that every new flavor had to impress before being offered to the public. George Mallory didn't reign as king very long as owner of the first Burger King restaurants in New York City. He died at age 52. Jim Cantalupo made his exit from this world – and his position as CEO of the world's most recognizable fast food chain, McDonald's, – at only 60. Maybe it's just coincidence that these high-profile corporate leaders died at such early ages … but then again, maybe not.

TRANS FAT

About 20 years ago, trans fat was fabricated by scientists to protect us against the saturated fat in butter. It was made by hardening vegetable oils into stick margarine or shortening. In order to get a stiffer fat (think of Crisco), hydrogen atoms were added to liquid vegetable oil and then pressurized – a process called "hydrogenation" – hence the term "hydrogenated oils". But it turns out that this fat is worse than the saturated fat found in butter, cheese, and coconut oil. There were no studies about the side effects of trans fat when it was first introduced. Later, however, research showed that trans fat was even worse for the heart than lard.

Trans fat, as it happens, is the whale of fats because it increases LDL levels, lowers HDL levels, and may cause major clogging

Trans fat is even worse for your heart than lard.

of arteries, type 2 diabetes, and other serious health issues. Pseudo names that clever marketers use on the Ingredient List are partially hydrogenated oils, hydrogenated oils, and vegetable shortening.

Partially hydrogenated oils are found in foods like peanut butter, with the exception of the all-natural kinds. The purpose is to prevent separation so the oil doesn't have to be stirred every time it's used. This is just another example of how lethargic Americans have become. We need to think of mixing the oil in natural peanut butter as a way to burn a few extra calories for the day!

Although trans fat was invented to address concerns that lard could lead to heart problems, it was quickly discovered that trans fat was also much cheaper to produce. Later, food manufacturers further discovered that trans fatty acids increase product shelf life. Have you ever wondered what's in a Twinkie that can make it last for 50 years? Some other foods that have trans fat lurking within are fried foods (French fries, chicken-fried steak), crackers, pastries, potato chips, icing, doughnuts, many popular cookies (Oreos, etc.), cereals, waffles, and even international and instant latte coffee beverages. And there isn't just a *little* trans fatty acid in most of these foods – usually it's in the 30%-50% range.

They're everywhere ....

Today, trans fat is found in 40% of the products on supermarket shelves. Look for trans-fat-free margarines such as Promise and Smart Balance.

The general population isn't aware of these vile fats because companies weren't initially required to list them on nutrition labels. On January 1, 2006, the Food and Drug Administration (FDA) mandated that food manufacturers must list trans fatty acids on Nutrition Facts Labels. I strongly encourage you to start reading Food Labels and Ingredient Lists, as we discussed in Chapter 2. Look for these fancy names on the Ingredient List: partially hydrogenated oil, hydrogenated oil, or shortening. Remember, the closer they are to the top of the list, the more trans fat there is in the product. In fact, if trans fat is listed in the top three ingredients, the food is mostly trans fat. We don't *need* any of this bogus fat. The only reason it exists is because food manufacturers want to have a longer shelf life for their products. That is the *only* reason. There are absolutely no health benefits. In 2002, the National Academy of Sciences concluded that **no amount of trans fat is healthy.**

NO amount of trans fat is healthy!

christopherSASHA

According to the comprehensive Nurses' Health Study – the largest investigation of women and chronic disease – trans fat doubles the risk of heart disease in women.

The Good Fats

Now that we've discussed the evil fats, let's focus on the beneficial fats, the ones that add flavor to our fare and help prevent disease. These are the unsaturated fats: polyunsaturated and monounsaturated. They come mostly from plant sources and have not been altered or damaged by food processing. Some of the benefits of the good fats include the flavor they provide, and the fact that they're filling and contribute to healthy blood vessels. But remember, even though they're good for us, from a caloric viewpoint too much fat is bad. Like all types of fats, they should be *eaten in moderation*. The body can survive getting 10% of total daily calories from fat. The National Heart, Lung and Blood Institute recommends between 25% and 35%. As for me, I try to stay around 30%, focusing primarily on monounsaturated fats because they are the best for us.

POLYUNSATURATED FATS

Polyunsaturated fats are healthier than saturated fats because they lower LDL cholesterol levels, the "bad" cholesterol that deposits plaque in our arteries and may eventually lead to heart attacks and strokes. However, unlike monounsaturated fats, polyunsaturated fats are believed to also lower HDL cholesterol levels (cholesterol that is believed to help remove LDL cholesterol from the blood and arteries). Polyunsaturated fats are found in vegetable oils like soybean, corn, sunflower, and safflower. They're responsible for healthy skin and the development of body cells.

Polyunsaturated fats supply a special group of "essential fatty acids" (EFAs) that cannot be synthesized by the body and therefore must be furnished by foods we consume. The two types of essential fats are called Omega-3 and Omega-6 fatty acids. EFAs are required for normal growth and for healthy skin and hair. They help regulate blood pressure, blood clotting, and the immune system. They're also vital to the operation of the brain and

For every one Omega-3, 1-4 Omega-6s are required for a healthy diet.

central nervous system. It's important to sustain an appropriate balance of Omega-3s and Omega-6s because the two work together to maintain and even improve health. It's recommended that for every one Omega-3, roughly one to four Omega-6s are required to make up a healthy diet.

An imbalance could contribute to the development of disease. For example, recent research published in the journal *Circulation* linked high levels of Omega-6s to heart problems. And an overload of Omega-3s may produce a risk for hemorrhagic stroke, a potentially fatal type of stroke in which an artery in the brain leaks or ruptures. Because today's standard American diet (SAD) tends to contain 11-30 times more Omega-6 fatty acids than Omega-3 fatty acids, there should be no need to supplement your diet with Omega-6s. On the other hand, Omega-3s could probably be supplemented with fish oils. Unfortunately, there is no "formally" established recommended daily intake for Omega-6 fatty acids. However, world expert on fats, Udo Erasmus, recommends a significant reduction in Omega-6 consumption in favor of more Omega-3s.

> The normal American gets 37% of his/her calories from fat.

ESSENTIAL FATTY ACIDS (EFAs)

Omega-3

Omega-3s have a myriad of benefits for preventing heart disease, lowering high blood pressure and high cholesterol, reducing inflammation, helping prevent osteoporosis and rheumatoid arthritis, and possibly helping with mood disorders like depression. Preliminary research suggests that Omega-3s might play a role in improving bipolar disorder, schizophrenia, attention deficit disorder, asthma, and many other conditions. Omega-3 fatty acids are found in whole grains, fruits and vegetables, olive oil, garlic, and fish. Like anything else, if overdone, Omega-3 fatty acids can be bad for you. High doses of Omega-3s from concentrated sources (fish oil supplements) can affect the blood's ability to clot appropriately. Fish oil supplements can also cause flatulence and diarrhea (and that stinks!).

Most experts still advise getting Omega-3s directly from fish, but try to limit your consumption of swordfish, king mackerel, and shark. They're most likely to be contaminated with mercury according to the FDA. In general, larger, older fish have more mercury than smaller, younger fish. And wild or line caught fish is usually healthier than farm raised fish. Also, try alternating the days you eat these oily fish. For example, if you eat wild salmon one day, the next time you consume fish, have sea bass, followed by rainbow trout. Varying your options will reduce your exposure to any one contaminant.

Varying your fish options will reduce your exposure to any one contaminant.

As far as mercury is concerned, chunk light tuna (in water) is better than white albacore. An even better option is canned salmon, which contains less than a quarter of the mercury found in tuna and is a better source of Omega-3 fatty acids, according to a recent study from Purdue University.

Always consult with your healthcare provider before including Omega-3 fatty acid supplements in your diet. Also, be sure to buy from established companies who certify that their products are *free* of heavy metals. Mercury, in particular, may increase blood pressure. Check out www.consumerlab.com for a list of mercury and PCB-free fish oil supplement brands.

Eating at least two servings of fish per week can reduce the risk of stroke by as much as 50%. You're probably thinking that if you radically increase your fish consumption your risk of stroke would be reduced even more. That way of thinking could cause risks for a hemorrhagic stroke, which could be fatal. People who eat *three servings of fish per day* may be at risk for hemorrhagic stroke. Once again, moderation is the key.

Besides fish oils, Omega-3 fatty acids can be found in plant oils such as flaxseed oil, pumpkin seed oil, walnut oil, and soybean oil. Walnuts, hazelnuts, cashews, and almonds are excellent sources of Omega-3. Also, don't forget pumpkin seeds, sunflower seeds, sesame seeds, and pine nuts as ways to add Omega-3 fatty acids to your diet. Most importantly, try to balance a healthy ratio of between one to four Omega-6s for every Omega-3 fatty acid.

ESSENTIAL FATTY ACIDS IN OILS			
OMEGA-3s (100grams)	(g)	OMEGA-6s (100grams)	(g)
Flax Seed Oil	24	Flax Seed Oil	6
Walnut Oil	11.5	Walnut Oil	58
Soybean Oil	7	Soybean Oil	51
Grapeseed Oil	<1	Grapeseed Oil	68

ESSENTIAL FATTY ACIDS IN NUTS			
OMEGA-3s (100grams)	(g)	OMEGA-6s (100grams)	(g)
Walnuts	5.5	Walnuts	28
Hazelnuts	<1	Hazelnuts	4
Cashews	<1	Cashews	8
Almonds	<1	Almonds	10

ESSENTIAL FATTY ACIDS IN SEEDS			
OMEGA-3s (100grams)	(g)	OMEGA-6s (100grams)	(g)
Flax Seeds	24	Flax Seeds	6
Pumpkin Seeds	7-10	Pumpkin Seeds	20
Pine Nuts	1	Pine Nuts	25
Sunflower Seeds	<1	Sunflower Seeds	30

Omega-6

The counterpart to Omega-3s are the Omega-6 fatty acids. Unfortunately, the standard American diet (SAD) is loaded with Omega-6s at the expense of Omega-3s. To maintain their status as "good" fats, you have to somewhat balance the two. If you look back at the "Essential Fatty Acids" tables, you'll notice that Omega-6s overpower Omega-3s tremendously. Remember, the ideal ratio is one to four Omega-6s for every Omega-3.

The Mediterranean diet has a good balance between Omega-3 and Omega-6 fatty acids. It doesn't include much meat (high in Omega-6s) and puts more emphasis on foods high in Omega-3s. Next time you go to a

Mediterranean restaurant, pay attention to the meal. They include lots of whole grains, fresh fruits and vegetables, fish, olive oil, and garlic – ingredients for health.

Some of the benefits from Omega-6 fatty acids are that they regulate inflammation and blood pressure, as well as help with gastrointestinal, heart, and kidney functions. They may also be helpful in reducing uncomfortable menstrual-related symptoms, such as breast tenderness, bloating, or cramps. Cereals, eggs, poultry, vegetable oils, and whole grain breads are excellent sources for Omega-6 fatty acids.

Monounsaturated Fats

The savior in the battle of the evil fats is monounsaturated fat, considered to be one of the healthiest types of fat because there seem to be no adverse effects (unlike trans fat, saturated fats, and Omega-6 fatty acids found in polyunsaturated vegetable oils). According to the study Dietary Effects on Lipoprotein and Thrombogenic Activity (DELTA), replacing saturated fats with monounsaturated fats will improve cholesterol levels by increasing HDL levels, decreasing LDL levels, and decreasing triglycerides, which are fatty materials that circulate in the blood. Triglycerides come from calories that aren't used immediately. They're transported to fat cells to be stored and used later for energy between meals. Excess triglyceride levels are a risk factor for coronary artery disease even if your total cholesterol level is normal.

Monounsaturated fats are typically high in vitamin E and may protect against certain cancers like breast and colon cancer. They're also essential for brain development and function, they promote healthy skin and hair, and they're crucial for the development of body cells. Although monounsaturated fats are good for us, we need to remember that they are still fats and still have nine calories per gram, *so use them in moderation.* Sesame seeds, pumpkin seeds, hazelnuts, Brazil nuts, almonds, cashews, avocados, rapeseed oil, and olive oil are terrific sources of monounsaturated fats.

> Monounsaturated fat is considered to be the healthiest type of fat.

PERCENTAGE OF MONOUNSATURATED FATS	
OLIVE OIL	73%
RAPESEED OIL	60%
HAZELNUTS	50%
ALMONDS	35%
CASHEWS	28%
BRAZIL NUTS	26%
SESAME SEEDS	20%
PUMPKIN SEEDS	16%
AVOCADO	12%

Spot Reduction

The body needs fat to perform many functions – and to survive. Like anything in this crazy world, fat needs to be consumed in moderation. An acceptable percentage of body fat for a male is between 11%-17%, while an acceptable percentage for a female is between 15%-23%. Women are naturally higher in body fat because they have breasts, hips, and thighs to protect and nourish in case of pregnancy. Estrogen is the culprit directing fat to these areas.

Some people become obsessed with getting body fat down to unhealthy levels. I find a lot of this with amateur bodybuilders at local gyms. You may be able to get your percentage of body fat down to 3%-4%, but you cannot maintain it that low for very long. It's not good for your health. The *essential amount of body fat* for a male is 2%-4%. Women need a bit more – 10%-12% *essential* body fat. When you get below these levels, you start getting sick all the time. Your immune system needs some fat to function properly. A few years ago, an amateur bodybuilder got his body fat down to a little over 1%. His organs started shutting down, including his brain, and he died. We *need* fat – just not an overabundance of it.

Men should shoot for 11%-17% total body fat. **Women** should aim for 15%-23% total body fat.

Many people don't realize that stored fat isn't necessarily from only excess fat calories. Excess calories from any source, including protein and carbohydrates, are stored as fat. The only way to lose body fat is through proper diet and EXERCISE. Many studies have proven time and again, the only way – *the only way* – **to lose weight and keep it off long-term is through proper diet *and* exercise.**

The spot reduction concept went mainstream about 10 years ago as people started going to the gym to start exercise regimes to get rid of fat just around their midsection. They wanted "six-pack" abs and thought they could work for an hour or so, three times per week, to burn the fat in just that specific area to get the abs they wanted. This misconception has become so popular that it's been given a name – spot reduction. ***The concept of spot reduction is an outright fallacy!*** It's impossible to reduce fat in only one area of your body, whether it be your stomach, arms, legs, butt, whatever. It is physiologically impossible.

Genetically, we are all created differently. Two people could implement the same high-repetition abdominal training technique (combining abdominal training with cardio), perform hundreds of reps for 35 minutes every morning – and get totally different results. One person may "burn" the fat from his/her midsection and achieve great abs, while the other may notice that his/her legs are much more defined. Only one thing is sure – they'll both have impressively strong midsections. The size of fat cells is different throughout each body. Some people may have larger fat cells in their face

It's physiologically impossible to spot reduce body fat.

than in their midsections, while others may have larger adipose cells in their midsections than in their legs.

When the body retains excess calories, all the fat cells get larger at the same time. Furthermore, when the body expends more calories, all the fat cells diminish at the same time. If you have larger adipose cells in your face, you'll notice a weight gain or loss in your face first. Unfortunately, only those genetically blessed with smaller adipose cells in their abdominal region will see results there the quickest.

Hopefully by now you have a much different perspective on the word "fat" than what you might have had before you started this chapter. Now let's see if we can clear up a few more misconceptions and learn some new things about a nutrient every bit as important: protein.

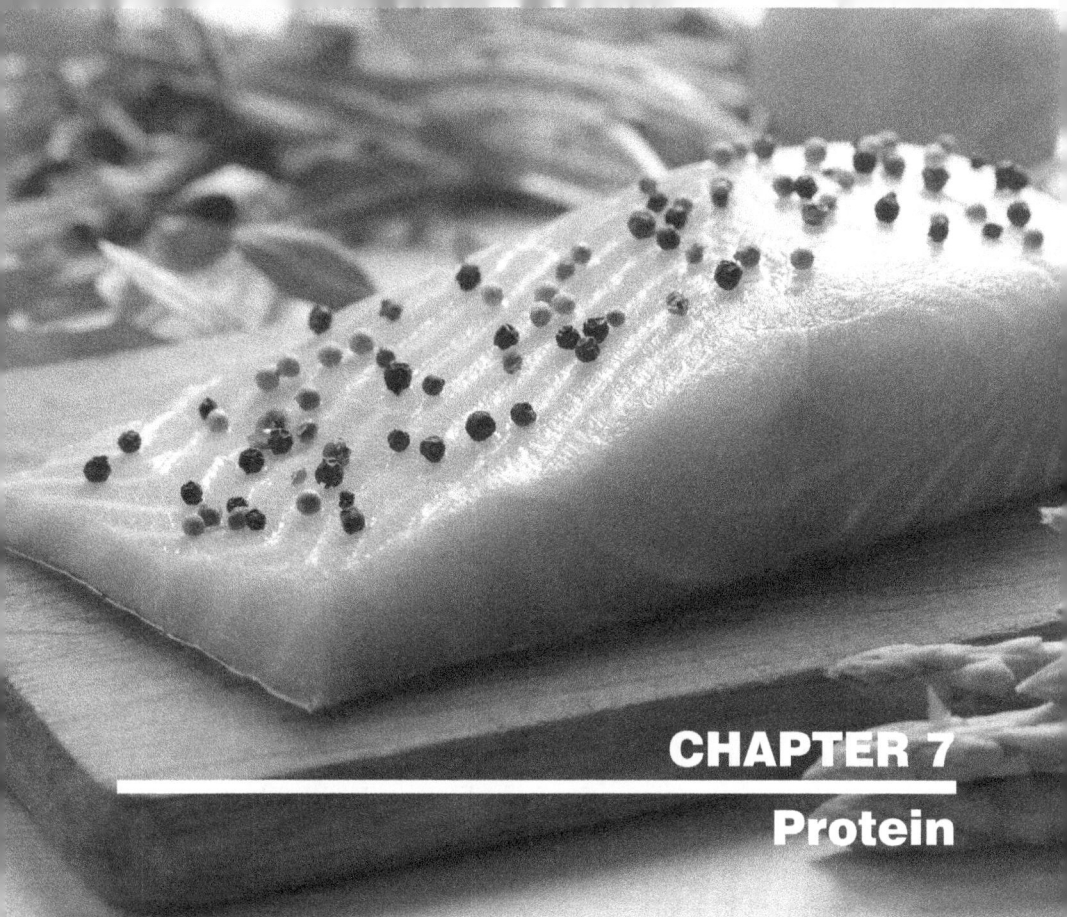

CHAPTER 7
Protein

Protein is the main element of muscles, organs, glands, blood, skin, hair, and nails. It makes up between 20%-45% of the material in your body (depending on who is reporting the statistic!) It's the second largest percentage of body matter; the first being – *what a shocker!* – water. Protein is essential in regulating your metabolism. It's needed for a healthy immune system and supports the growth and maintenance of your muscles, tissues, and bones. Protein functions range from creating the pigmentation in your skin to making up the bulk of your hair and nails to acting as a carrier to transport elements like oxygen through your bloodstream to your muscles. It would take almost a library of books to cover all the responsibilities of this macronutrient.

We require a continual supply of protein because our bodies can't store it like fats and carbohydrates. Our bodies convert fat into fatty acids, carbohydrates into glucose (blood sugar), and protein into amino acids. Carbs are broken down to glucose for the body to absorb and use as energy, and protein is broken down into individual amino acids, the building blocks of human protein and life. Unlike fats and carbohydrates, our bodies can only store excess amino acids in our bloodstream for several hours. Therefore, we require a continual supply of protein. This is one reason why I suggest eating every 2-3 hours, with protein in every meal.

AMINO ACIDS

While there are hundreds of different amino acids in nature, there are only 20 common amino acids that combine to produce all the protein our bodies need to survive. We don't need to get bogged down in the scientific technicalities of amino acids, but it might be worth gaining at least a general understanding.

Out of the 20 amino acids, 8 are considered "indispensable amino acids" (formerly known as "essential amino acids") because our bodies can't synthesize them, meaning, therefore, that we have to acquire them in food. Without them we would eventually die. Foods that are balanced with all of the indispensable amino acids are called "complete proteins." They can be found in all animal meats (beef, fowl, pork, lamb, fish), eggs and dairy products (milk, cheese, yogurt). If a shortage of these amino acids becomes habitual, the building of protein will stop and the body will suffer.

> Our bodies can't make indispensable amino acids so we have to acquire them through foods we eat.

The other 12 amino acids are "dispensable amino acids" (formerly known as "nonessential amino acids") because our bodies can produce them from the indispensable amino acids. They're just as important as the indispensable amino acids, however. Grains, fruits, and vegetables are called "incomplete proteins" due to the lack of one or more indispensable amino acids. However, often if two or more incomplete proteins are combined (peanut butter and whole wheat bread), they can create a complete protein and a high quality substitute for meat, a vegan's dream.

> Combining two or more incomplete proteins can create a complete protein.

IMMUNE SYSTEM

During our lifetimes, we'll develop millions of cancer cells which are taken care of by our immune system. The immune system is a network that produces various white blood cells and antibodies to defend our bodies from infectious organisms (bacteria, parasites, viruses.) It has the unique ability to distinguish between our own organisms and foreign organisms. Its function is to find and destroy invaders like cancer cells. When the immune system weakens, the body can't defend itself as well, making it easier for these foreign invaders to attack cells and our health.

During our lifetimes, we'll develop millions of cancer cells which are taken care of by our immune system.

I first experienced the importance of the immune system in my first "real" job at a funeral home when I was sixteen. The mortician and I became friends, and he proposed that I might choose a career as a mortician one day. As I became more serious about his suggestion, he occasionally invited me to help pick up the deceased from hospitals and nursing homes.

As time passed, I became more comfortable being around dead people. … at least until the night we picked up a body that had been found hanging from a tree in the nearby woods. Apparently, this person had been missing for more than a week. As I was helping put this poor soul into the body bag, I could see the decomposition of the skin. When the body dies, so does the immune system, making it open season for foreign organisms to strip the body away until there's nothing remaining but a skeleton.

ENZYMES

Enzymes are a very special type of protein found in every living cell, plant, and animal. They regulate almost every biochemical reaction in our bodies and are needed for the digestive system to work. Enzymes help
- purify the blood
- digest food and move muscles
- deliver nutrients to every cell
- operate organs properly (heart, brain, kidneys, muscles, lungs)
- build new proteins
- rid our bodies of toxic waste.

These are just a few things that contribute to a healthy immune system and healthy body. Without enzymes we couldn't exist.

Enzymes are made from amino acids, which means they're also proteins. They're found in all tissues and fluids, and are responsible for healing injuries (including training-induced microtrauma) and keeping us healthy. Enzymes do

Enzymes may be the essential agents in preventing chronic illnesses and increasing our lifespans.

everything from building cells to producing new enzymes to breaking foods down into glucose for energy. In fact, they may be the essential agents in preventing chronic illnesses and increasing our lifespans.

Each enzyme has a very specific function. They're like tools used on an assembly line at an automobile factory. Each worker in the factory uses a specific tool to perform his job to help achieve the collective end result – the automobile. When a worker has utilized his tool for an extended period of time, the tool begins to wear down, which will eventually prevent the tool from fitting the nuts and bolts it was intended to tighten, ultimately stopping the production of the car itself. The tool needs to be replaced, and so it is with enzymes. Each enzyme has a specific function during its lifetime. It continues to do its one specific job until it's transformed to a point that it doesn't function anymore. Each enzyme must have the correct shape to perform its part in keeping the body alive and healthy.

There are three major classes of enzymes: *metabolic enzymes,* which make our organs and tissues function properly; *food enzymes,* which come only from raw foods that we consume; and *digestive enzymes,* which digest the foods we eat. For a better understanding of how enzymes work, let's take a look at digestive enzymes. Digestive enzymes have only three functions: digesting protein, digesting fat, and digesting carbohydrates. Each enzyme digests only one macronutrient and that's all it does – always. Or at least until it becomes useless from transformations.

ENZYME	Substance It Digests
Protease	Proteins
Lipase	Fats
Amylase	Carbohydrates
Lactase	Lactose
Maltase	Maltose

The only way a carbohydrate can be digested and broken down into glucose for energy is if an amylase enzyme collides with it. If a protease enzyme encounters a carbohydrate, it won't do anything because it doesn't "fit" the structure of the carbohydrate. Consider your car key. It unlocks your car. Your car key is a carbohydrate and your car locks are amylase enzymes. Different enzymes break down different foods, so if your car key was a protein, your car locks wouldn't be able to be opened being amylase enzymes. They would need to be protease enzymes to perform the task.

Enzymes have a lifespan just like every other living organism. While they are alive, they're used and re-used, performing their own specific jobs. After they die, they're gone forever which is why we have to continually replenish these crusaders in our bodies with the protein in the foods we eat. Some enzyme-rich foods include sprouted seeds (alfalfa sprouts, peas, broccoli, cabbage), grains, and legumes.

Temperatures 118° and above will kill enzymes.

The problem with enzymes is that they die when heated, which is why we can't obtain enzymes from cooked foods, including processed foods. Temperatures 118 degrees and above will kill enzymes, so any food you cook will have no enzymes remaining by the time it gets to your table. Even steaming or microwaving the food will destroy its enzymes. Freezing foods, however, will not affect them.

A deficiency of enzymes could eventually create conditions like arthritis, high cholesterol, high blood pressure, type 2 diabetes, etc. As we get older, we gradually use up our enzymes and we become more and more enzyme deficient. This puts us at risk for chronic ailments like allergies, skin disease, and other diseases including cancer. This is why it's imperative to continuously consume foods high in enzymes, or protein. Another alternative is to take enzyme supplements. As always, consult your health care provider before consuming any type of supplement.

As we age, we become more and more enzyme deficient, which puts us at a higher risk for chronic illnesses, including cancer.

As we discussed in Chapters 5 and 6, there are good carbohydrates and bad carbohydrates and good fats and bad fats. Well the same goes for proteins. Animal meats (beef, poultry, pork, fish) have a huge amount of protein, but the downside is that they also have saturated fats – the bad kind of fat. So how do we get protein-rich meats while being conscious of saturated fats?

You could do a little research and an analysis on the nutrients of meats, but why don't I take that cumbersome task off your hands? It seems the skinless chicken breast is the benchmark of high quality protein with little fat. But did you know that some lean beef has only one more gram of saturated fat and has higher amounts of other nutrients than the glorified skinless chicken breast?

Every nutrient is important in a well-balanced diet and in lieu of listing them all, I'd like to mention three that I think are especially important: zinc, iron, and vitamin B-12. All three nutrients vary in concentration in animal meats which is why I feel it's important to vary the types of meats you eat. For example, beef is an excellent source of zinc, but just an average source of thiamin. Pork is superior for thiamin and iron, but mediocre in zinc.

> Every nutrient is important in a well-balanced diet.

Zinc

Pound for pound, oysters provide the most zinc of any food, but red meat and poultry are also excellent sources. Whole grains, beans, nuts, and dairy products are good sources of zinc too. Zinc is the most influential mineral in a healthy immune system. Our bodies need this vital mineral to form enzymes and insulin, synthesize DNA, heal wounds, help control our appetite, and assist in the development of certain types of white blood cells that fight infections. Zinc also helps increase our metabolisms and stabilizes blood sugar levels. A deficiency in zinc may result in decreased muscle strength and endurance.

There's a controversial myth about increasing your zinc intake to fight off a common cold, but the jury is still out on this one. Until more research is done, don't believe it. If you consume too much zinc, adverse effects may include reduced immune functions and decreased levels of HDL (the good cholesterol). According to the American Academy of Anti-Aging Medicine, 50 milligrams (50mg) per day is the highest amount of zinc that is considered safe.

Iron

Iron is another essential mineral. It's the most copious mineral in our blood and has the major responsibility of producing hemoglobin, a protein that transports oxygen in red blood cells from our lungs to the rest of our bodies, including our brain and muscles. If it wasn't for this mineral, our muscles wouldn't work. Our cells wouldn't be able to function properly without oxygen. Iron is also responsible for brain development, energy production, and supporting our immune system.

Although iron can be stored in the liver, iron deficiency is still the most common nutritional deficiency in America. It's possible for men to be deficient in iron but premenopausal women are at greater risk for two reasons. First, they typically eat less than men so they're not as likely to get the required amount through their diet. Second, premenopausal women lose blood during menstruation. Also, for healthy pregnancies, pregnant women need up to twice as much iron per day. The unborn child needs iron as well and could deplete the mother's iron stores if she doesn't have an iron-rich diet or supplementation. Iron deficiency could lead to symptoms like muscle fatigue, weakness, and lethargy.

Generally, men need 8mg of iron daily, and premenopausal women need 18mg. Most men are able to attain their daily amount of iron without even trying, so they need to be cautious not to get too much of this mineral because it could cause free radical damage to their muscle tissue, leading to premature aging.

Foods that are rich in iron include whole grains, dark green leafy veggies, lamb, fish, poultry, beans, and red meat, particularly liver. Even though pork and *lean* red meats are leaner than ever before, generally speaking lean red meats should be eaten no more than three times per week. Alternatives to red meat are venison, buffalo, elk, and other wild game.

So what are you waiting for? Explore your horizons and try something different. You just may find that you like wild game more than you thought.

Vitamin B-12

The function of vitamin B-12 is to synthesize normal red blood cells and help maintain the insulation that protects nerve fibers, which is paramount for a healthy central nervous system. B-12 is also needed to help produce DNA and metabolize fats, carbohydrates, and proteins. The most common sources of vitamin B-12 are meats, fish, eggs, and dairy products.

Unlike other water-soluble vitamins, our bodies don't excrete B-12 through urine very quickly. Instead, like iron, we store it mainly in the liver where bile reabsorbs it for future use. It's possible to become B-12 deficient which may result in excessive fatigue, infections that may take longer than usual to heal, and breathlessness. If you're B-12 deficient for an extended period of time, it could lead to irreversible neurological damage.

Lean Meats

BEEF

Most people think they have to eliminate red meat when they're trying to maintain a healthy diet because they associate beef with high fat and cholesterol. It's true that beef used to be extremely high in fat, but in the last decade beef producers have heard Americans cry for a meat low in saturated fat that isn't bland. Once fat is trimmed from lean beef, some cuts of lean beef can provide as few as 4g of fat compared to 3g in a chicken breast. Further, half the fatty

> Some cuts of lean beef can provide as few as 4g of fat compared to 3g in a chicken breast.

acids are the heart-healthy monounsaturated fats. Beef contains a fatty acid called conjugated linoleic acid (CLA) which has proven to decrease body fat and increase lean muscle mass in animal studies. Also, beef has a powerhouse of nutrients in every bite. According to the *Journal of the American Dietetic Association,* beef is the #1 source of protein, zinc, and vitamin B-12. It has all 8 indispensable amino acids and is an important dietary source of iron. Lean beef has 8 times as much vitamin B-12, 6 times the amount of zinc, and 3 times the amount of iron than the marvelous skinless chicken breast. Ask your local butcher for any cut of beef with the words "loin" or "round" in the name. For example, eye of round, sirloin tip, top round roast ... you get the picture.

> Beef contains a fatty acid called conjugated linoleic acid (CLA) which has proven to decrease body fat and increase lean muscle mass.

Go ahead and enjoy some flavor in your diet... and don't feel guilty.

SKINLESS CHICKEN BREAST VS. LEAN BEEF
Per 3 ounce, cooked (85 Grams)
UNITED STATES RECOMMENDED DAILY ALLOWANCE (USRDA)

*Based on a 2,000 calorie diet. Please consult with your physician on any matters regarding your health.

MEAT	CALORIES	PROTEIN	TOTAL FAT	SAT. FAT	ZINC	IRON	VITAMIN B-12
Skinless Chicken Breast	140	26g	3g	1g	6%	5%	5%
Top Round Roast	160	31g	3.5g	1g	39%	14%	37%
Eye of Round Steak	150	25g	4.5g	1.5g	39%	14%	37%
Top Sirloin Steak	150	26g	4.5g	2g	39%	14%	37%

PORK

Now known as "the other white meat" because it's low in fat and calories, pork provides a high level of nutrients and is an excellent source of quality protein. Twenty years ago, pork was a high fat, high calorie food, but through better breeding and feeding, pork is now 29% lower in saturated fat, 14% lower in calories, and 10% lower in cholesterol. According to the National Pork Board, some cuts of pork have 31% less fat than they had just 20 years ago. What's more, the Canadian's Heart and Stroke Foundation's Health Check Program includes lean pork as a wise food choice.

> The Canadian's Heart and Stroke Foundation's Health Check Program includes lean pork as a wise food choice.

The pork tenderloin is the leanest cut of pork with only 4g of fat, comparable to a skinless chicken breast. The one extra gram of fat converts to 9 calories, so that's easily justified. Remember, we need a variety of foods so that we can have a change of taste, rather than eating boring chicken breasts all the time. Cuts from the "loin" ensure the leanest meat.

Word to the wise...

Watch out for sausage and anything "cured" or "smoked." They're full of nitrates, which convert to nitrites while you're chewing, then convert to nitrosamines in your stomach. Nitrosamines are cancer-causing chemical compounds, so please limit your consumption of these types of foods. Also, when you're in the mood for ham, look for fresh ham and check the ingredients to make sure that it's not smoked, rather uncured and nitrate-free.

SKINLESS CHICKEN BREAST VS. PORK
Per 3 ounce, cooked (85 Grams)
UNITED STATES RECOMMENDED DAILY ALLOWANCE (USRDA)

*Based on a 2,000 calorie diet. Please consult with your physician on any matters regarding your health.

MEAT	CALORIES	PROTEIN	TOTAL FAT	SAT. FAT	ZINC	IRON	VITAMIN B-12
Skinless Chicken Breast	140	26g	3g	1g	6%	5%	5%
Pork Tenderloin	140	24g	4g	1.5g	15%	7%	33%
Ham	130	21g	4.5g	1.5g	15%	7%	33%
Loin Chops	170	26g	7g	2.5g	15%	7%	33%
Butt Half Leg of Pork	180	26g	7g	2.5g	15%	7%	33%
Boston Butt Roast	180	26g	7g	2.5g	15%	7%	33%

christopher SASHA

LAMB

While lamb is not very popular in the United States, it's a favorite in many other countries in the world. Lamb used to have a high amount of saturated fat, but, like pork, through better breeding and improved butchering methods, the fat content in lamb has been greatly reduced. In fact, 50% of the fat in lamb is monounsaturated, which is good for you. It provides twice as much iron as pork, three times the amount of the skinless chicken breast, and up to eight times more than fish. Lamb is a little higher in cholesterol than beef and pork. The 2010 U.S. government guidelines suggest only 300mg of dietary cholesterol per day, so remember that a 3 ounce (cooked) serving of lamb is between 70-80mg.

SKINLESS CHICKEN BREAST VS. LAMB
Per 3 ounce, cooked (85 Grams)
UNITED STATES RECOMMENDED DAILY ALLOWANCE (USRDA)

*Based on a 2,000 calorie diet. Please consult with your physician on any matters regarding your health.

MEAT	CALORIES	PROTEIN	TOTAL FAT	SAT. FAT	ZINC	IRON	VITAMIN B-12
Skinless Chicken Breast	140	26g	3g	1g	6%	5%	5%
Lamb Shank	150	24g	6g	2g	30%	17%	37%
Lamb Leg (top round)	150	24g	6g	2g	30%	17%	37%
Leg of Lamb	160	24g	6.5g	2.5g	30%	17%	37%
Loin of Lamb	170	23g	8g	3g	30%	17%	37%
Lamb Tenderloin	170	23g	8g	3g	30%	17%	37%

FISH

Finfish and shellfish are excellent sources of protein and other important vitamins and minerals, and they also provide the heart-healthy Omega-3 fatty acids. Fish get their high levels of Omega-3 from the foods they eat, like algae. Algae are one of the primary producers of fatty acids. Omega-3s are part of the polyunsaturated fat group and have been proven to help reduce risk for coronary heart disease along with a myriad of other health problems.

Approximately 250,000 Americans die each year due to cardiac arrest. According to a recent study at the University of Washington, eating a modest amount of salmon (one to two servings per week) can reduce the risk of primary cardiac arrest.

christopherSASHA

The drawback to eating fish and other seafood is that they almost all contain traces of mercury. Mercury is a natural element in the air, water, and soil. However, it eventually settles in water. The general rule of thumb is that larger fish that have lived longer contain more mercury.

The danger in consuming high levels of mercury is that it could harm the brain, heart, lungs, kidneys, and immune system. Unborn babies, young children, and the elderly seem to be most susceptible to these perils. If you're like me and would rather be safe than sorry, try to limit (or eliminate) shark, swordfish, tilefish, and king mackerel because they're usually loaded with mercury, and even halibut which borders on containing high levels of mercury. And speaking of limiting certain types of fish, try to limit processed seafood like smoked, cured, and – believe it or not – most canned fish (including canned light tuna) because salt is added during the processing which skyrockets your sodium intake. *Sorry!*

> The larger fish that have lived longer contain more mercury.

Still, there's no doubt that fish is an excellent change of pace in your diet. Try to include fish one to four times per week. Additionally, try to vary the types of fish since some contain more vitamin B-12, others have more iron, still others have less fat… you get the idea. Here's a bonus fact: protein in seafood is easier for our bodies to break down and absorb than protein in red meats and poultry. This means our bodies will utilize more of the protein and less will be excreted through our digestive system without being used.

SKINLESS CHICKEN BREAST VS. FISH
Per 3 ounce, cooked (85 Grams)
UNITED STATES RECOMMENDED DAILY ALLOWANCE (USRDA)

*Based on a 2,000 calorie diet. Please consult with your physician on any matters regarding your health.

MEAT	CALORIES	PROTEIN	TOTAL FAT	SAT. FAT	ZINC	IRON	VITAMIN B-12
Skinless Chicken Breast	140	26g	3g	1g	6%	5%	5%
Tuna (light, canned in water)	90	21g	1.5g	0g	4%	7%	42%
Orange Roughy	89	19g	1g	0g	2%	5%	7%
Shrimp	90	17g	1g	0g	6%	11%	16%
Sea Bass	105	20g	2g	1g	3%	2%	4%
Salmon (pink)	127	22g	4g	1g	4%	5%	49%
Rainbow Trout	144	21g	6g	2g	3%	2%	70%

EGGS

The World's Most Perfect Food. When I was a teenager, I didn't realize what that meant. I was really more interested in going to the neighborhood pizza joint, which provided everything a teenager needed – carbs, fat, protein, and people-watching with my friends. Now that I'm (somewhat) more sophisticated, I finally understand the message. Eggs are one of the best sources of protein and essential vitamins and minerals. In fact, eggs have a higher quality of protein than meat and fish, and are used as the reference standard for protein in assessing all other foods.

Whole eggs contain most minerals required for a healthy body. Women are more prone to osteoporosis, making eggs almost perfect in their diets. Eggs provide phosphorus and calcium for healthy bone growth which will help prevent the softening of bones. The egg contains a yolk (vitamins and minerals) and albumen, commonly known as the "white" (mostly protein). Sometimes you have to take the good with the bad. The yolk has all the indispensable amino acids but also has fat and cholesterol. The albumen has the highest quality of protein and vitamin B2 (riboflavin). I have high cholesterol, due to genetics, so I sacrifice the vitamins and minerals (along with the fat and cholesterol) and focus on the white and its protein. I'll get my vitamins and minerals from other food sources.

> Eggs have a higher quality of protein than meat and fish, and are used as the reference standard for protein in assessing all other foods.

Rocky's Raw Egg Shakes...

Raw eggs contain avidin, a protein that binds to biotin (a member of the vitamin B complexes) and prohibits our bodies from absorbing the vitamin biotin. Biotin helps in the biosynthesis of fatty acids and glucose, fuel sources for our bodies. It's also a catalyst to metabolize carbohydrates and proteins. A diet rich in avidin for an extended period of time could lead to biotin deficiency. This is rare, but it could happen, leading to conditions like skin rashes, hair loss, high cholesterol, and heart problems. When the egg is cooked, the heat denatures avidin, making it prone to digestion.

And not only that, but keep in mind the dangers of salmonella, always a potential risk with raw eggs. My recommendation? Unless you get paid $23,000 to drink raw eggs and star in a movie as a small-time boxer readying for a fight with the heavyweight champion (like Sylvester Stallone in the movie "Rocky"), stay away.

Deli Meats

In our crazy world of getting up at 5:00 in the morning to get to the gym, sprinting off to work, dashing to meetings, hustling the kids to soccer practice, spending quality time with the family, keeping in touch with friends, dealing with everyday debacles, it's no wonder we look for processed foods. These types of foods are our short-term saviors. For the sake of time and convenience, it makes sense to go to the deli, buy ready-to-eat sandwiches, and scarf them down quickly in order to rush to the next meeting. Why would we want to spend an hour in the kitchen preparing dinner when we can grab a hot dog, sausage, or deli meats from the grocery store and have dinner on the table within minutes?

I know in the short term it sounds logical, but when you consider the long term effects on our bodies, eating processed foods is not a good habit to get into. Studies have suggested that large quantities of processed meats such as deli meats, hot dogs, and sausages have been linked to increased risk of cardiovascular disease, colorectal cancer, and type 2 diabetes.

Listeria

Deli meats have been traced to Listeria infections. Listeria (Listeria Monocytogenes) are bacteria that cause food poisoning in our intestines. Food contaminated with it can cause Listeriosis, which can be fatal. According to the U.S. Department of Agriculture, it's unlikely for healthy individuals to catch Listeriosis. Infants, pregnant women, the elderly, and individuals with weakened immune systems are more susceptible. Only *thorough* cooking can kill Listeria bacteria.

Therefore, the USDA's Food Safety and Inspection Service advises that if you are going to eat deli meats, luncheon meats, or hot dogs, make sure to reheat these foods until they are steaming hot. The issue with Listeria is that if not all the bacteria are killed during the cooking process, the bacteria that did survive will reproduce. They're tough little buggers that can not only resist heat, but also resist salt and nitrite. They're also capable of surviving and multiplying in temperatures as low as 24 degrees, surviving even refrigeration.

According to the National Food Processors Association, 37% of the typical American's diet is comprised of ready-to-eat foods.

Sodium Nitrites

The other problem with deli meats is the chemical preservative that manufacturers use to keep their meats pink and vibrant in color ... a preservative that fools consumers into believing these meats are fresh. Sodium nitrite is in almost every processed, cured, and smoked meat. Its original purpose was as a food preservative to fend off dangerous bacteria that caused botulism, which could lead to paralysis and death. But sodium nitrates are now known to increase the development of nitrosamines in the body, which assist the proliferation of cancer cells, specifically in the pancreas and the colon.

The fact is our bodies do require a *small amount* of nitrates to perform a few biological functions like fighting bacteria in the stomach and protecting against bacterial illnesses. Sodium nitrate is converted to sodium nitrite during our digestive process. In the stomach, nitrite, combined with stomach acids, forms nitric oxide, which helps heal wounds and burns, aids in controlling blood pressure, assists in blood clotting, and enhances brain functions. However, these are dietary nitrates that are found in drinking water and vegetables and fruits – not chemical preservatives. Nitrates are naturally found in soil when nitrogen combines with oxygen. Nitrogen can be derived from chemical fertilizers and animal waste. Plants absorb the nitrates, which is how we get nitrates from fruits and vegetables. Then whatever the plants don't absorb gets carried back to the soil in groundwater, and is brought back to the surface via well pumps.

Fears about sodium nitrites began in the 1970s when research showed that laboratory animals developed cancer from high nitrate dosages. The study correlated the consumption of cured meats with illnesses in children. At that point, the USDA tried to ban sodium nitrite, but the ban was prevented by the food processing industry because by then they depended on it to keep meats looking visually appealing. If deli meats, as well as other meats like salami, pepperoni, fish, ham, hot dogs, bacon, bologna, corned beef, some sausages, etc., don't have sodium nitrite injected into them, they turn a putrid grayish color. They aren't the bright reddish-pink color you see in the grocery stores. If you saw these meats in their true color, would you still buy them? The food industry is geared to sell, sell, sell. The majority of people buy based on cosmetic appearance – and food manufacturers know that.

Instead of banning it, the FDA and USDA authorized a comprehensive review of sodium nitrite as a food additive. Two scientific reports were produced by the National Academy of Sciences (NAS). In the end, the NAS stated that nitrate does not cause cancer and nitrite does not act directly as a cancer-causing agent in animals. The NAS also recommended that nitrate and nitrite supplementation be reduced as low as possible without endangering protection against botulism. Furthermore, the NAS has searched for nitrate alternatives for foods, but unfortunately has not yet been successful.

According to the Environmental Protection Agency (EPA), the primary danger associated with nitrates is that they are converted into nitrites during digestion and nitrites can poison humans, particularly infants and children. More importantly, according to the U.S. Surgeon General, nitrites can combine with amines (a by-product of protein digestion) to form cancer-causing nitrosamines. Nitrosamines can cause malignant tumor growth over a long exposure period, such as a lifetime of eating nitrite-added deli meats.

> Nitrites can combine with amines to form cancer-causing nitrosamines.

However, some food manufacturers believe chemical additives and preservatives, including nitrates and nitrites, are no longer needed. To some companies these chemicals are dinosaurs, originating in a time when meat was neither heat-treated nor pasteurized and nitrites were the only way to prevent botulism. They believe that the time and temperature of cooking are key factors in preventing bacterial growth in meats, and that better production and food storage methods have decreased the potential for food-borne illness. They argue that the only purpose for using nitrites in cooked meats today is to keep the traditional pink color and cured flavor. Today, they say, nitrites act more as a convenient cover for lower standards of production.

The USDA keeps this quiet, but a proven strategy to counteract foods with sodium nitrite is a fairly large amount of vitamin C. This inhibits the conversion of sodium nitrite to nitrosamines, which are potent carcinogens. But the only fool-proof way to avert the side effects of sodium nitrite is to completely eliminate the chemical from your diet.

Nitrite in its raw chemical form is considered a highly toxic chemical and the USDA acknowledges its primary function as a color fixative – it makes old, dead meats appear fresh and vibrant. The USDA also encourages the addition of antioxidants to nitrites, such as sodium ascorbate, sodium erythorbate, and vitamin C which inhibit the formation of nitrosamines. The problem with relying on the added vitamin C to protect from cancer threats is that two-thirds of the added vitamin C is destroyed during cooking. So cooking the meats mostly defeats the vitamin's purpose.

> Sodium ascorbate, sodium erythorbate, and vitamin C inhibits the formation of nitrosamines.

Now, if the USDA accepted the results of the two reports issued by the National Academy of Sciences stating "nitrates do not cause cancer and nitrites do not act directly as cancer-causing agents in animals," why would they lower the amount of nitrates and nitrites as low as possible without endangering the protection of botulism? Furthermore, why would the USDA encourage the addition of antioxidants that inhibit the formation of nitrosamines, which are known to cause malignant tumor growths? Are they telling us everything we need to know to make healthy food decisions? Or is the USDA protecting the industries they were supposed to regulate?

Whey Protein

With my insane schedule, I don't always have the time to sit for a meal so I constantly have protein shakes in thermoses just for those occasions. It takes about two minutes to whip up a few servings of shakes, which is less time than it takes to go to the grocery store to buy a sandwich. I put the thermoses in my briefcase or gym bag so I have them by my side whenever I may need a quick snack.

With all the different types of protein powders, it's hard to determine which ones are best. Even after being in the business for more than 13 years (where does the time go?), I still feel a little overwhelmed by all the companies vying for my business. Walking into a health food store, I'm bombarded with aisles and aisles and shelves and shelves of different protein powders. Remember, this is a multi-billion dollar business and every company wants a big slice of the pie.

The question is which protein will satisfy my individual needs? Soy protein is cheaper. If you're just trying to get the required daily amount of protein, this might be the right protein for you. However, if you're trying to build muscle and recover quickly after a workout, whey protein might be a better choice.

If you decide on whey protein, you have to continue to narrow your choice … hydrolyzed, concentrate, isolate, or bioactive whey fraction protein? It goes on and on. If you choose a whey protein isolate, you further have to decide if ion-exchange is better for your individuals needs or if micro-filtered is advantageous.

Whey protein comes, believe it or not, from the cheese industry. It's a high quality protein from cow's milk with all the indispensable amino acids the body needs every day. Whey protein provides a whole array of benefits like potentially reducing blood pressure and cancer cells, improving liver function and immunity, suppressing hunger, boosting the burning of fat (more calories are used to digest protein than any other macronutrient), and supporting strong and healthy bones. Many experts consider whey protein to have the highest nutritional values of all proteins. They base their consideration on the Biological Value (BV), a criterion to measure the quality of a protein. The BV measures the amount of usable indispensable amino acids, dispensable amino acids, and Branched-Chain Amino Acids (BCAAs) contained in a particular protein. Consequently, the higher the BV, the better the protein is digested, utilized, and retained in the body.

> Whey protein comes from the cheese industry.

BCAAs are small chains of proteins called peptides, which are vital for growth. They're composed of three of the indispensable amino acids (leucine, isoleucine, and valine) needed for the maintenance of muscle tissue and to preserve stores of glycogen in the muscle. If you remember from Chapter 5, glycogen is a form of glucose that can be converted to

christopherSASHA

energy. Athletes prefer BCAAs over all other amino acids because they're not metabolized by the liver, but rather rush directly into muscle tissue. They're the first to be used during resistance training, which is theoretically why these good guys need to be consumed before and immediately after a work-out.

Unlike other amino acids, BCAAs aren't metabolized by the liver. They're rushed directly into muscle tissue.

Whey is a by-product of cheese made when milk goes through the heating process. The proteins that are filtered out during this process are damaged by heat and used to be thrown away. Then scientists found that the "damaged" proteins could be quite beneficial nutritionally – creating a whole new industry... *whey protein.*

Let's review the most popular whey proteins to help decide which one, or ones, might work best for you.

First, hydrolyzed proteins are broken down into peptides of different lengths. Because the protein is broken down, your digestive system doesn't have to work as hard and it's absorbed into your bloodstream more quickly. Hydrolyzed proteins have never really received much public attention because they taste like chalk, they're expensive, and their benefits were never scientifically proven.

The first generation of whey protein powders are called "whey protein concentrates." They're between 35%-85% pure protein. The rest of the contents are fat, lactose, and minerals. So if you're lactose-intolerant, you might want to dodge this type of whey protein. Concentrates are usually processed the least of all whey proteins, making them cheaper than isolates. They're also cheaper because they aren't as pure. If you're on a budget and looking for a respectable amount of protein and don't mind a little extra fat and lactose, whey protein concentrate may be for you.

The second generation is whey protein isolates. There are two methods of separating out the whey in these types of whey protein isolates: ion-exchange isolates and micro-filtered isolates. Due to the filtering process, whey isolates are more expensive than whey concentrates. Ion-exchange isolates are around 90%-96% pure protein with less fat and lactose than concentrates. They have the highest protein content but lose many of the peptides that provide all the health benefits mentioned above. So if your goal is to find a powder supplement with the highest protein levels per gram and you don't care about the health benefits, ion-exchange isolates is your protein.

In my opinion, the best whey protein on the market today is micro-filtered isolates, particularly Cross Flow Micro Filtered (CFM). They're over 90% pure protein and, because the cold-temperature micro-filtering process doesn't destroy all the peptides, you also enjoy most of the health advantages these peptides possess. Here's the bonus: micro-filtered whey isolates also have more branched-chain amino acids that are crucial for building and retaining muscle tissue. Unfortunately, the benefits of this protein come at a cost. These whey proteins are the most expensive.

The next generation, which recently hit the market, is Bioactive Whey Fraction (BAWF) protein. Whey is an extremely complicated protein composed of smaller protein subfractions or peptides. Each peptide, like Lactoferrin and Lactoglobulin to name a couple, has its own unique biological properties with its own unique health benefits. Only through new filtering techniques could these protein subfractions be separated from whey.

BAWF protein is going to be hugely superior to the whey proteins we currently have on the market. Not only will these BAWF proteins contain high levels of quality protein, but they will also possess strikingly heightened levels of bioactive health-promoting compounds. Even the whey protein isolates today, though highly concentrated with protein, only have a minute amount of these potent peptides. Ion-exchange isolates, incidentally, are the worst offenders when it comes to filtering out these vital peptides. Studies are currently concentrating on the effects these new proteins will have on athletes' muscle mass and performance. I don't know what results BAWF proteins will actually provide, but I do know one thing – they are expensive. Until there's more research and evidence that BAWF protein works better than any other whey protein on the market today, I'll stick with what works for me.

Whey is excellent for many reasons, but it won't make you look like Arnold Schwarzenegger by just supplementing your diet with it. A defined, chiseled, Greek-god-like physique takes hard work, determination, and persistence. If you don't have the body you desire in a month, don't give up. Body sculpting takes long hours in the gym, eating the right foods at the right times, and plenty of rest. I assure you, as each strenuous workout passes, you will get that much closer to your goal.

> If you don't have the body you desire in a month, don't give up.

Protein Overload

Thirty percent of your daily caloric intake should come from high quality protein. However, recent research has proposed that a healthy diet should have only around 10%-15% of your calories coming from protein, while the Institute of Medicine suggests no more than 35%. The World Organization of the United Nations recommends 4.5%, 6% according to the Food and Nutrition Board of the U.S. Department of Agriculture, and the U.S. National Research Council proposes 8%! So whose guidelines do you follow? The answer (if there is any one answer) is difficult to discern.

The amount of protein you should consume depends on factors like your age, genetics, amount of lean body mass, activity level, and medical conditions. For example, athletes trying to build muscle can consume 1g-1.5g of protein per pound of body weight, which is more than the average person because they burn through more calories. Although protein is responsible for a myriad of functions, it doesn't require an overkill to get the job done. Generally, the more sedentary your lifestyle, the less protein you need. However, our bodies demand a perpetual supply every day for a healthy, balanced diet. The United States Recommended Daily Allowance (USRDA) suggests 2-3 servings (6-9 ounces) per day. One steak at your favorite restaurant should cover that requirement. I, along with most Americans, get more than the recommended amount without even trying, so I concentrate more on good fats and some complex carbohydrates like raw vegetables.

Raw foods have the enzymes to utilize the protein to build muscle and fight chronic illnesses and disease. I also include a very limited amount of fruit. When it comes to fruits, I believe fructose (sugar in fruit, among other places) is one of the culprits in our obesity epidemic. Fructose is a double-edged sword. On one side, it's good (especially for diabetics) because it doesn't raise insulin levels, but on the flip side, without an increase in insulin levels, the appetite suppressing hormone leptin isn't secreted. Leptin signals our brains that we're full and without that signal, we'll overeat, which is the road to obesity and all the chronic illnesses that come with it.

Athletes and very active people (construction workers, personal trainers, shipping and receiving laborers) might want to consume a little more protein to repair and build body tissue, to transport nutrients, and to make muscles contract. But beware of too much protein. On one hand, dieticians and some scientists warn that high protein diets can lead to a host of problems, like dehydration, calcium deficiency, osteoporosis, and kidney stones. On the other hand, professional bodybuilders say, "hogwash."

There is no scientific evidence that a high protein diet will cause damage to a healthy kidney or liver.

As for me, I truly believe that everything in this world is for us to enjoy in moderation. Except in the case of pre-existing kidney or liver disease, there's no scientific evidence that a high protein diet will cause damage to a healthy kidney or liver. The only valid problem with a high protein diet is that protein needs more water, calcium, magnesium, and vitamins D3 and K2 to metabolize than carbohydrates and fats.

Magnesium regulates calcium transport while vitamins D3 and K2 take the calcium out of the bloodstream and allow it to be absorbed into your bones. Without these two vitamins, you can take as much calcium as you want and it won't help prevent you from falling victim to osteoporosis, osteopenia, and calcification of your arteries. So if you take in extra protein, it would be wise to increase your water, calcium, magnesium, and vitamins D3 and K2.

Our bodies can't store protein like they can store fats and carbohydrates, which is why we need to have a constant supply. Whatever excess protein we eat gets converted to glycogen for later use as energy, converted to fat, or expelled through our urine and feces. When we eat too much protein, excess nitrogen is excreted as a toxic byproduct of protein breakdown called urea, which is formed in our liver and discharged through our kidneys and expelled from our bodies through our urine. It's our kidneys' responsibility to flush out the excess urea and unprocessed proteins from our bodies through our urine.

Without vitamin K2, you become susceptible to osteoporosis, osteopenia, and calcification of arteries.

This is why drinking plenty of water is so important. We need the water to help our kidneys filter the urea out of our bloodstream. The more protein consumed, the higher the levels of urea and uric acid (another toxic by-product of protein metabolism) in our blood. Our bodies get rid of these two toxic substances by driving water into the kidneys to help flush them out. The general rule is the more protein we digest, the more water we need to drink.

When more protein in relation to the amount of calcium is ingested, calcium and other minerals like magnesium are depleted from our bodies (including our bones) through our kidneys. However, more studies need to be conducted to determine the proper ratio of protein to calcium. When we eat meat, our blood becomes more acidic which requires calcium to neutralize the acid. The calcium, along with the acid, is then filtered through our kidneys and is forever lost in our urine. Because Americans eat too much protein, we require higher amounts of calcium in our diets. If we don't increase our dietary calcium intake, our bodies will excrete it from our bones which will eventually cause the bones to become weak, potentially resulting in osteoporosis.

Because protein breakdown products are eliminated from our bodies through our kidneys, excessive protein consumption puts extra demands on them. This becomes more of a problem as we get older because our organs become less efficient. The most common kidney stones (calcium stones) are made up of calcium and oxalate. Oxalate is a salt of oxalic acid that can link up with calcium, called calcium oxalate, which is virtually insoluble. When high amounts of calcium oxalate are present in our kidneys, they can harden and crystalize helping to form kidney stones. They're very tiny but very painful, and can cause a blockage, stopping the flow of urine. My father had this happen to him and he cried like a baby. In his case, the kidney stone had to be surgically removed.

Where's the irony in this?…

Eskimos have the highest rate of osteoporosis even though they also consume the highest amount of calcium of any of the world's population. Studies suggest their high protein intake (mainly from their diet of fish) may contribute to the bone-weakening disease.

In case excessive protein intake does lead to problems down the road, I try to limit my overall protein to 30% of my daily calories. I also try to get a good mix of proteins in my diet by limiting meat consumption and getting some protein from vegetables, very few fruits, and whey protein shakes. I always drink plenty of water and increase my calcium, magnesium, and vitamins D3 and K2 to limit my odds of developing any of the aforementioned health problems.

And speaking of drinking plenty of water, let's not overlook what turns out to be the most important element of all. As we'll see, hydration is more than just quenching your thirst; it's mandatory for proper health.

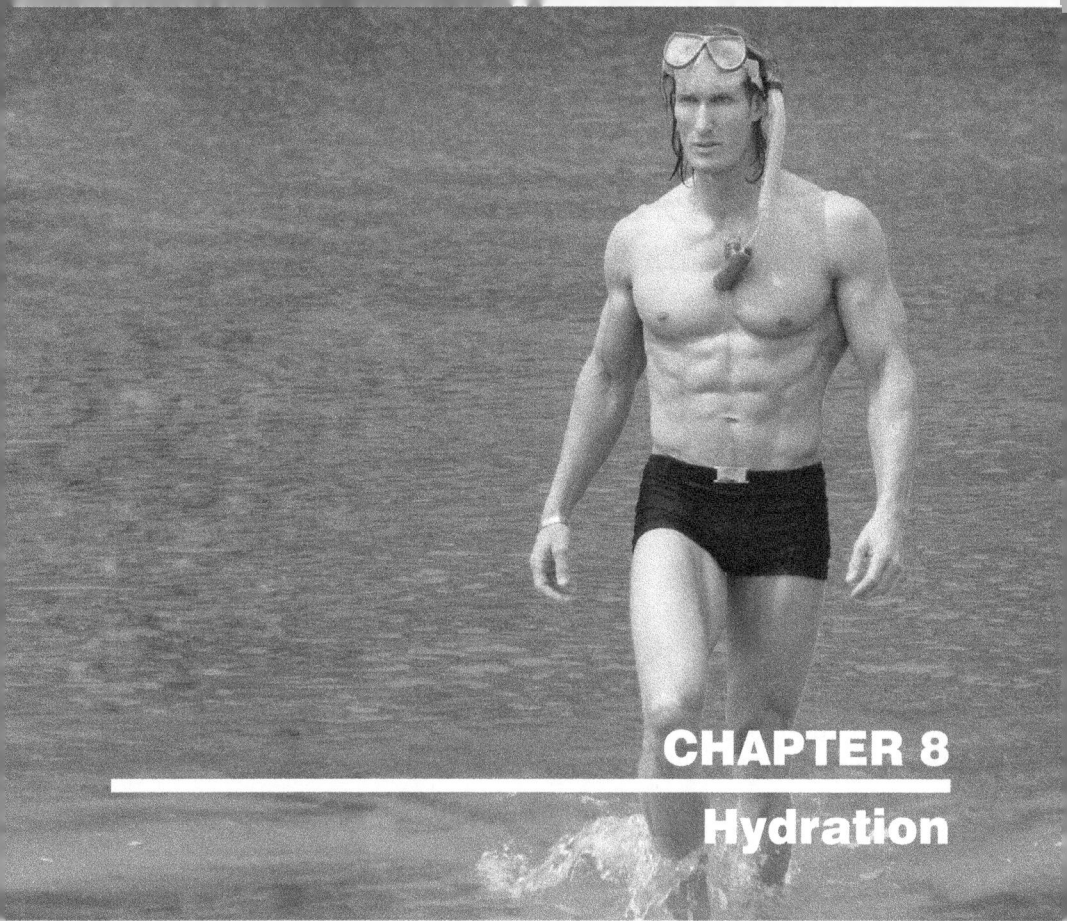

CHAPTER 8
Hydration

Of all the substances our bodies crave, water is the most important. Our body tissues consist of between 55%-75% water. Protein is right behind with about 45% of total body composition. We can survive about a month without food, but, without water, we'd have to cash in our chips within 5 to 7 days. Consuming water is probably the most important thing we can do to maintain good health.

We can also get our daily water intake from foods we eat, like fruits and vegetables. Watermelon, for example, is over 90% water (hence the name) and fresh tomatoes are about 93% water. Of course we can obtain water from many alternative sources like milk, juice, tea, coffee, and sports drinks. But the best way to hydrate our bodies is to drink good old-fashioned water because it has no calories, no additives, and no preservatives. It's pure.

Water is crucial to our bodies because it's involved in just about every bodily function. The water in our bodies helps metabolize fats, maintain

> Consuming water is probably the most important thing we can do to maintain good health.

proper muscle tone, regulate body temperature, lubricate joints, digest food, transport nutrients and oxygen to cells, and remove toxic waste from our bodies. Our blood, as well as our lungs, muscles, and brains, are composed mostly of water and require water to perform their functions properly.

Drink More Water

It seems to me that almost everyone who comes to me for weight loss training has the crazy notion that they must *decrease* their water consumption to lose weight. In a way, they're right. If they decrease their water intake, they *will* lose weight, but mostly water weight and muscle – exactly what they shouldn't be losing. When you lose muscle, your metabolism slows down. This is detrimental for anyone, especially people trying to lose weight the correct way.

People looking to lose weight should be *increasing* their water consumption…that's right, *more* water. "But won't I retain water doing that?" is always the question I hear. No, I say. Once we have all the water we need to hydrate our cells and organs, our bodies get rid of excess water via urination and sweat. Our bodies only retain water when deprived of it.

> Our bodies only retain water when deprived of it.

After I coax clients into drinking more water, most come back to me with concerns about frequent urination. They feel uneasy having to constantly run to the washroom. It's true … when guzzling more water than you're used to, your bladder becomes stretched. It's more frequently stimulated, causing you to urinate more often. But try to last this out just a few weeks while your bladder becomes accustomed to the change. In time you'll urinate in larger amounts, but less often.

Carbohydrates and too much sodium will also cause water retention. In fact, carbs trigger our kidneys to store sodium. Our bodies try to maintain balance between sodium and water. So when we consume carbs, our bodies have to retain water to offset the sodium being held. Every gram of carb retains about 3 grams (3g) of water. In other words, 464g of carbs *retain* about three pounds of water. This is one reason we weigh more during the day as opposed to

> 464g of carbs retain about 3 pounds of water.

when we first wake up – we eat carbs throughout the day which retain water. This is also the main reason the South Beach Diet claims that you can lose up to 13 pounds in the first 2 weeks. On this particular diet, carbohydrates are very limited during the first phase and so water loss occurs. In fact, the first phase of this diet omits bread, potatoes, fruit, and rice which are all carbohydrates that retain water. Since there are fewer carbs, the kidneys store less sodium resulting in excess water and sodium being expelled by urination.

The result is that you lose weight (sometimes a lot of weight) during the initial phase. Don't be fooled. Your scale registers a lower total body weight, but it doesn't tell you that the weight you lost was mainly water and muscle.

To verify this, get a body fat test before you start the diet and again two weeks later. You'll find that your body fat percentage will be almost identical. It may be slightly lower – but certainly not 13 pounds lower. Furthermore, if you're not resistance training, you're going to lose even more muscle.

> Your scale registers a lower total body weight, but it doesn't tell you that the weight you lost was mainly water and muscle.

The South Beach Diet also boasts that you *"lose belly fat first."* As explained in Chapter 6, it's physiologically impossible to reduce fat from any one particular area of your body. All fat cells increase and decrease at the same time. Genetics and hormones determine where your largest amount of fat cells are going to be. So how can everyone lose belly fat first?

The best way to get rid of water retention is to reduce sodium intake. If you consume too much sodium, drink more water to dilute it. A little tip to burn a few extra calories: ***try drinking ice cold water.*** It burns more calories, because our bodies utilize energy warming the water to body temperature. If you can't refrigerate your water, drink whatever water is available to you. The point is, drink more water.

I once heard that it was healthy not to drink fluids while eating a meal. So being the dweeb I can often be, I gave it a go. When I was getting ready for a photo shoot, I needed to drop a few pounds so I reduced my fluid intake, especially during meals. I had a hard time choking down food (a whole new meaning to the term *force feeding*) and I developed heartburn during this stint, a sign of water deprivation in the upper gastrointestinal tract.

I didn't know it at the time but water is critical when you eat because it aids in the digestion process and absorbs and transports nutrients into cells. After a few days experimenting with this theory, I lost about three pounds but the destruction I did to my body was not worth the three pound loss. I was tired all the time, I couldn't focus on anything (except when the photo shoot was going to be over), and my workouts were mediocre at best. I'm happy to say that today I drink plenty of water, especially during meals.

Coffee & Soda Thwart Weight Loss

The other concern voiced by individuals trying to lose weight is about the types of fluids to drink. When my clients keep a food diary (discussed in Chapter 3) of everything they eat and drink throughout the day, I can see why they're not losing weight. Most people become fixated on what they're eating, but drop the ball on what they're drinking. Many people feel tired and weak when they first start dieting (due to the body not getting the amount of calories it's used to getting, which will adjust in time), so they increase their coffee and soda consumption during the workday to stay awake. When they exercise, they down sports and energy drinks which are loaded with sugar. Coffee and soda have caffeine in them which stimulates the central nervous system, making most people stay awake and more alert. Not only does caffeine stimulate the brain, it also releases insulin and often causes disarray with blood sugar levels. The result is that you fly high for a while, but once your blood sugar level drops, you become tired again and itch for more caffeine stimulation.

> Sports and energy drinks are loaded with sugar.

> The USDA reports that the consumption of soft drinks has increased 500% in the past 50 years, and studies have linked the rise in obesity in children to the overconsumption of soda and sweetened drinks.

The average soda has about 36g of sugar in one can! Remember, 4g of sugar equals 1 teaspoon of sugar so most soda (12 ounces) contains about 9 teaspoons of this psychologically addicting white poison. And if soda is your drink of choice for a caffeine fix, you could be drinking a lot more than you think to get your adrenaline pumping. The body eventually adapts to the amount of caffeine so more is needed to get the same effect. This could be why many caffeine addicts are overweight.

Some argue that caffeine is a diuretic, a substance that drains water from your body by increasing the number of times you urinate. And though caffeine is a mild diuretic, it's not worth the insulin reactions that it stimulates. You might want to consider abandoning caffeine if you're dieting and not losing weight.

> The average can of soda has about 36g of sugar—about 9 teaspoons of psychologically addicting white poison.

How Much Water

Here's the million dollar question – *"How much water do we need?"* The standard answer used to be that it was healthy to drink eight glasses of water every day. But this was never scientifically proven. No one really knows how this myth originated, but some say it started in the 1940s when the National Academy of Sciences recommended 1 milliliter of fluid for every calorie burned.

Then dietician gurus came up with the idea that we should consume approximately half the number of ounces of water as body weight. For instance, if you weigh 200 pounds, then you should consume about 100 ounces of water daily. But is this universally true? What about 2 people who both weigh 200 pounds but live in different climates? Maybe I weigh 200 pounds and live in Alaska and another guy, who also weighs 200 pounds, lives in Florida. Do we both require the same amount of water? When you consider that Florida is a lot hotter and more humid than Alaska, it would be logical to assume that the guy in Florida needs more water to remain hydrated. Obviously there are other variables to take into consideration.

As more research is done in the fitness and nutrition arena, we learn more about what we need, and how much water we need to maintain optimal health. Things aren't as cut and dried as they once were thought to be. Factors like age, activity level, lean body mass, climate, and the amount of protein consumed are some of the factors that need to be considered instead of taking the old one-size-fits-all approach. Generally, an active person will demand more water to stay hydrated than a person with a sedentary lifestyle. When it comes to perspiration, the people who sweat and can wring out their gym clothes after a workout should guzzle more than the people who only mist their clothes. If you have a stomach bug and are vomiting, have diarrhea, or are sweating profusely, all of these circumstances involve the loss of fluids that need to be replenished.

> Factors like age, activity level, lean body mass, climate, and the amount of protein consumed determine how much water you should consume.

The new and improved formula specifically designed for each and every person is to drink enough water so your urine looks almost clear. No calculations, no measuring. Just look before you flush. However, there is an exception to this guide. Regardless of how much your fluid intake may be, an overabundant amount of vitamins C or B2 (riboflavin) will make your urine bright yellow and glow in the dark…well, almost.

CELLULITE

Drinking more water also helps with cellulite appearance. When you're dehydrated, your cells shrink which increases the appearance of cellulite. Cellulite is the term used to describe the adipose (fat) cells under the skin that give a bumpy or dimpled look in areas like the hips, thighs, and butt. Although it's more common in women, some men get cellulite too. A huge majority of people think that cellulite is caused by being overweight because it's most obvious in obese women. The fact is that cellulite appears in 90% of all women, and develops in overweight ladies as well as in normal weight and thin women.

Fat is stored in compartments and separated by collagen. Then strands of tissue connect your skin to deeper tissue layers to form pockets of fat cells. It's the connective tissue separating around the fat cells that creates the cottage cheese look. When fat cells increase in size, the more dimply the skin looks, and vice versa. Unfortunately, cellulite is predetermined by genetics.

> There's no way to get rid of cellulite.

There's no way to get rid of cellulite so don't believe anyone who says they can. Sure, you can do a few things to diminish its appearance. You can keep your skin moisturized to make it look smoother, or use a self tanner. Pale skin has a more cottage cheese-like appearance than tan skin. Also, if you have money to burn, there's a treatment called endermologie.

When I first started my personal training career I worked for a narcissistic bloke who insisted his wife have at least three endermologie sessions weekly. The instrument the endermologie technician used had a suction attachment that would lift the skin. The theory was that the skin under the vacuum-like suction attachment would lift due to the suction, thus creating circulation in the area of the cellulite. By creating circulation, the skin would appear smoother. Hence, the cellulite would look as though it had disappeared. The process did eventually produce some results, but the client didn't see any effects before at least a dozen sessions. And even though it seemed the cellulite was diminishing, the treatment had to be on-going, otherwise the cottage cheese appearance would come back. And it cost $125 a pop!

A cheaper route to go is to stay well-hydrated to diminish the dimply appearance.

Also, cardio and weight training (specifically leg exercises like lunges) have long been proven to diminish the appearance of cellulite.

Dehydration

Not drinking enough water could lead to dehydration, a condition that occurs when people lose more water and salts, like potassium and sodium, than they take in. Of course, there are different severities of dehydration and our bodies have a simple defense mechanism to help prevent us from becoming completely dehydrated – it's called thirst.

Feeling thirsty is usually the first sign of dehydration, but as we age our thirst-defense mechanism diminishes so we need to be aware of other indicators.

Symptoms signaling that we need a quick swig of water might include lethargy, headaches, constipation, and dark yellow urine with a distinctive stench. If you have any of these symptoms, you might be slightly dehydrated. Try drinking a little more water.

Dehydration could lead to health problems if you don't listen to your body and replenish lost fluids. Cells could dry out and eventually malfunction if you don't consume the water your body needs to function properly. When you're sick as a dog and can barely move because every muscle in your body aches and you can't keep anything in your system, I know it can be extremely difficult to drink. But that's when you especially need water. Otherwise you could become so dehydrated that your blood pressure could drop to a point that could damage your brain, liver, and kidneys.

Feeling thirsty is usually the first sign of dehydration.

Hyponatremia

Just as severe dehydration can happen, so can hyponatremia, or water intoxication. Hyponatremia usually happens when a person's sodium level is very low ... maybe they're sweating copiously and losing both water and electrolytes, but they only replenish with water. Their sodium concentration then gets very diluted.

Sodium is an electrolyte that helps distribute water throughout the body. The lower the sodium levels are, the harder it is for water to move from the gut to the bloodstream. Actually, if our sodium levels are too low, we become dehydrated even if drinking a lot of water. This is why the symptoms of hyponatremia and dehydration are so similar even though they're completely opposite conditions.

The symptoms of hyponatremia and dehydration are quite similar even though they're completely opposite conditions.

Electrolytes are minerals in our blood and other body fluids. They're essential for our bodies to maintain proper fluid balance within cells, muscle actions, and other processes. Electrolytes like sodium, potassium, and chloride are lost when we sweat, breathe, urinate, etc., so we need to continually replace them by eating a balanced diet and drinking plenty of water.

In order for our cells to function properly, we need a constant balance between water and electrolytes in our blood. Drinking too much water can seriously dilute electrolytes, which could lead to brain swelling, putting pressure against the skull and leading to symptoms like dizziness and disorientation. This is probably how hyponatremia earned its nickname "water intoxication." A person with hyponatremia resembles someone who's drunk. If the condition goes untreated, it can result in convulsions, coma, and, in extreme cases, death.

According to the World Health Organization (WHO), the best combination of electrolytes mixed in 32 ounces of water is:
- 20g glucose
- 3.5g sodium chloride
- 2.9g trisodium citrate
- 1.5g potassium chloride

If like most people you don't happen to have a laboratory handy where you can quickly mix large batches of this combination, you could try Pedialyte, a product that, though geared more towards children, has the correct balance of sugars and electrolytes to quickly replenish fluid and electrolytes when you've been sweating a lot. Also, some say that ¼ teaspoon of sea salt for every quart of water will help your body regulate water consumption properly.

A healthy person (without kidney disease) can flush approximately 2 ½ gallons of fluids through his/her kidneys per day, so it's with difficulty that people become water intoxicated. Hyponatremia is most often associated with high endurance activities like marathons and Ironman triathlons, which take hours to complete. A recent study showed that some runners in the 2002 Boston Marathon were actually on the edge of hyponatremia. The faster these participants ran or the longer the race took to complete, the more heat their bodies created. When our bodies go above their normal temperature, we sweat (a combination of water, sodium, potassium, and chloride) to bring our temperature back to normal. Yet some runners actually drank so much water without also replacing these important electrolytes, that they were *overly* hydrated.

Healthy kidneys can flush approximately 2 ½ gallons of fluids per day.

Those of you in high school or college…

Please don't fall prey to a popular hazing ritual that has made news most notably in California. As an initiation, fraternity members forced a panel of pledges to drink 5 gallons of water within a short amount of time. Most stopped when they began to vomit, but one was so eager to be accepted that he continued to drink the water even after vomiting. He became disorientated – and eventually died from hyponatremia. Eight fraternity members in charge of the initiation were found guilty of misdemeanor hazing and four of them were also charged with felony involuntary manslaughter charges and are serving time in jail.

Tap Water versus Bottled Water

Controversies arise about the safety of both tap and bottled waters. Some believe tap water is safer than bottled water, while others believe the marketing claims of the companies who sell bottled water. But did you know that many bottled waters are actually tap waters pitched into plastic containers and sold at a premium price for the sake of convenience? There are all types of waters on the market today ... from sparkling water to bottled water to tap water, and everything in between. The cost of water can range from almost nothing to a liter costing more than a gallon of gasoline. So, which one is the best for you?

> Many bottled waters are actually tap waters pitched into plastic containers and sold at a premium price.

TAP WATER

The drinking water in the United States is known to be the cleanest in the world. But what does that really mean? Our tap water is contaminated with pesticides, parasites, heavy metals, nitrates and nitrites, along with other vile pollutants that could be hazardous to our health. To lower the level of these contaminants, a large number of poisonous chemicals, like chlorine, are added to the water to kill bacteria and other microorganisms. Chlorine is a pesticide that annihilates living cells. Have you ever noticed when you get out of the shower that your skin, especially your face, feels tight? That's the aftereffect of chlorine, killing the living skin cells on your body. A report in the *American Journal of Public Health* stated that up to two-thirds of the harmful exposure to chlorine came from skin absorption and inhalation while showering. Our bodies are like sponges, so whatever we put onto the surface eventually gets absorbed into our bloodstreams. This is why chlorinated water has been linked to heart disease, birth defects, and certain types of cancer like colon and bladder cancer.

> Chlorine is a pesticide that annihilates living cells.

The National Academy of Sciences (NAS) estimate that 200–1,000 people die in the United States each year from cancers caused by ingesting the contaminants in tap water.

METROPOLITAN WATER SUPPLIES

Tap water is regulated by the Environmental Protection Act (EPA). Metropolitan water supplies seem to be cleaner than rural water supplies, which may be subjected to fertilizers, pesticides, and soil erosion contaminating ground water supplies. In most major U.S. cities, hundreds of organic chemicals can be found in the drinking water at any time, but water utilities only test for about 75. According to a Ralph Nader report, over 2,300 chemicals that could cause cancer have been detected in U.S. tap water.

Another concern is the amount of fluoride added to tap water. Fluoride was originally added in an attempt to reduce tooth decay. However, an over-abundance of fluoride can cause osteosarcoma, a form of bone disease seen primarily in males under the age of twenty. A better attempt to promote healthy teeth would be to concentrate on the teeth themselves by brushing with fluoridated toothpaste. That way the chances of exposure for the rest of the body to this toxin would be greatly reduced. About 50% of the fluoride we swallow every time we drink tap water accumulates in bones, making them more brittle and eventually leading to fractures. This doesn't happen overnight. It takes a long period of time, but still it happens. Ethical questions also arise about whether the government has the right to put fluoride in tap water without our consent.

If you're worried about the amount of fluoride or any other contaminant in your tap water, have your water tested and buy a water filter that will correct the problem.

RURAL WATER SUPPLIES

Small town residents have to be even more cautious with their water. Major cities test their water more often than rural areas. Private wells have the same fluoride issues as large city water supplies, and sometimes even more because high levels of fluoride can occur naturally. And pollutants like E. coli, salmonella, hepatitis A, arsenic, copper, lead, mercury, radium, just to list a few, are more plentiful in rural water supplies. Rural water can also be threatened by other chemicals and pesticides that farmers use for crops. One of these pesticides is atrazine, a highly-used weed killer. Of all

christopherSASHA

Atrazine is responsible for the majority of health standard violations.

the chemical contaminants in tap water regulated by the EPA, atrazine is responsible for the majority of health standard violations. Adverse health effects of atrazine can range from heart congestion and low blood pressure to reproductive disorders and cancer.

Considering all the water available to Americans, tap water is by far the cheapest and most accessible. It can't be beat for low cost and convenience. Unfortunately, tap water often contains pesticides designed to take away life, and, when used in large amounts, can even take away human life. Healthy individuals with strong immune systems probably don't have to worry much about these contaminants. However, to be on the safe side, homes with infants, children, pregnant women, the elderly, and those with weakened immune systems might want to get their water supplies inspected for contaminants that might harm their health. If you're concerned about your tap water, ask your water company for a copy of their Annual Water Quality Report and consult a health department official or call the EPA's Safe Drinking Water Hotline (800-426-4791).

It's imperative to drink clean water. So if you're concerned about your water quality, install a water filtration system in your house. Be careful which filter you purchase because some are only designed to make the water look clearer and taste better. You'll want a filter that will take out the pollutants that could affect your health. Look for filters that meet NSF/ANSI standard 53 certified to eradicate the pollutants in your water.

Look for filters that meet NSF/ANSI standard 53 certified to eradicate the pollutants in your water.

BOTTLED WATER

There's a deluge of bottled waters on the market jostling for your business, including mineral water, sparkling water, spring water, Artesian water, distilled water, carbonated water, fluoridated water, and even vitamin water. These are just a few. The list goes on and on. Water used to just be a necessity to sustain life. Now it's the latest, most fashionable fad. Lots of people want to be socially accepted and politically correct while quenching their thirst with the hippest bottled water, so they gladly pay a premium to be "in the groove." In doing so, an estimated $60 billion a year is being forked out globally for bottled water, according to Forbes.com.

Twenty-one gallons of bottled water is consumed by each American each year.

It's crazy. We complain about the price of a gallon of gasoline, but have no problem shelling out an average of $3 for a liter of bottled water! A liter is approximately ¼ of a gallon. So our trendy water costs about $12 a gallon. What would we think if gas stations were charging $12 for a gallon of gasoline?

And what are we paying this premium for? A lot of it is just tap water. Approximately one-third of bottled water in America comes from the same supply as your kitchen sink.

Our trendy water costs about $12 a gallon.

Check the label on your bottled water. Dasani, a product of Coca-Cola, is tap water that has been filtered a few times with a final reverse osmosis process. Basically, you're paying up to ***10,000 times more for a gallon of bottled water than one that came from the same source as the water from your faucet.*** Is that absurd? If you want to make sure you're not drinking bottled tap water, look for waters labeled "natural spring water" or "mineral water." These waters cannot come from a public water supply but must instead come from a potable underground source.

To add to this absurdity, regulations for bottled water are *less* strict than for tap water. Bottled water is considered a food according to the government and, therefore, regulated by the FDA. But there's a dearth of funds for bottled water regulatory programs on both the state and federal levels. Inspections are only done annually and don't get as persnickety as inspections for tap water. If you think bottled water is safer than tap, think again. Studies have shown that a random selection of bottled waters from retailers and manufacturers still contained chlorine, fluoride, bacteria, nitrate, arsenic, and lead. Doesn't that sound tasty? The fact of the matter is, bottled waters don't have to be 100% contaminant-free. Even though you're paying a premium for bottled water, there is no law stating that it has to be safer than tap.

So far, we've only been concerned about the safety of the water itself, but what about the plastic bottles containing the water? Many companies recycle the plastic bottles. But how diligent do you think they are when it comes to sanitizing them? And let's not forget the chemicals used to produce the

It can take up to 1,000 years for a buried plastic bottle to biodegrade in a landfill.

bottles in the first place. Chemicals like vinyl chloride, which is a carcinogenic compound, are used to hold the water until the consumer drinks it. Frequently, people will also refill their bottles and often without cleaning them first, so the bottles can become contaminated with mold. Another obvious problem is that plastic bottles are not environmentally friendly. It can take up to 1,000 years for a buried plastic bottle to biodegrade in a landfill.

If you're going to buy bottled water, here are some tips to remember:

- Look for waters that have some type of ozonation, carbonation, or disinfection process (ozone or ultraviolet disinfection) that will eliminate harmful bacteria.
- Buy waters that were bottled at the source.
- Look for the NSF Mark on the label or contact the NSF Consumer Affairs Office (877-867-3435). The NSF Mark assures you that the product has been tested by one of the most respected independent certification companies in existence today – NSF International.
- Refrigerate immediately after purchasing bottles of water because bacteria form at room temperature after prolonged periods of time. Think about how long those bottles of water might have been sitting in inventory and on the store shelf before you bought them.

Whether you drink tap or bottled water, play it safe by getting the most contaminant-free available. Bottled water isn't cheap and it hasn't been scientifically proven to be any cleaner or safer than tap water. If you choose to gulp down bottled water, try spring or mineral water. However, tap water is just as good if you do your homework by getting a list of possible pollutants and following up with the purchase of a water filtration system that removes those contaminants.

Changing our beliefs about the foods we eat is only part of *transforming your lifestyle*. We also need to change our beliefs about physical activity. Aside from poor

Bottled water isn't cheap and it hasn't been scientifically proven to be any cleaner or safer than tap water.

nutritional habits, our obesity epidemic is also due partly to our modern lifestyle – conveniences like automobiles and computers. Years ago, people walked to work. They worked in the fields or engaged in physical labor in manufacturing plants. Since America has entered into more of a service age, few of us perform manual labor. Most of us have become more sedentary. But our bodies are designed to move! So let's move on to the core of our bodies, where almost every movement we make originates: *our abdominal muscles*.

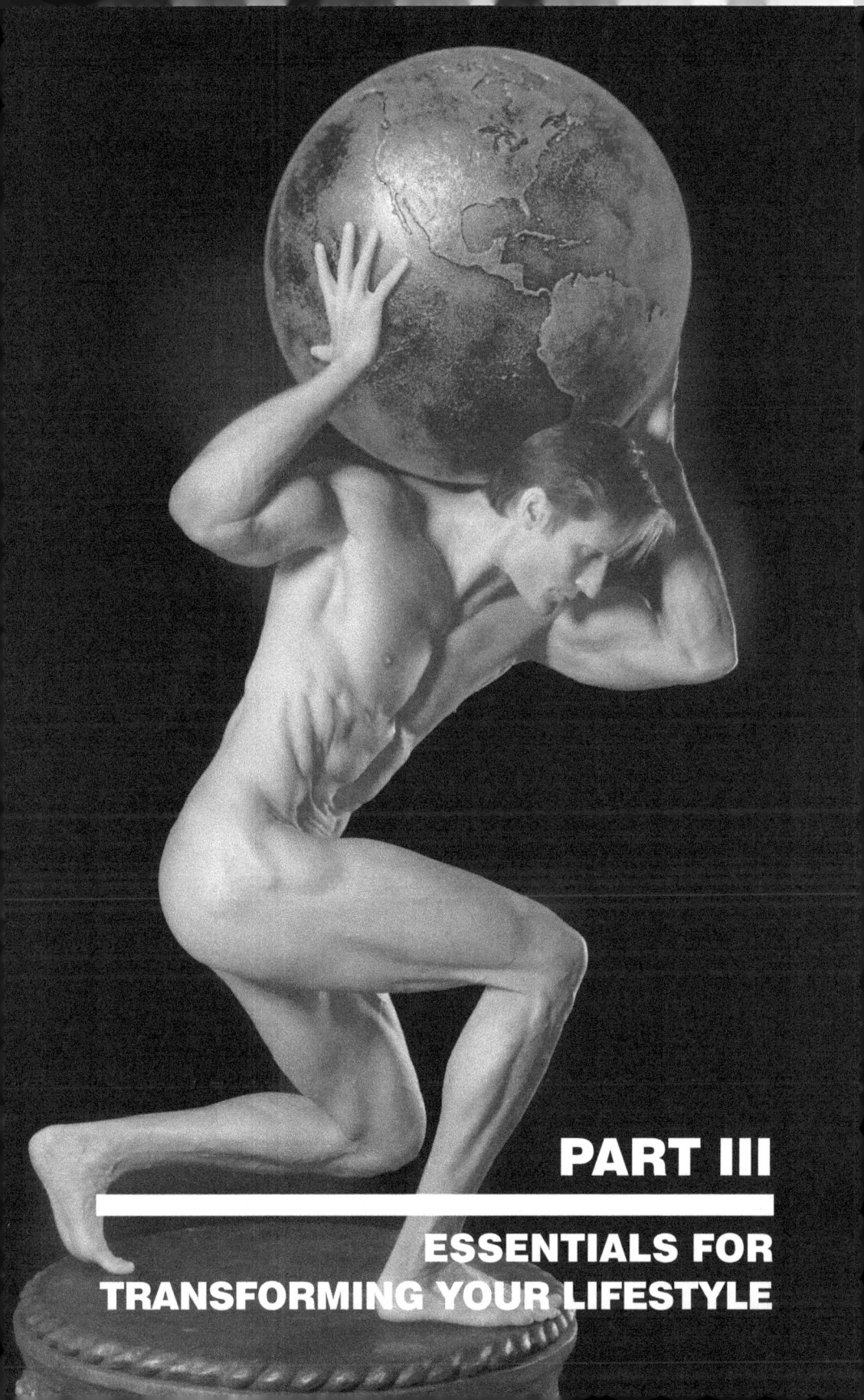

PART III

ESSENTIALS FOR TRANSFORMING YOUR LIFESTYLE

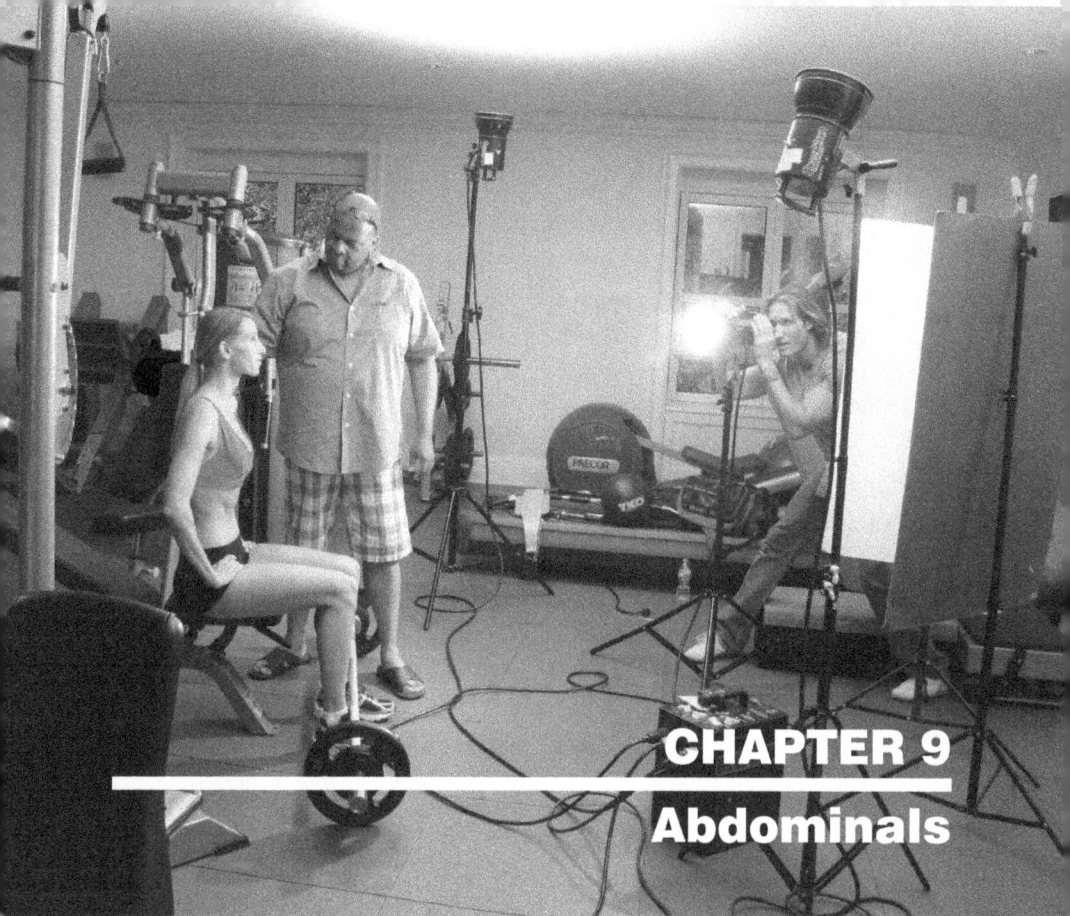

CHAPTER 9
Abdominals

Plenty of gym-goers have impressive arms, chests, backs, shoulders, and legs, but few have the discipline to achieve perfection in what can be the most impressive muscle group ... the abdominals. I believe it's the midsection, and not the biceps or chest, that tells the story of one's overall health. Generally speaking, a well-defined set of abs proclaims to the world, "I am healthy and in smashing shape!" On the flip side, if you're a little soft in the midsection, chances are you're a little soft everywhere, which could become a health problem later in life.

The abdominal muscles are probably the most controversial muscle group of our anatomy. Everyone has a different theory as to what works the best for creating an awe-inspiring midsection. Does there exist a single theory that's best for everyone? Or does a person have to discover what's best for him or her individually? You may find that one person's approach to ab training works well for you while another person's doesn't work at all. We all have different anatomy blueprints bequeathed by our parents, which were handed down from their parents, and so on and so on. It would be impossible, therefore, for a cookie-cutter ab training program to work 100% effectively for all of us.

christopherSASHA

Health Benefits

There are a multitude of health benefits we may obtain through general exercise, but additional benefits can be derived by directly targeting our midsections. General exercise can help prevent many chronic illnesses, like heart disease, stroke, high cholesterol, type 2 diabetes, osteoporosis, and hypertension. Exercise has also been shown to reduce mental stress and strengthen the heart muscle, improving oxygen delivery and resulting in a lower heart rate. But exercises for the abdominal region specifically further these benefits. Strong stomach muscles help stabilize the pelvis in its neutral position (a slight forward tilt). They promote alignment for proper posture, while weaker abs allow the pelvis to tilt backward, putting pressure on the lower back and leading to chronic back aches.

Most exercisers don't realize the countless functions of our abdominals. They focus on aesthetic rewards like confidence in their physiques and attracting objects of their affection. I'm all for any type of motivation. If thoughts like these get you to exercise, then go for it!

Weak abs allow the pelvis to tilt backward, putting pressure on the lower back and leading to chronic back aches.

But let's look beyond vanity to get a better understanding of why abdominal training is so valuable. Your stomach muscles have more influence than any other muscle group in your body because they're involved in almost every movement you make. In fact, even when you're doing nothing but standing, they help stabilize your body. They're the cornerstone of power and strength. Everyone has abdominals. Most people can't see them because they're hidden under a layer of fat. Many people work their midsections to extremes but can't find one ripple to reward their efforts because they have too much body fat. The sad truth is that fat doesn't flex, no matter how much you squeeze and twist your body.

The stomach muscle group (core) is responsible for promoting intra-abdominal pressure to help stabilize your spine and help

- alleviate lower back pain,
- internal organs to function properly,
- prevent injuries,
- assist in sports performance,
- maintain body posture, keeping the back straight.

If these aren't good enough reasons to include abdominal training a few times every week, then defer to the aesthetic results you can achieve by incorporating an ab regimen to your weekly routine. My point is to use whatever strategy works for you. Just be sure to include exercise as a part of your lifestyle. You'll create a happier, healthier you.

Abdominal Anatomy

Let's discuss the structure of the midsection and explain the importance of how it's used by our bodies to perform everyday activities. I focus on the main 5 muscles in the midsection (rectus abdominis, internal and external obliques, transverse abdominis, and erector spinae) to enhance support in this area and, of course, to sculpt the *transforming your lifestyle* physique.

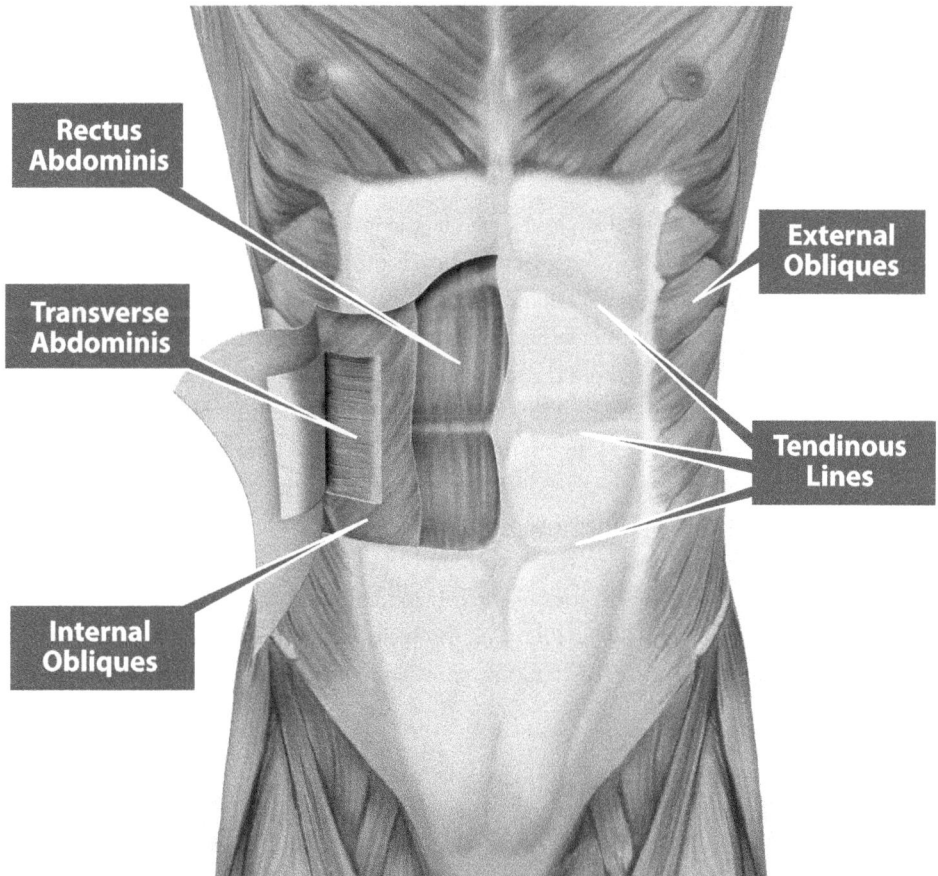

RECTUS ABDOMINIS

The king of all abdominal muscles is the *rectus abdominis*, commonly known as the "six-pack." But did you know that we actually have an "eight-pack?" Very few of us (myself included) will ever be able to see the last row of the rectus abdominis. It just isn't in our genetic blueprint because the bottom tendinous line isn't wide enough to separate the lower section of the rectus abdominis.

The rectus abdominis is a single muscle divided by 1 vertical and 3 horizontal fibrous bands called tendinous lines. When the rectus abdominis is developed and defined, it protrudes between these lines and it looks like bubble wrap. It attaches your pelvic girdle to the lower part of your sternum (xiphoid process), enabling your torso to bend forward. This assists in proper posture by stabilizing the pelvis in a neutral position. The primary function of the rectus abdominis is to enable our hips to bend forward (lower region) and our torso to bend forward (upper region) – technically called spinal flexion.

> The rectus abdominis, (commonly called the "six-pack") is actually one muscle.

EXTERNAL & INTERNAL OBLIQUES

External and internal obliques are deeper muscles located at either side of the rectus abdominis. They crisscross each other. The *external obliques* run diagonally downward (in a V-shape) from the side of the ribcage to the front part of the rectus abdominis while the *internal obliques* run diagonally upward (in an inverted V-shape) from the side of the hip to the lower front part of the ribcage. They work in conjunction with the opposite side, meaning that when the internal oblique is working on one side, the external oblique is working on the opposite side to help perform the same function. For example, to perform a twisting crunch (explained on page 220), your left elbow must come up and cross over your body to reach your right knee. Your *left* external oblique contracts and works with your *right* internal oblique to perform this one maneuver. These muscles enable your body to rotate the torso, bend from side to side, assist the rectus abdominis in spinal flexion, and help stabilize the pelvis.

TRANSVERSE ABDOMINIS

The *transverse abdominis* is the deepest of the major abdominal muscles and the most overlooked. These muscle fibers run horizontally and wrap around our abdominal wall to hold all of our internal organs in place, very much like a girdle. It's the primary muscle used to force air from our lungs when we cough, sneeze, and lift heavy things – like weights. Most importantly for women, this is the main muscle used in labor and delivery.

The more you condition and tighten your transverse abdominis, the smaller your waistline will appear because it will compress all your internal organs into a smaller space.

ERECTOR SPINAE

Finally, the *erector spinae* completes the "core" circle by encasing the rear of the midsection. The erector spinae consists of 3 different muscles (iliocostalis, spinalis, longissimus) that extend from the pelvis to the back of the skull. It's this group of muscles that allows our spine to extend and gives major support to the spinal column to keep it erect. Muscle groups have other muscle groups that counteract or resist each other. For instance, our tricep muscle group counteracts our bicep muscle group (and vice-versa), our upper back muscles counteract our chest muscles (and vice-versa), and our erector spinae are the antagonistic muscles to our abdominal muscles (and vice-versa).

Erector Spinae Muscles

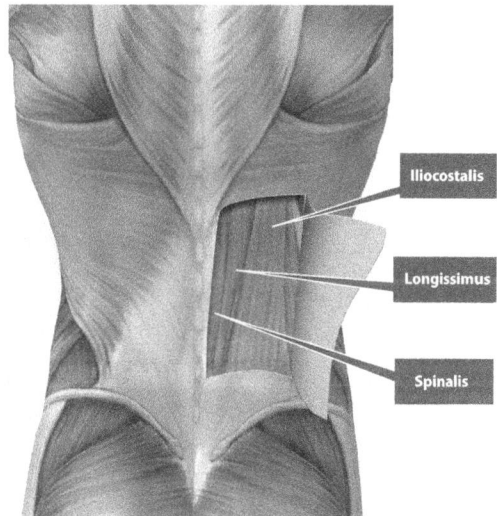

Iliocostalis

Longissimus

Spinalis

Antagonistic muscles pull against the prime movers to slow them down. This is imperative in preventing joints from hyperextension (extending beyond the joint's normal range), maintaining balance between opposing muscle groups, and keeping your joints aligned for proper posture. For example, while doing bicep curls (agonist muscles or prime movers), your triceps (antagonist muscles) slow the movement down and stop your elbow joint from going beyond its normal range of motion. Without your erector spinae, your torso would flop forward and down to the floor instead of standing upright and perpendicular to the floor.

Genetics

If your primary goal is to sculpt your body to become a top fitness model, I believe this is the most important part of the book for you. Read and reread this section to remind yourself that there are some things in life that are simply beyond one's control. Everyone has a genetic code predetermining what our muscles will look like once developed. Some people will have a thick, rippling, defined eight-pack abdomen. Others will create a flat, smooth muscular surface, and still others will be somewhere in-between. No matter how hard you train your abs or perform cardio, and no matter how diligent you are with your diet, *you cannot change the shape of your muscles*.

I found this out the hard way. I spent a year focused on trying to develop a set of rock hard abs. I wanted to be able to hide my fingertips between abdominal rows. I wanted abs that would make Arnold Schwarzenegger envious. I was obsessed with my goal – only to be disappointed despite all my determination and sacrifices. At the time, I thought I had failed. For an entire year, I kept an impeccably clean diet, I trained my abs every other day (unless they were still sore from the previous ab workout), I did cardio twice a day, alternating my intensity levels, and I used diuretics often. In the end, I was down to 3.9% body fat and armed with an extremely strong midsection. But in no way did I have the set of abs I thought would inspire people.

In the end, it's genetics that determines the shape and appearance of your muscles.

I couldn't understand why I didn't produce the stomach muscles of my dreams. I did everything I was supposed to do. Delving into more research about muscle composition and physique sculpting, I experimented with many different theories, spawning countless trial and error techniques. It took me over 6 years to realize that in the end, it's genetics that determines the shape and appearance of your muscles.

Fast- and Slow-Twitch Muscle Fibers

The size and shape of muscles are determined by factors like types of muscle fibers (fast-twitch versus slow-twitch), the amount of muscle fibers within each muscle cell, how your nervous system relates to recruiting fibers to move resistance, the shape of the muscle belly, and cell volume capacity.

Every muscle in your body has varying amounts of fast-twitch and slow-twitch muscle fibers. Technically speaking, muscles have two categories of fast-twitch fibers and only one category of slow-twitch fibers. However, we'll generalize muscle fibers as only fast-twitch and slow-twitch.

Fast-twitch muscle fibers are power muscle fibers that are activated when intense force is needed, such as when lifting heavy objects, both in and out of the gym. They have less blood flow, which means less oxygen delivery, so they fatigue quickly and are slow to recover. Therefore, they're not designed for endurance but rather for quick, powerful contractions for a short period of time. Slow-twitch muscle fibers, on the other hand, are designed for endurance. They fatigue slowly because they have more blood flow and oxygen delivery to remove more waste by-products from the muscle. They aren't designed for mass, but rather to give muscle fibers the energy to contract for long periods of time.

> Fast-twitch muscle fibers are power muscle fibers when force is needed.

So which muscle fiber is better to have? Both. We need both fast-twitch and slow-twitch muscle fibers for our bodies to function properly. Some muscles, like the heart and abdomen, contract every second of every day. If we didn't have slow-twitch muscle fibers, the muscles wouldn't be able to perform their necessary jobs. We all know why the heart has to perpetually contract, but did you know that our stomach muscles are continuously contracting as well? Slow-twitch muscle fibers stabilize our bodies, keeping us from collapsing due to the force of gravity.

> Slow-twitch muscle fibers are designed for endurance.

In a world concerned with vanity, we would love to have mainly fast-twitch muscle fibers in our abdominal region so that we would all have perfect six-packs. But slow-twitch muscle fibers are vital for all-day movement. How much fun would it be to develop a set of washboard abs if you had to lie down every minute because your muscles couldn't hold your body up?

Resistance training forces your nervous system to recruit muscle fibers (both slow-twitch and fast-twitch) to handle extra weight. The heavier the weight, the more fast-twitch muscle fibers are recruited. It's important to know that your nervous system always recruits *both* types of muscle fibers in *all* activities. At the beginning of the movement, slow-twitch muscle fibers are mostly used but if the movement requires more force than the slow-twitch muscle fibers are capable of handling, then they ease off while the fast-twitch muscle fibers carry more of the responsibility. Most people think that muscle size and strength develops only when they perform very low repetitions with heavy weight. True, muscles will get stronger because muscles learn to adapt to heavier weight by recruiting more muscle fibers, but they will not necessarily get bigger.

In order for the muscle to get bigger, it has to be strained for long periods of time, and the time it takes to perform 4 repetitions isn't enough for all muscle fibers to play in the game. Also, contractile proteins in muscle cells need enough tension for a longer period of time in order to be demolished. This is the point where you actually cause tiny micro-tears in your muscle fibers. Only then will they repair themselves by making fibers stronger and thicker, resulting in an increase in size.

Periodization

Our muscles react differently with varying amounts of weight, repetitions, and rest periods. There are a multitude of abdominal routines on the market today – each promising to deliver a Greek-god midsection. One program that's been around for centuries is called "periodization." Although a type of periodization was used by ancient Greeks readying for the Olympic games, modern day periodization was reinvented in the 1960s by Leo Matveyev, a Russian physiologist. Alas, a new training method was born, only to be modified again and again, tailored to strength training and power athletes. Periodization doesn't allow the exerciser to do the same exercises with the same amount of weights and number of reps every time. These variables are constantly changing so the body doesn't have much time to adapt, which results in a stronger body.

Humans are creatures of habit, and exercise is no different than any other activity in our lives. Most people who work out find a routine they like and stick with it… indefinitely. The problem is that your body will quickly adapt to this routine, so you plateau until you change the routine and shock your body again. I see people do the same routine every time they come to the gym. They do 1 set of 10 repetitions of squats, leg curls, chest press, lat pulldowns, bicep curls, and tricep extensions, with the same weight, every single time. Then they wonder why they're bored and not making any progress. This is where periodization steps in to do wonders for you, both physically and psychologically.

Periodization is a training program designed to target both types of muscle fibers by utilizing varying amounts of weight (intensity), which dictates the number of repetitions and rest periods (volume), based on your *personal* 1-repetition maximum lift. These programs can vary from extremely complex to extremely simplistic. I like to play it safe by staying somewhere in the middle.

OVERTRAINING

Periodization also advocates the importance of rest because that's actually when our muscles grow. Many exercisers erroneously think their muscles grow while they strain to lift the weight. Just the opposite is true.

Protein synthesis is a bodily function that breaks proteins into amino acids, then reforms them into proteins your body can utilize for repairing tissue, including muscle tissue. When muscles are recovering (resting), protein synthesis nearly doubles, slowly creating a bigger and stronger you. Bodies require rest to properly perform protein synthesis.

> Protein synthesis nearly doubles when our muscles are resting, which slowly creates a stronger you.

Like other muscle groups in your body, your abs demand time between workouts to recover and rebuild. But unlike many other muscle groups, your abdominals contain a high percentage of slow-twitch muscle fibers, enabling them to recover more quickly than other muscle groups. I suggest taking a day or two off between ab workouts to fully recover. After a day or two, if you still feel a tightness or soreness in your midsection when you cough, laugh, get out of bed, or stretch, then your body is telling you that the muscles haven't quite yet recovered.

Always listen to your body!

If you exercise your abs before they completely recover, you'll be thwarting your efforts by overtraining. You'll not be giving your abs the time

After a day or two, if you still feel a soreness in your muscles, your body is telling you that your muscles haven't recovered.

needed to fully repair. Overtraining actually does more harm than good because you'll be lifting the same amount of weight every day without benefiting your physical development. Or, worse, you'll lift less than you did a few days before. After all, to build bigger muscles you need to tax muscles to recruit more fast-twitch muscle fibers, and that can't happen if your resistance is less than it was the day before.

If you regularly experience muscle soreness, fatigue, injuries due to training, and/or reduced concentration, odds are that you're overtraining. Train hard, but train smart.

Periodization forces you to take time off. Whether it's active or passive recovery, your body needs rest to heal and rebuild. The weeks you rest will ensure you're not overtraining your muscles and will help prevent injuries.

THREE PERIODIZATION PHASES

The periodization method is always broken into cycles. Sometimes it's broken into cycles that last up to 4 years, like the Olympic cycle. To keep things simple, I will demonstrate the phases using my 6-month workout regimen.

There are 3 different phases involved in periodization: macrocycles, mesocycles, and microcycles.

Macrocycles are the largest period of time. In our case, the macrocycle will last 6 months, although it could last only a couple of months, or up to 4 years. Next is mesocycles. I keep them at 5 weeks myself, but you can do 3, 4, or 6-week periods if you want. The mesocycles, when combined, contribute to making up the macrocycle.

In each mesocycle phase, I focus on 1 particular goal in my training. For example, 1 mesocycle may be about increasing the size of my muscles. Another mesocycle might be about increasing strength. The next about power, and so on.

Finally, the microcycle is the shortest phase, lasting only 7 days. In the microcycle, I do 1 week of recovery. This is the time I give all the muscles in my body a break from resistance training and I concentrate on cardio training. Every other day I do some form of cardio with no exercise (passive recovery) in between those days.

This is also a time I need, psychologically, to prepare for the following week when I ease my way into the next mesocycle. After my 1 week of recovery, I get back into the swing of things by leisurely working on exercises for my next mesocycle. For instance, if the next mesocycle targets muscle size, I begin doing exercises that I will be doing for the next 5 weeks, but I begin in a gradual manner. If I complete only 2 sets of 15 repetitions for each exercise, that's okay. If I only complete 4 of the 6 exercises, that's okay, too. It's okay because my only objective is to get my muscles ready for the "real" work when I hit them hard for the next few weeks.

When this mesocycle is complete, I take another week off to recover. The following week, I ease my way back into the next mesocycle. These phases continue until I have completed all of my mesocycles – hence my one 6-month macrocycle.

Detailed Ab Periodization Program

Here's a detailed 6-month periodization program I am currently doing. Periodization can be used in the same manner for all muscle groups but, for the sake of simplicity, I will only detail my abdominal routine. *These mesocycles should be performed in the order I have them.* This way we progressively build the strength of our muscles and lower our risk of strained and pulled muscles. Remember….train hard, but train smart!

MESOCYCLE I (ENDURANCE)

The first mesocycle is based on *building endurance*, which means I do no weight and an extremely high amount of repetitions. Let's define a repetition: one full-range movement of a particular exercise. For example, one repetition for a traditional crunch is when you're lying on the floor and bend your torso upward as high as you can go then back down to your starting position. For this phase, I pick 1 exercise for each section of my abs – rectus abdominis (upper region), rectus abdominis (lower region), and internal and external obliques, and 1 exercise for my erector spinae (lower back).

> Always start with a number of repetitions you can perform in excellent form.

I begin with 4 sets of 60 repetitions of supported crunches (page 229), with 15-second breaks between each set. A word of caution: always start with a number of repetitions you can perform in excellent form. There's no point of doing 60 repetitions in lousy form because you'll risk injuring yourself. Play it safe by starting with 20 repetitions (or even 10 repetitions) in perfect form for each set and work your way up. Remember … train hard, but train smart.

After my fourth set of supported crunches, I take a 90-second break and then move on to flat bench knee bends (page 214). Again, I'll do 4 sets of 60 repetitions with 30-second breaks between each set. I take longer rest periods between these sets because it takes longer for my abs to recover from this particular exercise. After I complete all 4 sets, I take another 90-second break before I start my oblique exercise. For my obliques, I do twisting crunches (page 220). I don't take any breaks between these sets. I go from one side to the other until I wrap up all 4 sets of 60 repetitions. After a 90-second breather, I do only 2 sets of Good Mornings (page 241) for my erector spinae, lower back. I only do 15 repetitions per set with 60 seconds of rest between sets. Personally, I find that any more than this amount strains my erector spinae for days.

You don't have to do the same exercises that I do. You may choose to go to page 210 and pick 1 "beginner" exercise from each of the abdominal categories – lower rectus abdominis, obliques, and upper rectus abdominis. Then choose 1 of the erector spinae exercises to keep your midsection aligned. Again, I do 60 reps because I've been doing these exercises for years. You can do as few reps as you need to maintain proper form. Try starting with 10 reps per exercise and build from there.

Don't be surprised if it takes 30 minutes to complete this abdominal routine. I do this routine 3 times per week for 5 weeks (mesocycle I). Then I take 1 week off, not doing any type of direct ab exercise. During this time I also omit any form of resistance training, but I do 45-minute cardio sessions every other day. I vary my cardio – kickboxing, hitting the heavy bag, bike riding, power walking at my neighborhood park. The cardio helps my body recover quickly by delivering oxygen and nutrients to rebuild the muscle fibers I destroyed while working out.

Cardio helps the body recover quickly.

MESOCYCLE II (STRENGTH)

After my first recovery week, I ease my way into the second mesocycle, which focuses on *strength*. I select 3 ab exercises to target each region of my abs. This time I choose hanging straight leg raises (lower abs), lying side crunches (obliques), and weighted Swiss ball crunches (upper abs). I use light weights for the first week to get my abs ready for the following 4 weeks of heavier weights.

The second week of this mesocycle includes a 2 ½-pound dumbbell between my feet for my hanging straight leg raises (page 213). Each week I try to increase the weight a little more. I do 3 sets of 10 repetitions for this exercise with 60-second breaks between. Then I do very little weight for my lying side crunches (page 223). My preference is a tapered look (V-shape) so that my shoulders are wide and lead to a svelte waistline. Adding heavy weights to oblique exercises creates a blocky waistline. Therefore, I opt for no more than 10 pounds additional weight when training my obliques. *A final caveat when training your obliques:* use extreme caution while working these muscles because most lumbar (lower back) strains occur during these types of exercises. I stick to 3 sets of 15 repetitions for my lying side crunches, with no breaks between.

> Take extreme caution while working your oblique muscles.

I finalize my ab workout by doing 10 repetitions of weighted Swiss ball crunches (page 231). This is a hard exercise because balance plays a huge factor, which recruits more core muscles to be activated to stay atop the ball. Again, I do very light weights the first week to allow my muscles to adapt to the movement for the upcoming weeks as I consistently increase the weight.

While I have the Swiss ball at my side, I end my ab workout with Swiss ball prone leg lifts (page 240) for 2 sets of 15 repetitions. I do this routine 2-3 times per week for 5 weeks (mesocycle II). Then I take 1 week off from doing any type of direct ab exercises. By this time, I'm ready for a break! I take a week off from the gym to put it in neutral and recharge my batteries. I don't do any type of exercise, including cardio; it's called passive recovery. I want to give my body a break from all physical stress so it can recuperate. Then it's time to hit the gym with the next mesocycle.

MESOCYCLE III (POWER)

The third mesocycle is based on *creating power* which will help your body get used to activating its fast-twitch muscle fibers immediately. This phase of our periodization requires that we anchor one end of our body in order to push our muscles to the max. The only way to make our muscles work their

> The only way to make our muscles work their hardest is to anchor the opposing side.

hardest is to anchor the opposing side. For example, you'll work your biceps harder (leading to bigger and stronger biceps) if you utilize a preacher curl bench as opposed to standing bicep curls. The same holds true for abs. You'll be able to work your upper rectus abdominis harder if you do ab crunches with your feet anchored under a support bar than if you were to do the same exercise without your feet anchored under a support bar. Give it a try and you'll quickly notice how much more weight you can crunch with your feet anchored.

This mesocycle is all about maximum weight. Complete control the entire

> Complete control the entire time during these exercises is paramount.

time during these exercises is paramount. Again, train hard, but train smart. Initially use light weights the first week of any new mesocycle so that muscles get adjusted to the exercises they'll be executing for the next few weeks.

As always, when training the midsection, I choose 1 exercise for each of the 5 main areas – the lower rectus abdominis, internal and external obliques, upper rectus abdominis, and erector spinae. The first week of this mesocycle will be like every other first week of a new mesocycle. Use light weights for each of the exercises. This time I select high cross-cable reverse crunches (lower abs), bicycles (internal and external obliques), touch 'n go weighted crunches (upper abs), and Roman chair back extensions (erector spinae). I only do 3 sets of 4-6 repetitions for every exercise, except bicycles. Again, I use light weights, if any, for my oblique exercises because I don't want the blocky look.

I usually begin my ab workouts with lower abs because they're the section I see results in most slowly. I hit them first while I'm fresh, when my abs are raring to go. I use a flat bench and tightly secure a set of handles to my ankles so I can crank up the weight in a controlled manner. My first set is relatively light to get acclimated to the movement, but then I push myself. I cannot stress enough how important it is to be in complete control during the entire *power phase* of the periodization cycle. This is the mesocycle in which overly ambitious gym-goers most frequently get hurt. Please don't be one of them! Your efforts will be thwarted if you have to take time off because you tried pulling more weight than your body was ready for. Slow and steady always wins the race. This mesocycle requires more rest time between sets so I allow myself 3 minutes between sets. This gives my muscles time to produce more ATP (Adenosine Triphosphate), which will give them the energy to keep me going with heavy weights.

After 3 sets of lower abs, I give myself only 90 seconds before I hit my obliques. I use a 5-pound plate behind my head and do 30 bicycles on each side, 60 total twists per set. I take a 60-second break between each set until I have done all 3 sets. I don't need as long of a break between these sets. Again, I take a 90-second break before I hit my upper abs with touch 'n go weighted crunches. I place a weighted bar on the floor and anchor my feet under it allowing me to pull more weight. The first set is always the test run, with a fair amount of weight to get a feeling of where I should focus my muscle contraction. A muscle contraction is the physiological tension put on muscle fibers when they either lengthen or shorten. I then rest 3 minutes between each set, concluding my ab work. I go right into my erector spinae with Roman chair back extensions. I hold a 25-pound plate across my chest for the first set, rest, then use 35 pounds for the following set, with 3 minutes between each set.

The 5-week power mesocycle is a grueling phase of periodization. When this mesocycle is complete, you'll be ready for a week of active recovery. Have fun by playing your favorite sports. By now you should notice that your performance is better. You'll have more power in your movements and less injuries, if any. After a week off from resistance training, you'll be ready to complete the final phase of my 6-month periodization program.

MESOCYCLE IV (NEGATIVES)

The fourth, and final, mesocycle consists of *negative resistance training*. There are 3 types of contractions to build muscle strength and size – isometric contractions, concentric contractions, and eccentric contractions. Isometric contractions occur when muscles are activated in a position that doesn't allow the muscle to either shorten or lengthen. As an example, imagine you're on your last repetition of preacher curls and you get stuck in the middle. The weight wants to bring your arms down and you want to bring your arms up, so there's no movement. Your muscles are now at a fixed length; the weight pulling downward equals the force of you pulling the weight upward. At this point, your biceps are isometrically contracted.

> 3 types of contractions: isometric, concentric, and eccentric.

The most common muscle contraction is known as the concentric contraction, which is when the muscle shortens. Using the preacher curl example again, the concentric contraction occurs when you bring the weight up toward your chest. As you bring the weight up, your bicep muscles get shorter. The eccentric (negative) contraction occurs when you're fighting to keep the weight up but the weight is heavier than the force your muscles are able to generate to keep it up. As you relentlessly labor to keep the weight up, the weight slowly goes downward, which lengthens your bicep muscles.

The main reason I include negative resistance training in my periodization programs is because muscles can handle more weight eccentrically than they can concentrically – leading to an increase in strength.

Like the other 3 mesocycles, I choose 1 exercise for each component of the midsection. This time I'll do reverse crunches (lower abs), Roman chair side crunches (internal/external obliques), rope crunches (upper abs), and Good Mornings (erector spinae). I'm not as concerned about concentric contractions during this mesocycle but I'm careful to maintain proper form. The eccentric contraction is where my focus remains for the next 5 weeks. This means I focus on slowly returning to my starting position of each exercise. I do the fourth mesocycle differently than the prior 3 mesocycles by breaking each week into varying amounts of repetitions.

The first week consists of 10 reps of the same amount of weight for each of the 3 sets of each individual exercise. The second week includes 10 reps for the first set of each individual exercise, then drops to 8 reps with a heavier weight for the second set of each individual exercise. Then it drops again to 6 reps with an even heavier weight for the final set of each individual exercise. Week 3 involves 4-6 reps of the same amount of weight for each of the 3 sets of each individual exercise. Week 4 follows week 2 (10 reps, 8 reps, 6 reps), and the fifth, and final, week mimics the first week with 10 reps of the same amount of weight for each of the 3 sets of each individual exercise.

I want to remind you that I use only my body weight for the vast majority of oblique exercises. If I don't exhaust my obliques, I'll go up to a maximum of 10 pounds extra weight. That's it. No more than 10 pounds, because I don't want a blocky midsection.

When I complete the fourth and final mesocycle, which completes my 6-month macrocycle, I take 2 weeks recovery before starting the next 6-month macrocycle. The first week is passive recovery time in which I usually go on vacation somewhere and forget about exercise. Exercising is a lifestyle for me and after doing it for more than 20 years, I feel completely comfortable taking time off from the gym because I know I'll be eager to get back to my workouts before my 2 weeks of recovery come to an end.

However, for the fledgling exerciser, this rest period may be a curse. I know how easy it is to fall out of a workout routine. I did it myself when I first embarked on my health management regime. I only meant to take a couple weeks off from the gym to settle into a new house. After the second week off from my workouts, I told myself that I'd go back the following week, and then it was the week after that, and then the week after that. I was still telling myself I was going to get back to the gym the next week almost a year later. Please don't make the same mistake. The longer you put it off, the harder it is to get back into the habit of making your health a priority – *in other words, making YOU a priority!*

After my week of leisure, I take another week for recovery. This is an active recovery week. I start cardio every other day. I'll mix things up by doing traditional cardio (treadmill, elliptical, bike) with some kickboxing and other sports I enjoy. This is the week that gets my body ready to launch the next 6-month macrocycle. If you kept a daily log of the amount of weights and repetitions you did during the entire preceding macrocycle, you should notice that your lifts and repetitions have increased for the current macrocycle.

> I know how easy it is to fall out of a workout routine and put it on the backburner.

For example, let's say that 6 months ago, during the first mesocycle, you performed 10 crunches, 10 knee bends, and 10 twisting crunches. Now, 6 months later, you're performing 25 crunches, 25 knee bends, and 25 twisting crunches during your first mesocycle. This means that you're stronger than you were 6 months ago. You have more muscle and a higher metabolism so your body will utilize more calories to feed the extra muscle and store less as body fat.

No one said that you have to do the same exercises for each macrocycle, so feel free to mix it up. The point is to make your workouts as diverse as you want because if you get bored with your workouts, you'll have trouble sticking with the program. Personally, I do 2 consecutive macrocycles of the same exercises so I can validate my progress. If I get bored with the same exercises, I'll pick different ones and start a whole new competition with myself. As research continues in the fitness arena, new exercises will be introduced, leading to more options you can implement with the periodization method.

Now that we've broken down my ab regimen, it should be clear why a 6-minute ab routine won't give you a *transforming your lifestyle* midsection! Awe-inspiring abs require 3 crucial elements: midsection exercises, cardio, and diet, with diet being the greatest factor. In fact, a wise rule to follow for great abs is the 80/20 ratio. Spend 80% of your time fine-tuning your diet and 20% of your time torturing your abs.

80% diet, 20% exercise.

Remember …you could have the most impressive abs but no one will know if there's a layer of fat hiding them.

Focus and Form

Exercise requires focus. It isn't about going through the motions while thinking about your shopping list or what's on your weekend itinerary. In my experience, lack of concentration provides an environment for getting hurt. A pulled muscle, a pinched nerve, a torn muscle are some of the accidents I've seen people incur while not focusing on what they were doing while exercising. Slow down. Connect your mind with the muscles you're contracting and exercise complete control over every inch of every movement.

Connect your mind with the muscles you're contracting.

At the full exertion of each repetition, squeeze the muscle as hard as possible. If I'm distracted by my environment while working out, I close my eyes and concentrate on whatever muscle I'm working at the time. It really works. Give it a try.

Focus isn't the only important factor; form is also a must. I could go through proper form for each of the hundreds of exercises I put my clients through but the *transforming your lifestyle* focus is primarily about the core muscles. I believe the midsection is the foundation of our strength and power. Almost every movement originates from our abs, so let's focus on proper form.

- First, each repetition should have a 3-5 count exertion, 2 count hold and 3-5 count release (8-12 count pace) depending on the range of motion.
- Second, force the air out of your lungs while exerting and holding the movement. When I work my midsection, it's almost as if I'm trying to whistle during the exertion and holding phases.
- Third, your chin should be aligned with your sternum (your breastbone in the middle of your chest). It should always be about a fist's distance from your chest to help keep your neck in neutral position and avoid strain in the neck.
- Finally, any time you're doing an ab exercise requiring your back to be against something (floor, bench, Swiss ball), focus on pressing the small of your back against that object while performing the exercise. This will help avoid straining your back by putting the resistance on your abs, not your lower back.

There you have it. Now let's have some fun and get on the road toward a *transforming your lifestyle* physique!

Abdominal Exercises

The chart on page 210 are the core exercises I've counted on for the past 20 years to keep my *transforming your lifestyle* body. I've broken the exercises into "beginner," "moderate," and "advanced" levels to help distinguish which exercises may be best suited for your particular fitness level. Remember that proper form is imperative. A good rule of thumb is that if your form isn't up to par, choose a lower level until you maintain proper form for each repetition throughout the entire ab routine.

LOWER RECTUS ABDOMINIS	OBLIQUES	UPPER RECTUS ABDOMINIS	ERECTOR SPINAE
BEGINNER	BEGINNER	BEGINNER	BEGINNER
1. Lying Leg Raises (p.211)	1. Twisting Crunch (p. 220)	1. Supported Crunch (p. 229)	1. Supermans (p. 238)
2. Knee Bends (p. 214)	2. Lying Side Crunch (p. 223)	2. Supine Weighted Crunch (p. 232)	
3. Reverse Crunch (p. 217)	3. Seated Upper Body Rotations (p. 226)	3. Jackknife Crunch (p. 235)	
MODERATE	MODERATE	MODERATE	MODERATE
1. Captain's Chair Straight Leg Raises (p. 212)	1. Bicycles (p. 221)	1. Cross-Cable Crunch (p. 230)	1. Roman Chair Back Extensions (p. 239)
2. Running Man (p. 215)	2. Roman Chair Side Crunch (p. 224)	2. Touch 'N Go Weighted Crunch (p. 233)	2. Swiss Ball Prone Leg Lifts (p. 240)
3. High Cross-Cable Reverse Crunch (p. 218)	3. Lying Lower Body Rotations (p. 227)	3. Rope Crunch (p. 236)	
ADVANCED	ADVANCED	ADVANCED	ADVANCED
1. Hanging Straight Leg Raises (p. 213)	1. Corkscrews (p. 222)	1. Weighted Swiss Ball Crunch (p. 231)	1. Good Mornings (p. 241)
2. Hanging Bent Leg Raises (p. 216)	2. Hanging Side Crunch (p. 225)	2. Long-Arm Weighted Crunch (p. 234)	**TRANSVERSE ABDOMINIS**
3. Swiss Ball Reverse Crunch (p. 219)	3. Russian Twists (p. 228)	3. Decline Crunch (p. 237)	1. Cats (p. 242)

Choose one exercise from the lower rectus abdominis, obliques, upper rectus abdominis, and erector spinae categories - *in that order*. Perform 3 sets from each category before moving on to the next category. For example, do all 3 sets of reverse crunches (lower rectus abdominis), then all 3 sets of lying side crunches (obliques), followed by all 3 sets of supine weighted crunches (upper rectus abdominis). I always start with a lower rectus abdominis exercise because they're the hardest for me to notice results. I can work them harder when I'm fresh. After finishing your abs, don't forget to do 2 sets of an erector spinae exercise to keep your core muscles in balance. Consistency in all 4 categories is the only way to obtain optimal results and proper alignment with your pelvis.

Start

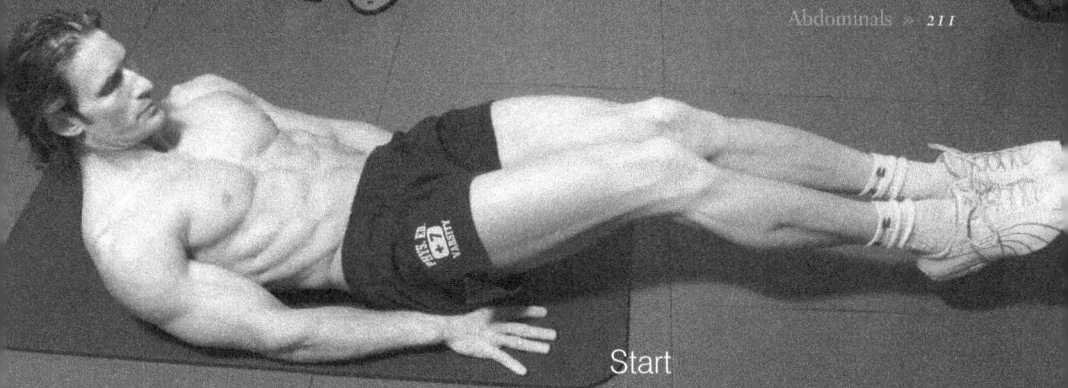

1. LYING LEG RAISES *(Lower Rectus Abdominis - Beginner)*

Lie supine on the floor with your legs together, knees slightly bent, and your feet about 6 inches off the floor. Put your hands on the floor by your hips and raise your shoulders slightly off the floor so that the small of your back is pressed firmly against the floor. This creates a 'C' shape in your midsection, called spinal flexion. **This is your starting position.** Using a 3 count, exhale while raising your feet off the ground about 2 ½ feet and pause for a 2 count. Again, use a 3 count and inhale while slowly lowering your feet about 6 inches and pause for a 2 count. Your range will start 6 inches from the floor and end 2 ½ feet from the floor. Remember to pause for a 2 count at each pivot. Repeat 20 repetitions for 3 sets with 30 seconds rest between each set.

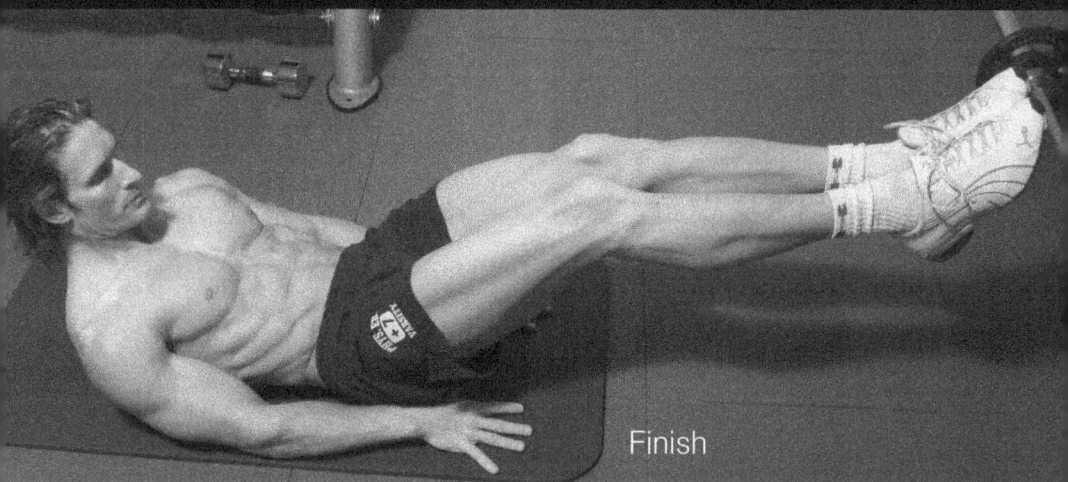

Finish

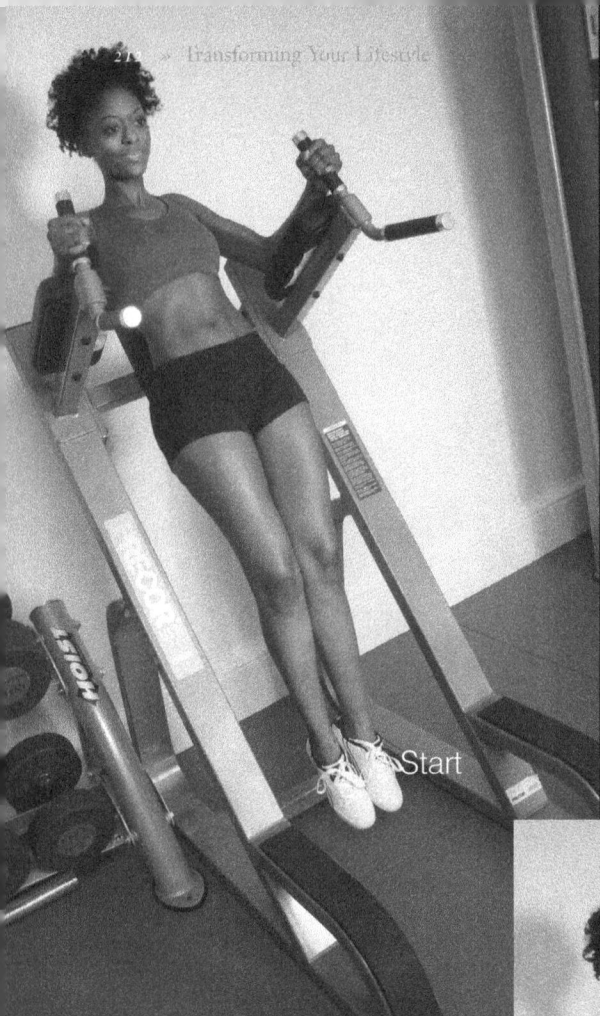

Start

2. CAPTAIN'S CHAIR STRAIGHT LEG RAISES
(Lower Rectus Abdominis - Moderate)

Holding onto the handles of a Captain's Chair, suspend your body and slightly tilt your pelvis so that the small of your back is pressed against the back pad. You'll be in a vertical and spinal flexion position. You should maintain a slight bend in your knees throughout this exercise. **This is your starting position.**

For a 3 count, exhale and raise your legs until they're parallel to the floor. Hold for a 2 count, then lower your legs toward the floor for a 3 count while inhaling.

Remember to stop just before you're completely vertical, so that you maintain spinal flexion to keep tension in your abs. This means you will not be completely relaxed until the exercise is finished. Perform 10-15 repetitions with 45 seconds rest between each of the 3 sets.

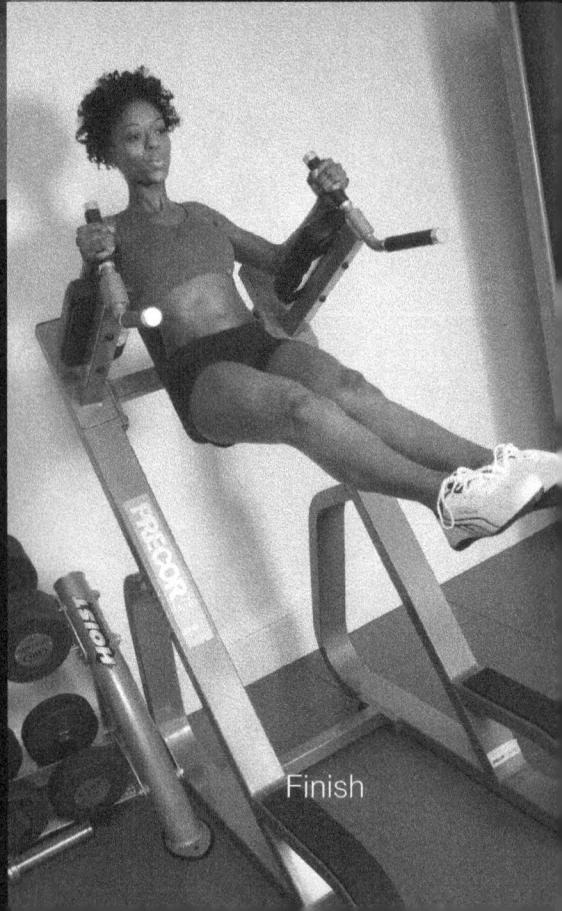

Finish

christopherSASHA

Start

3. HANGING STRAIGHT LEG RAISES
(Lower Rectus Abdominis - Advanced)

Hang from an overhead bar with an underhand grip about 2 inches wider than shoulder width. Again, keep your hips tilted forward a little to maintain spinal flexion. At this point, your feet should not be touching the floor. **This is your starting position.** Begin exhaling and raise your legs for a 3 count until your thighs are parallel with the floor.

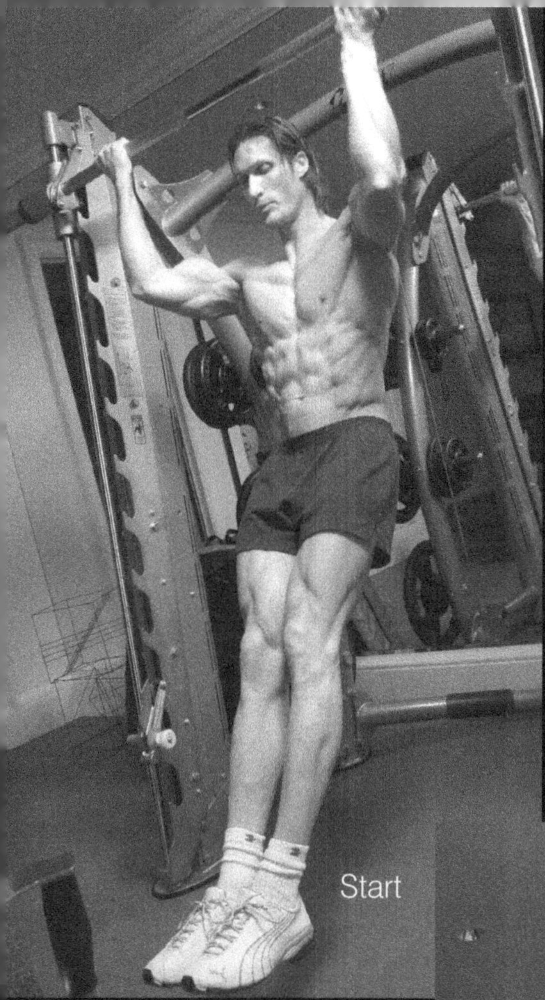

Hold for a 2 count then lower your feet toward the floor for a 3 count while inhaling. Again, do not completely relax at the bottom. You should always be in a slight 'C' shape at the bottom to keep tension in your abs. Also, your body should not swing while performing this exercise. If you're swinging, you're using momentum which can easily be stopped by slowing your movements in each direction. When done properly, this is a hard exercise. Perform 5-15 repetitions with a 60 second rest period between each of the 3 sets.

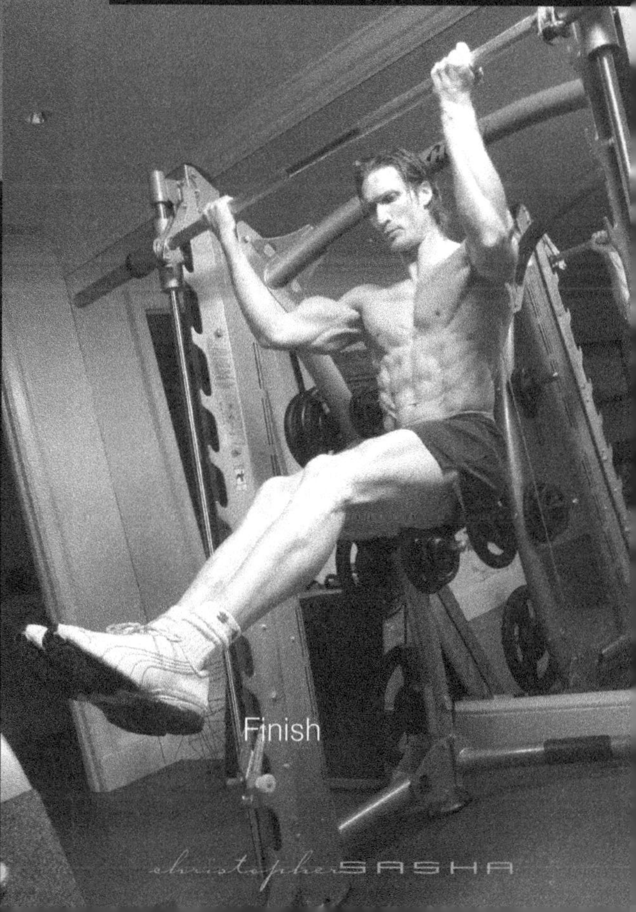

Finish

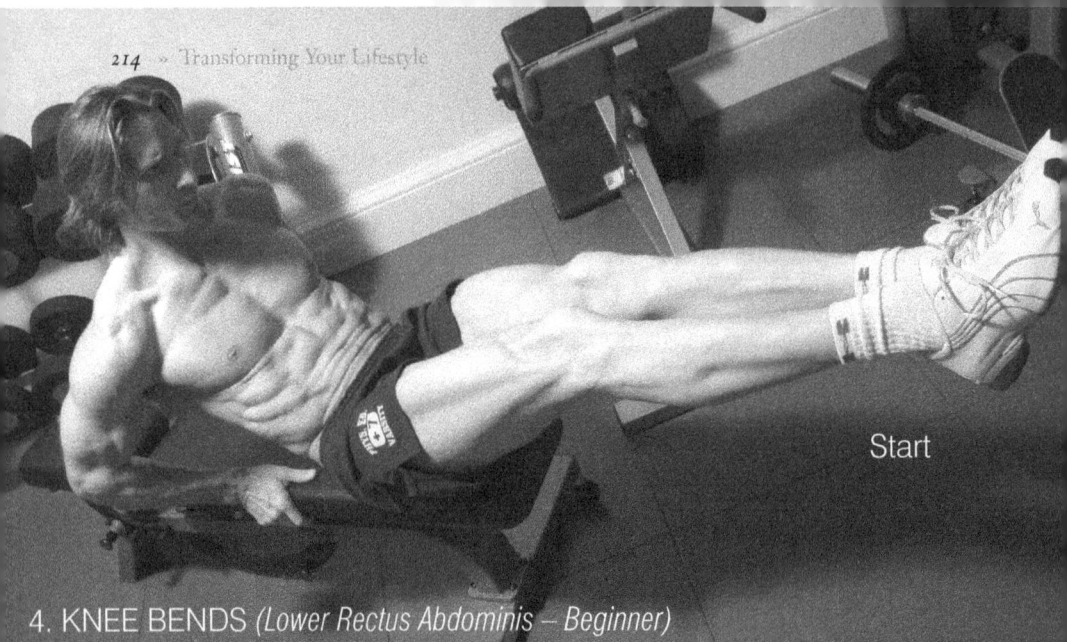

Start

4. KNEE BENDS *(Lower Rectus Abdominis – Beginner)*

Sit at the edge of a flat bench with your legs and feet together and extended in front of you. Your feet should be about 3 feet above the floor. The higher your feet are from the floor, the more difficult this exercise becomes. Grasp the sides of the bench about 12 inches behind you for support and lean your upper body back 45 degrees. **This is your starting position.** Begin exhaling for a 3 count while pulling your knees toward your chest as you simultaneously curl your upper body slightly forward. When you get to the point where your knees can't go any further toward your chest, exhale all the air out of your lungs and squeeze your belly button toward your spinal cord as hard as you can for a 2 count. Then extend your legs in front of you while inhaling. You should extend your legs so there is a slight bend in your knees without your heels touching the floor. Repeat for 10-15 repetitions with 30 seconds rest between each of the 3 sets.

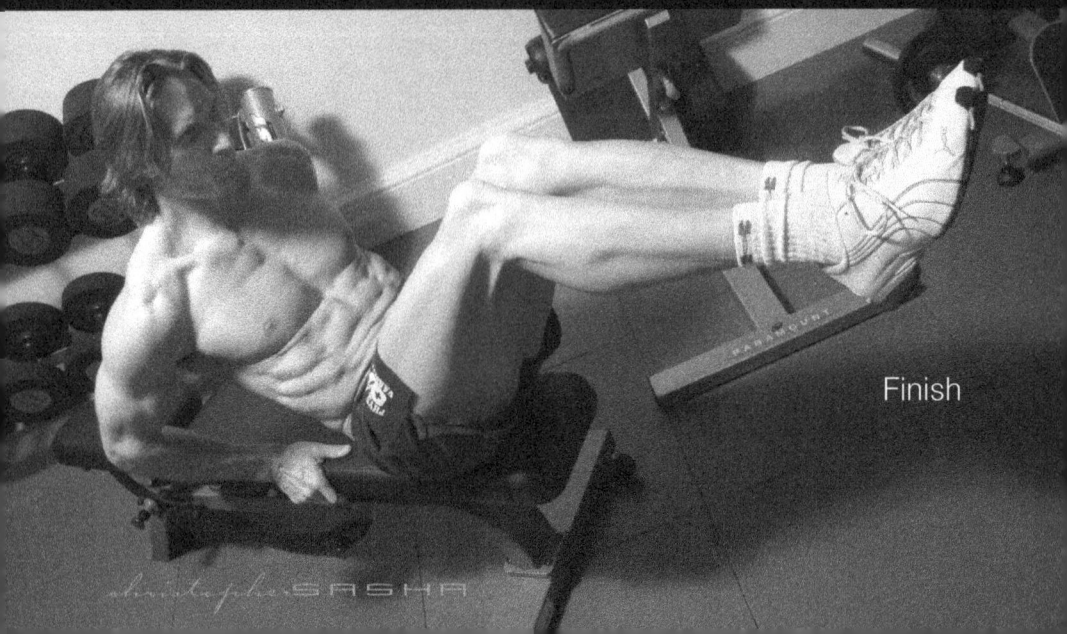

Finish

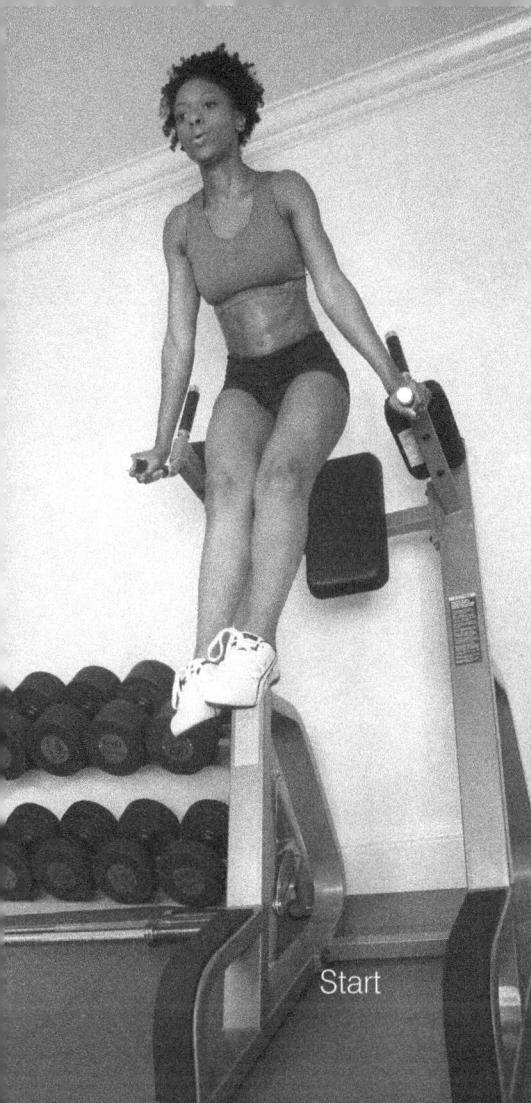

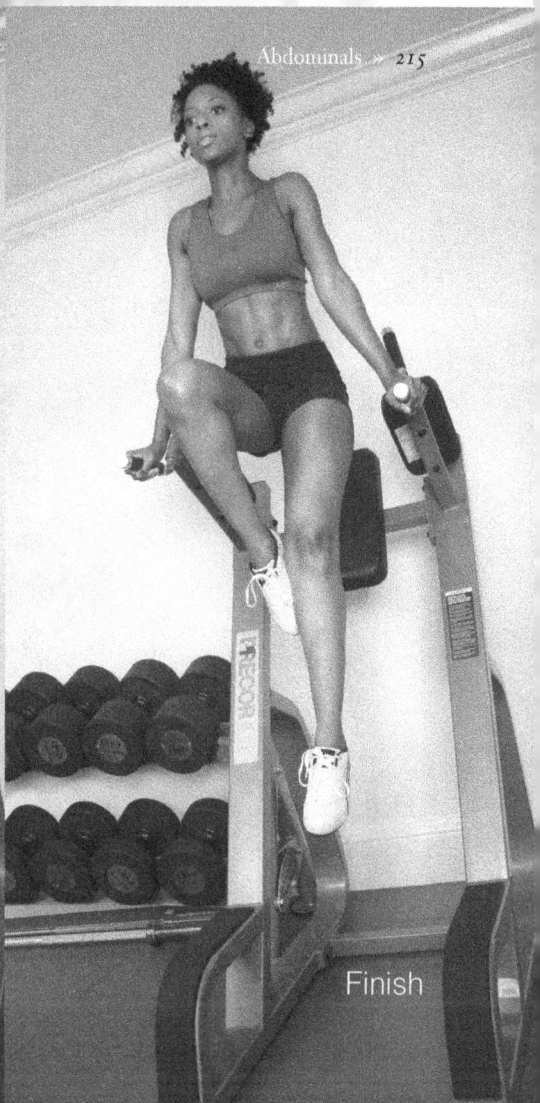

Start

Finish

5. RUNNING MAN *(Lower Rectus Abdominis – Moderate)*

Holding onto the handles of a Captain's Chair, lock-out your elbows to the sides of your body. Suspend with a slight forward pelvic tilt to position yourself in spinal flexion. **This is your starting position.** Raise your right knee up as high as possible. While lower your right leg toward the floor, simultaneously lift your left knee up as high as possible. While lowering your left leg toward the floor, simultaneously lift your right knee up as high as possible. Continue this motion for 30-60 revolutions. It should look as though you're running in place. There are no pauses but rather a continuous controlled motion.

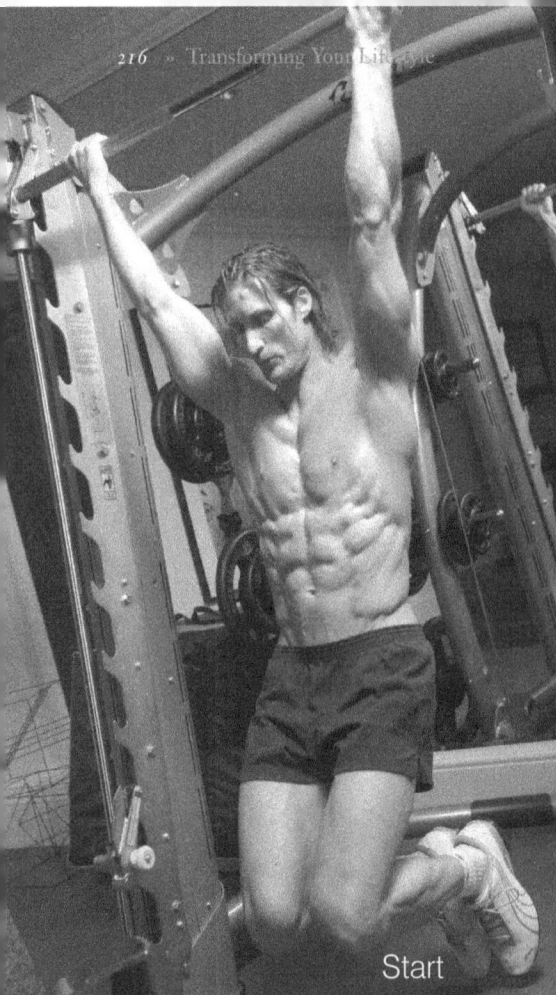

6. HANGING BENT LEG RAISES
(Lower Rectus Abdominis —Advanced)

Hang from an overhead bar with an underhand grip about 2 inches wider than shoulder width. Suspend with your pelvis tilted slightly forward so that your body creates a 'C' shape (spinal flexion). **This is your starting position.**

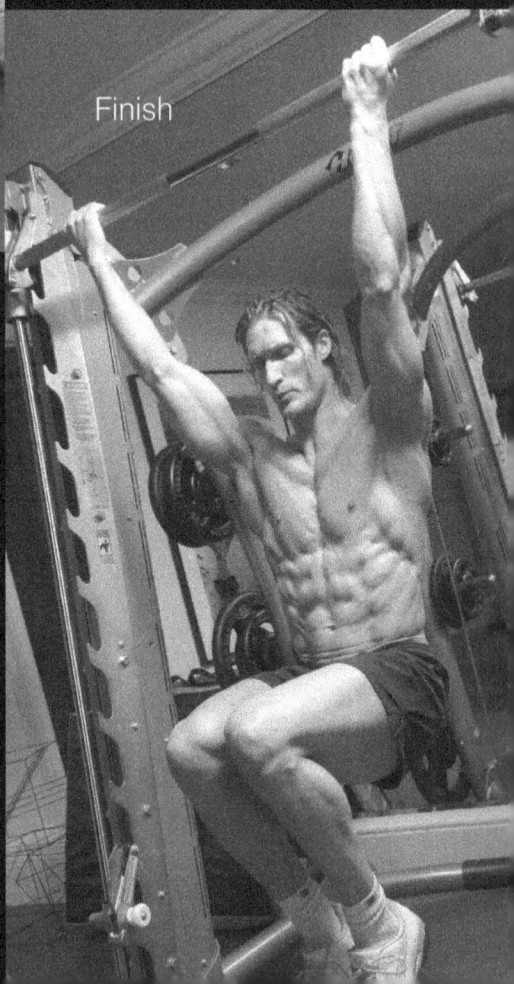

Start

Finish

Exhale while raising your knees as high as possible toward your chest for a 3 count. Hold your knees at the top for a 2 count, then lower your knees toward the floor for a 3 count while inhaling. Remember to maintain spinal flexion at the bottom (do not fully extend) to keep tension in your abs. Your body should not swing while performing this exercise. Should you find yourself swinging, slow down your movements. Perform 10-15 repetitions with a 60 second rest between each of the 3 sets.

Start

Finish

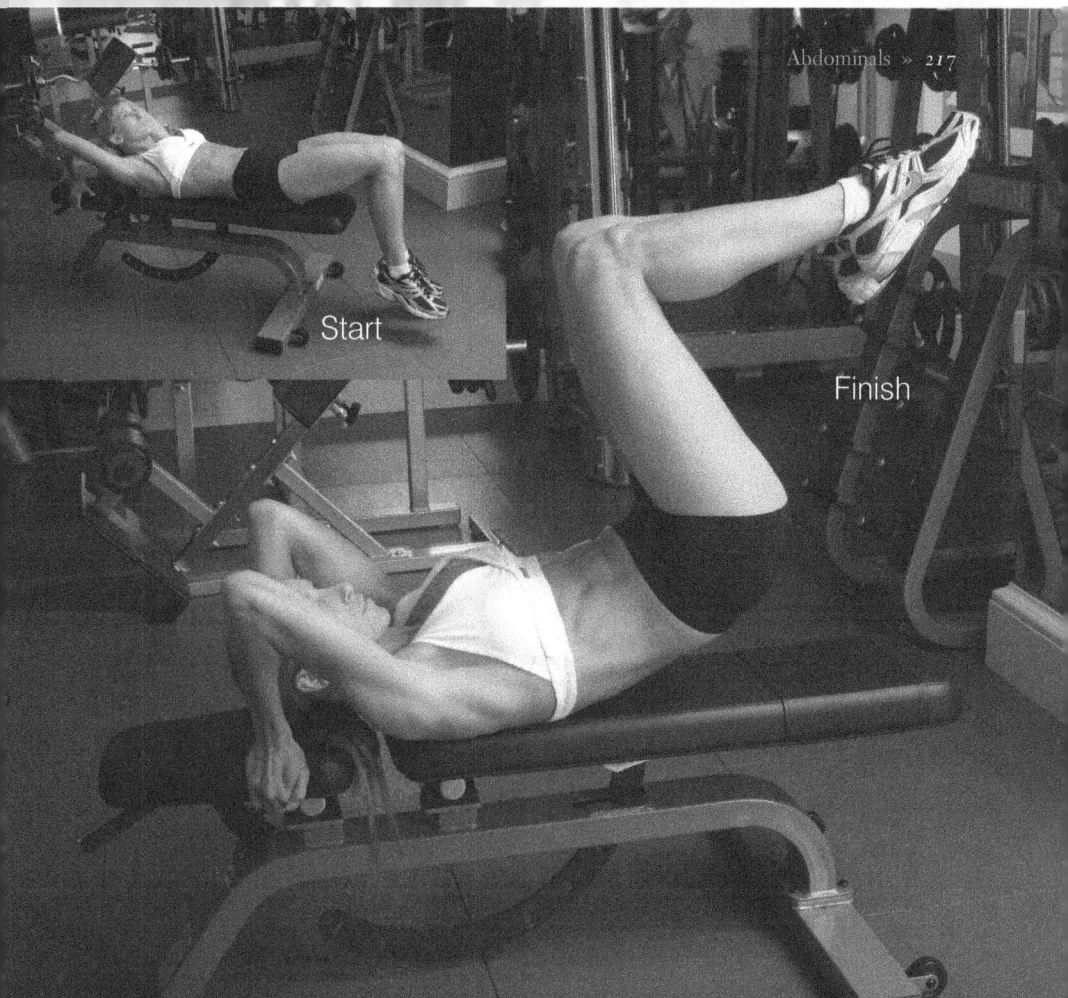

7. REVERSE CRUNCH *(Lower Rectus Abdominis – Beginner)*

Lie supine on a flat bench and grasp the sides of the bench by your ears to anchor your upper body. With your legs together and bent at a 90 degree angle at your knees, lower your feet toward the floor to the point where the small of your back is still firmly pressed against the bench to support your lower back. **This is your starting position.** Begin exhaling and rotate your knees toward your chest for a 3 count. Once you're up as high as you can go, squeeze your belly button in toward your spinal cord as you continue to force all the air out of your lungs. Then inhale as you lower your feet to your starting position for a 3 count. It's important to keep your lower back pressed firmly against the bench while at your starting position to maintain lower back support. Perform 20-30 repetitions with a 30 second rest between each of the 3 sets.

christopherSASHA

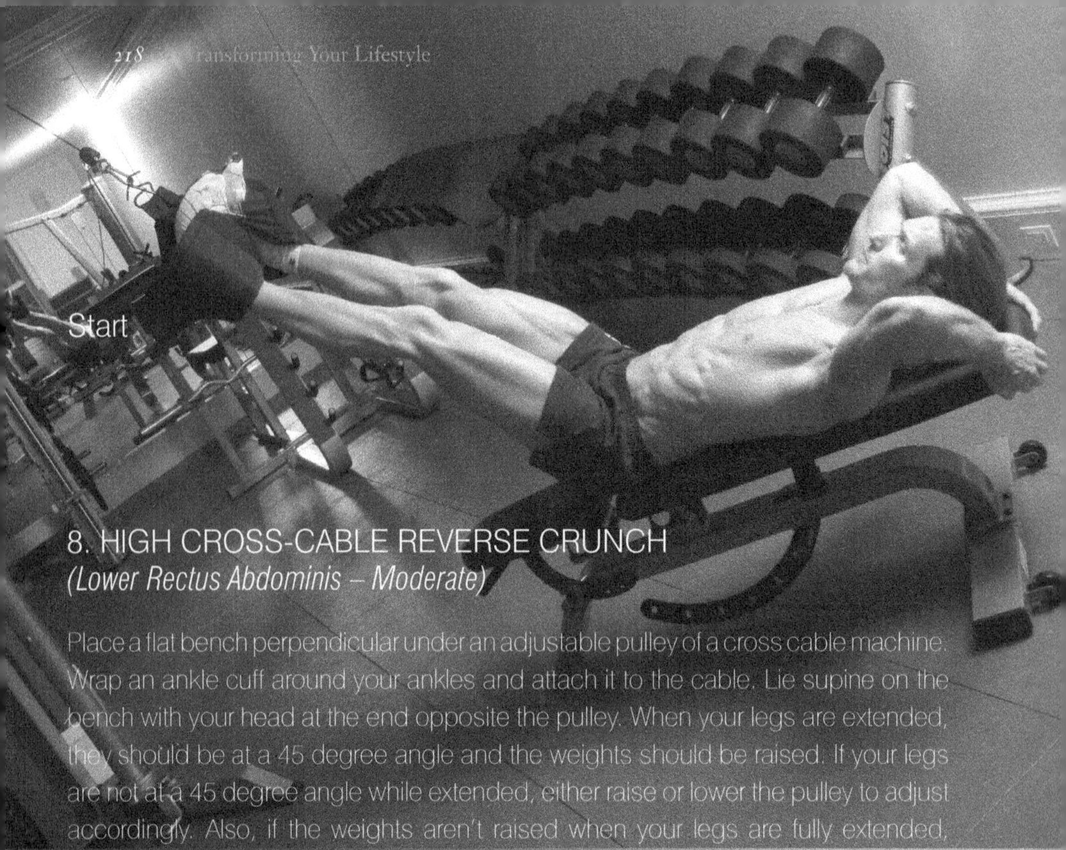

Start

8. HIGH CROSS-CABLE REVERSE CRUNCH
(Lower Rectus Abdominis – Moderate)

Place a flat bench perpendicular under an adjustable pulley of a cross cable machine. Wrap an ankle cuff around your ankles and attach it to the cable. Lie supine on the bench with your head at the end opposite the pulley. When your legs are extended, they should be at a 45 degree angle and the weights should be raised. If your legs are not at a 45 degree angle while extended, either raise or lower the pulley to adjust accordingly. Also, if the weights aren't raised when your legs are fully extended, move the bench further away from the pulley. Grasp the sides of the bench by your ears to anchor your upper body. **This is your starting position.** With your legs together, exhale and rotate your hips toward your chest (your knees approach your chest and your heels approach your butt) for a 3 count. Squeeze all the air out of your lungs then inhale while extending your legs to the starting position. Repeat 10 repetitions for 3 sets with 45 second rests between each set.

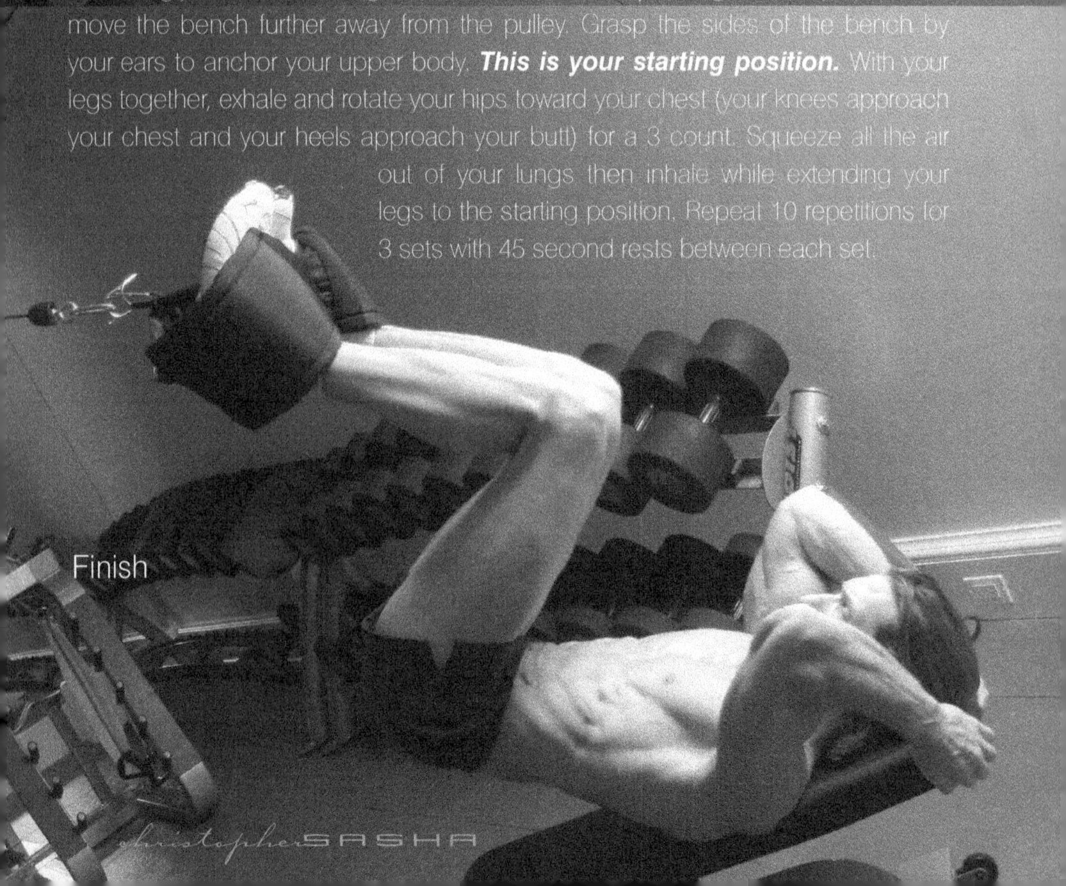

Finish

Start

Finish

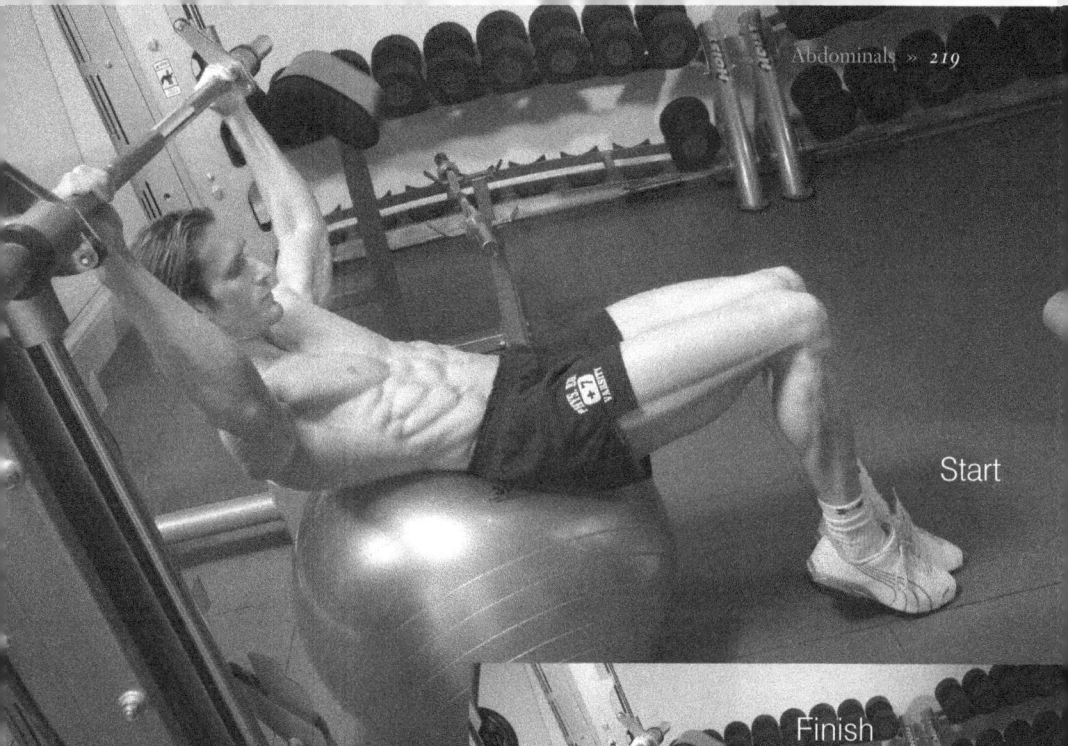

9. SWISS BALL REVERSE CRUNCH
(Lower Rectus Abdominis – Advanced)

Place a Swiss ball by the Smith machine and lie supine and perpendicular on the ball. Adjust the bar on the Smith Machine about 12 inches higher than your head. The small of your back should be on the pinnacle of the Swiss ball. Extend your arms behind your head and grasp the bar with both hands in an overhand grip to anchor your upper body. With your feet about an inch off the floor, your knees should be at a 90 degree angle. **This is your starting position.** Begin exhaling as you bring your knees toward your chest by rotating from your hips. Pull for a 3 count and stop when your thighs are perpendicular to the floor. At this point, your torso should be in a 'C' shape. Squeeze all the air out of your lungs then inhale as you lower your feet one inch above the floor. Don't touch the floor with your feet. This is an unstable exercise due to the Swiss ball which makes this exercise difficult. The bonus is that you'll recruit more core muscles to help stabilize while on top the ball. Perform 15-20 repetitions with 45 second rest periods between each of the 3 sets.

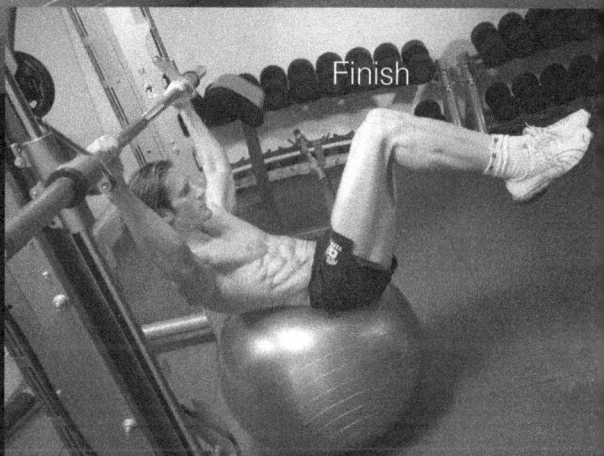

christopher SASHA

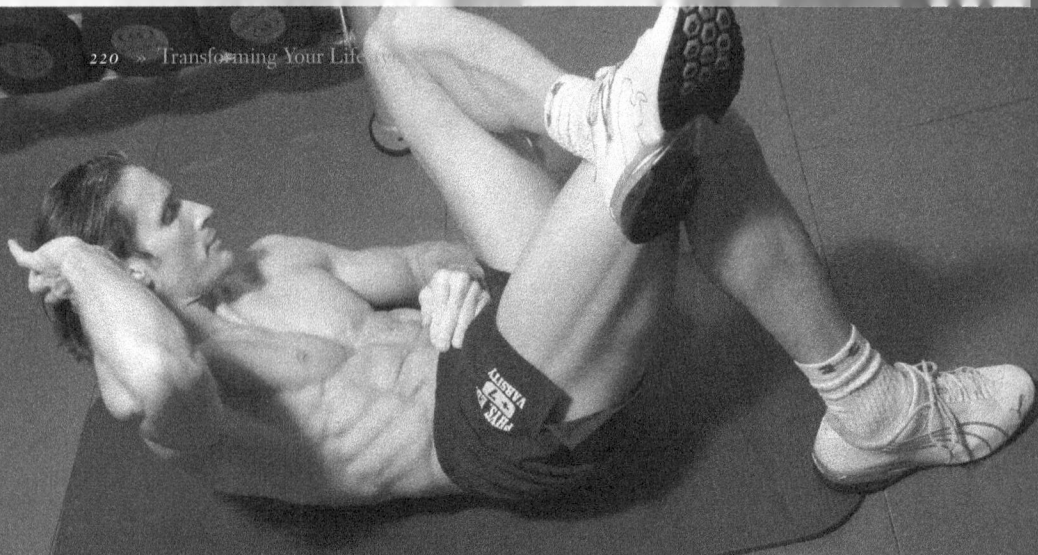

Start

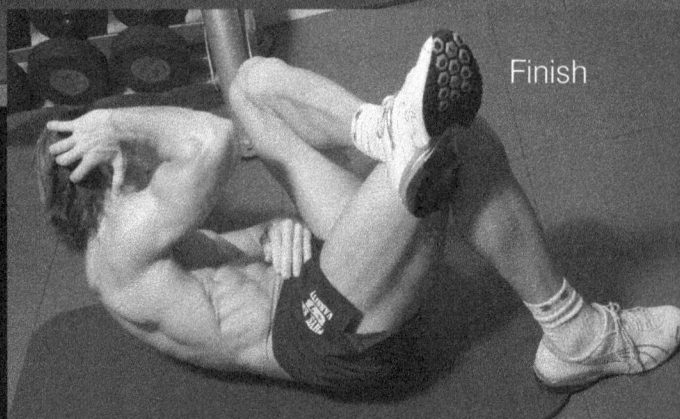

Finish

10. TWISTING CRUNCH
(Obliques – Beginner)

Lie supine on the floor with your right leg bent so that your right foot is flat on the floor. Cross your left leg over your right knee and rest your ankle on your knee. Place your left arm along your side with your hand on top of your abs. Apply a little pressure so that you can focus on the contractions as you perform this exercise. Hold just the fingertips of your right hand on the right side of your head. Using just your fingertips (instead of your entire hand) will drastically reduce the tendency to pull your head up during the exercise. **This is your starting position.** Begin exhaling and rotate your torso to the left for a 3 count. The object is to reach your right elbow to your left knee without changing the position of your elbow. Keeping your right elbow out wide will force you to rotate from your waist rather than swinging your elbow in and out to reach your knee. At the point where you can't rotate any further, squeeze all the air out of your lungs, force your lower back into the floor, and focus on the contraction by feeling the tension in your abs with your left hand. Hold for a 2 count then inhale as you rotate your torso to the right and back to the floor. Don't rest at the bottom. Continue 15-20 repetitions then do the same on the opposite side. There will be no rest between the 3 sets.

Start

Finish

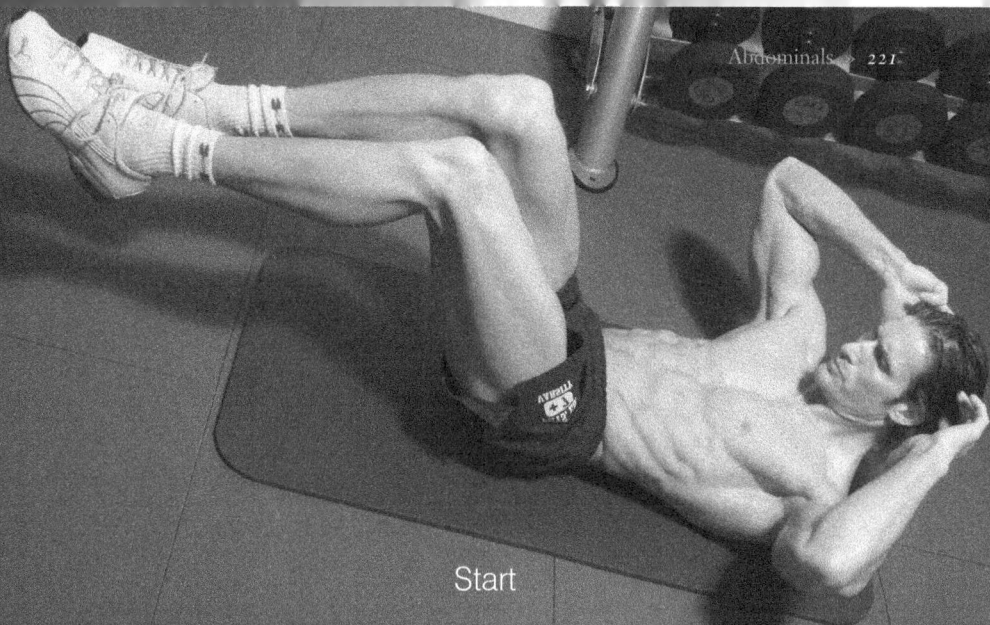

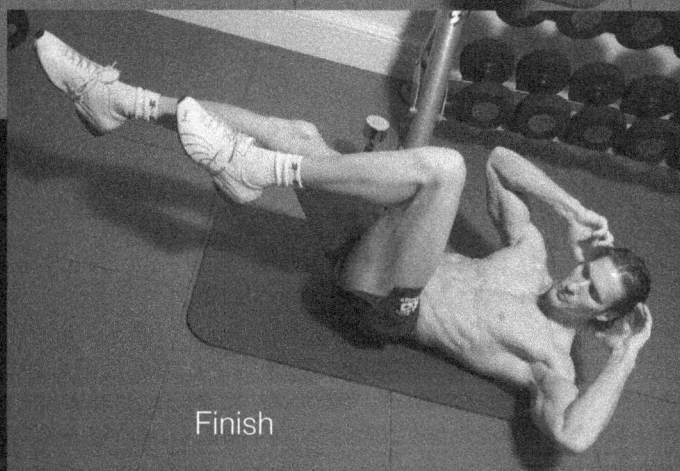

11. BICYCLES *(Obliques – Moderate)*

Lie supine on the floor with just your fingertips by your ears. Raise your feet up so that your hips and knees are bent 90 degrees. Now raise your shoulders slightly off the floor to create spinal flexion. Your lower back should be pressed firmly into the floor in this position. **This is your starting position.** Slowly rotate your torso to the left as you extend your right leg. Pause for a 1 count. At this point, your right elbow should be close to your left knee. Now reverse the rotation so that your left elbow is close to your right knee while your left leg is fully extended. Pause for a 1 count for each rotation. It should look like you're riding a bicycle while rotating your torso side to side. Continue this motion for 20-40 repetitions on each side. For example, if you did 20 repetitions for 1 set, you will rotate your torso to the right 20 times and to the left 20 times, counting a total of 40 rotations for the set. Take 45 second rests between each of the 3 sets.

Start

Finish

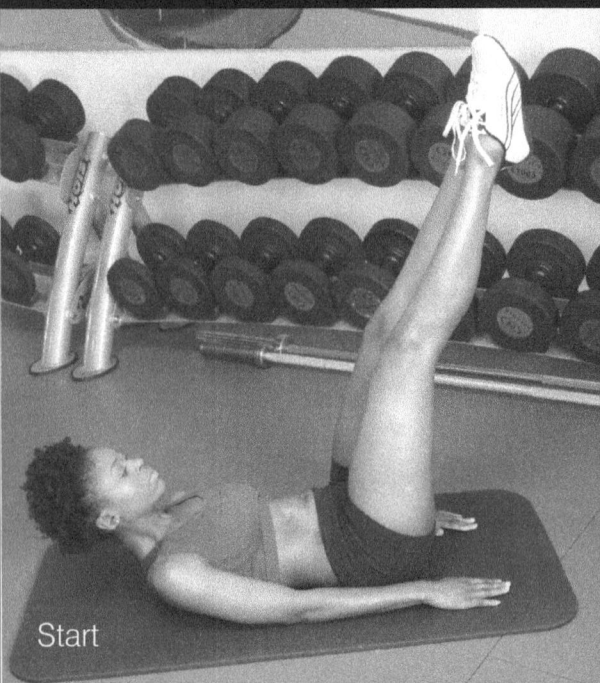

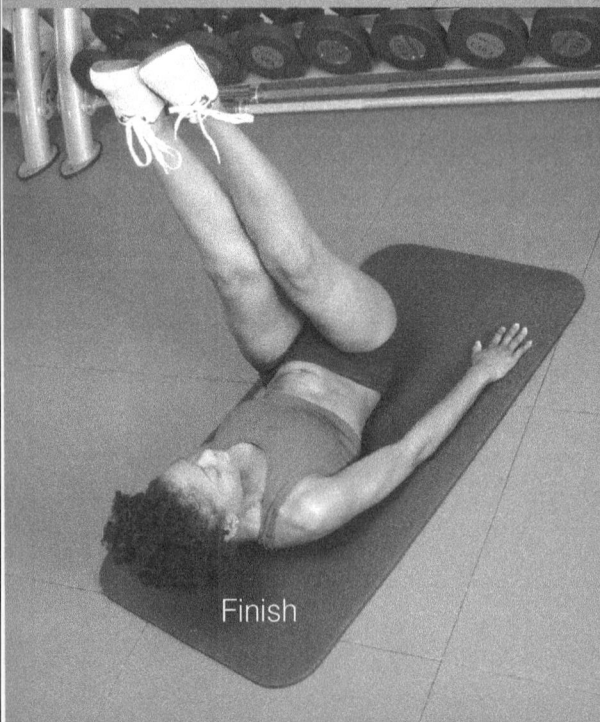

12. CORKSCREWS
(Obliques – Advanced)

Lie supine on the floor with your arms by your sides, palms on the floor. Raise your feet off the floor toward the ceiling so that your legs are perpendicular to the floor. Now slightly raise your head and shoulders off the floor. **This is your starting position.** Using your arms as your stabilizers, exhale and slowly curl your lower spine up toward the ceiling and rotate your hips as far to the left as possible. Pause for 1 count then rotate your hips as far to the right as possible. Again, pause for 1 count. Inhale as you slowly lower your spine toward the floor without touching the floor. This will keep tension in your abs the entire time. Without resting at the bottom, exhale and slowly curl your lower spine up toward the ceiling and repeat, rotating your hips as far to the left and right sides as you can, with 1 count pauses between for 10-15 repetitions. Rest for 45 seconds between each of the 3 sets.

christopher SASHA

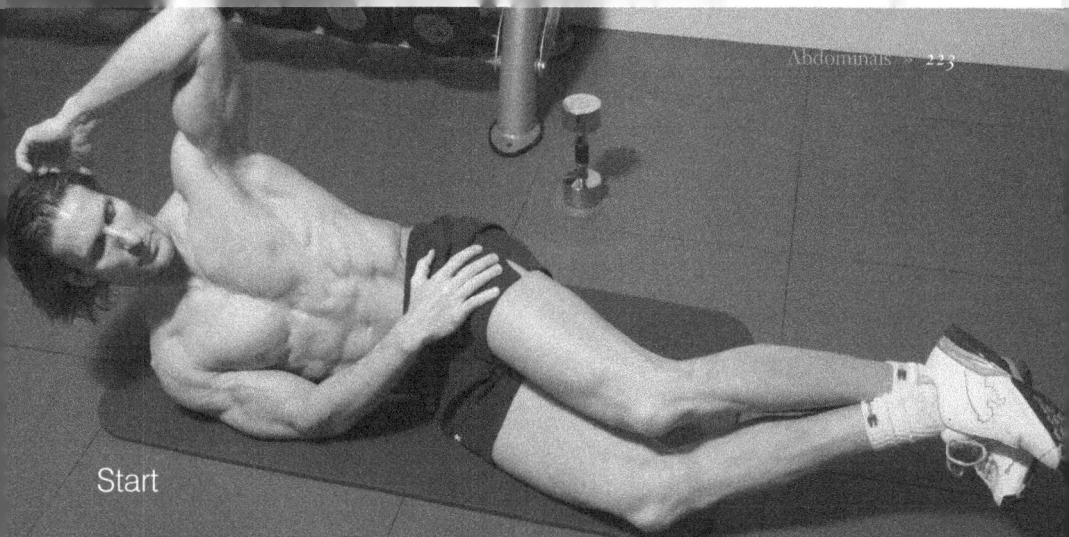

Start

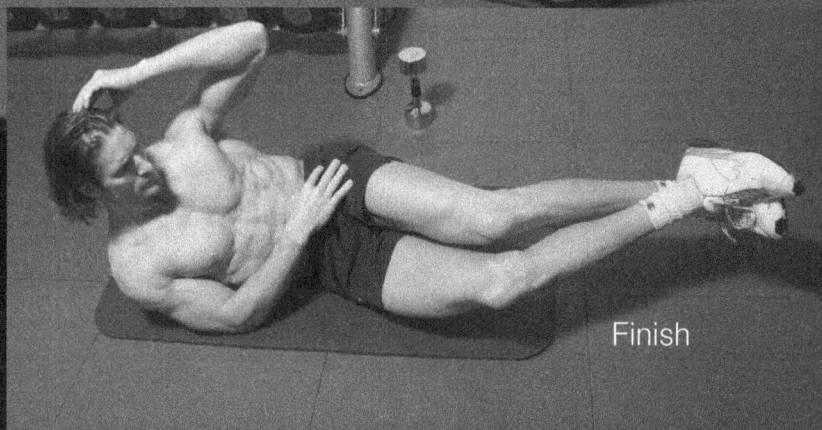

Finish

13. LYING SIDE CRUNCH *(Obliques – Beginner)*

Lie on your right side on the floor with your legs extended and crossed at the ankles. Raise your feet a few inches off the floor. Place your right arm along your body with your hand pressed against your left obliques (this is to help balance and focus on the muscles contracting as you perform the exercise). Place the fingertips of your left hand behind your head. You'll have more tendency to pull yourself up by your head if you place your entire hand behind your head. Remember, we're trying to work your abs, not your bicep and neck. **This is your starting position.** Keeping your feet a few inches off the floor the entire duration of this exercise, exhale for a 3 count while lifting your upper body up and toward your hips in a side curl movement. Pause and squeeze at the top until all the air is out of your lungs, then inhale as you lower your upper body toward the floor for a 3 count. Don't rest at the bottom until you've finished the set. Perform 15-20 repetitions then immediately roll over without a break to perform an equal number of repetitions on the opposite side. This is one set. Take 30 seconds between each of the 3 sets.

14. ROMAN CHAIR SIDE CRUNCH *(Obliques – Moderate)*

Using a Roman chair, lie on your left side so your left hip is on the pad with your legs crossed and feet supported by the foot roller. Have a slight bend in your knees for extra support. Adjust the hip pad so that your waist is about 2 inches higher than the pad. Fully extend your right arm above your head so your arm is beside your head. Your body should be at a 45 degree angle from the floor. **This is your starting position.** Be very careful and precise with this exercise so you don't pull any muscles. Exhale and pull your upper body up toward the ceiling for a 5 count. At the top, continue exhaling and squeeze your right side obliques until all the air is out of your lungs. Inhale as you lower your upper body down toward the floor for a 5 count. To maintain constant tension in your obliques, don't rest at the bottom. Perform 10-15 repetitions then switch sides for an equal number of repetitions. This is one set. Take 45-60 seconds between each of the 3 sets.

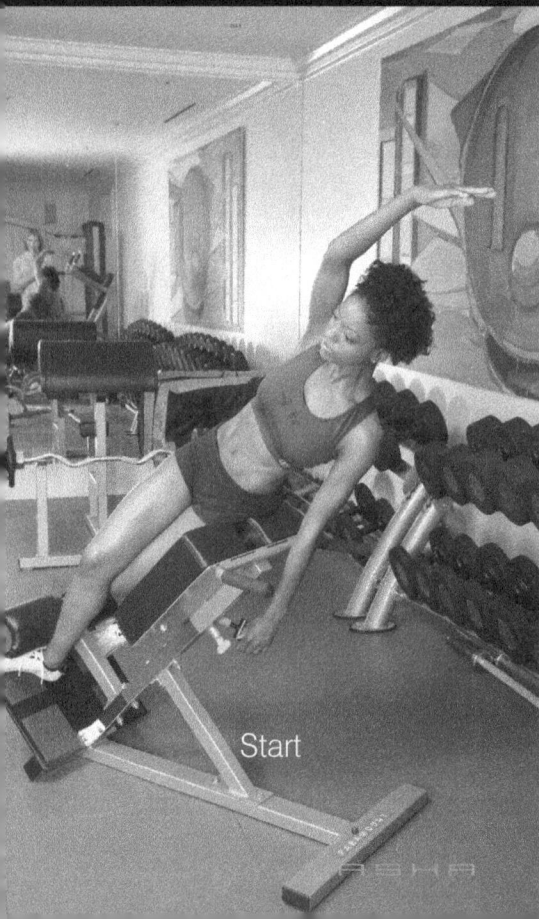

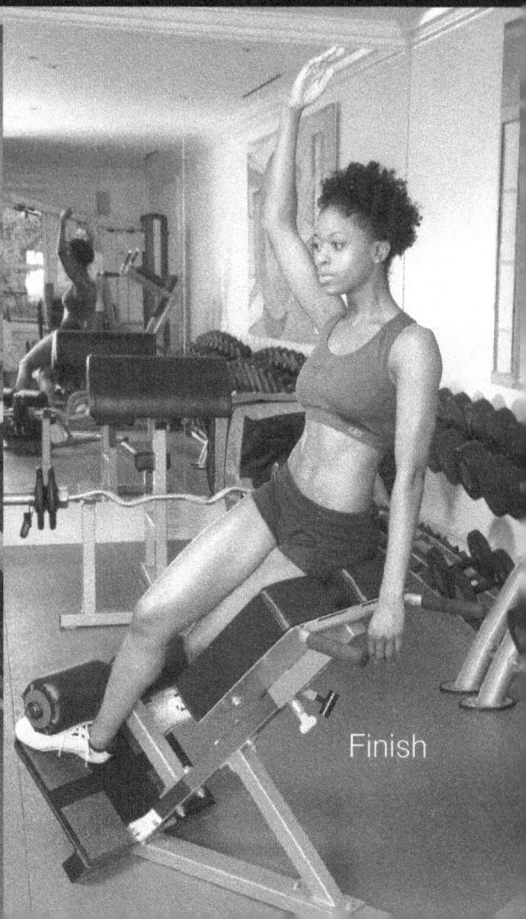

Start

Finish

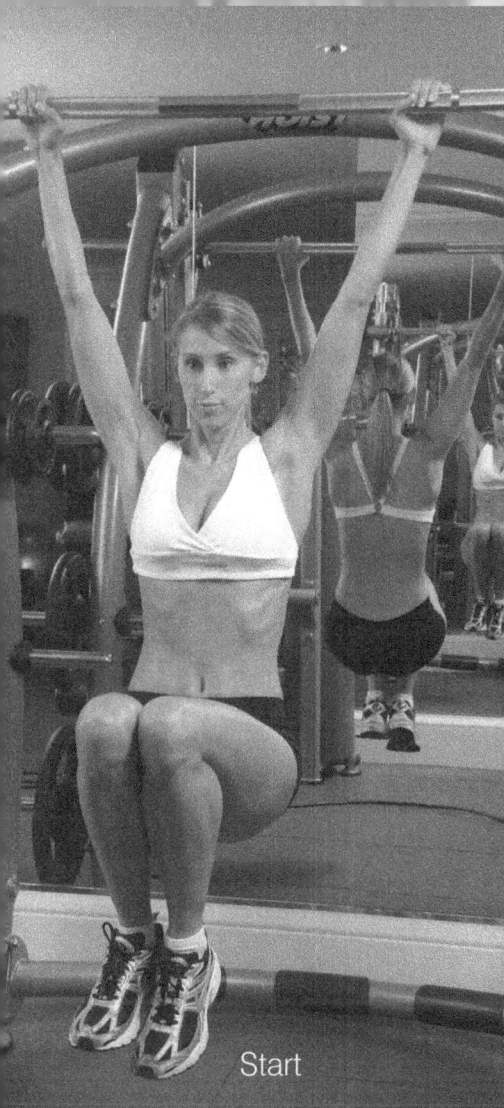

Start

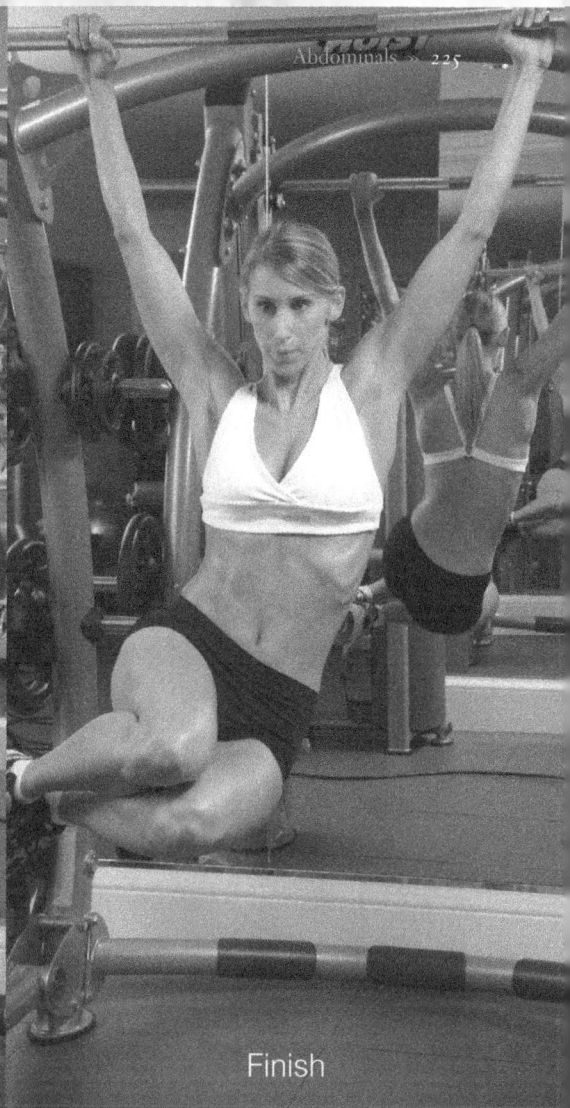

Finish

15. HANGING SIDE CRUNCH *(Obliques – Advanced)*

Hang from an overhead bar with an overhand grip about 2 inches wider than shoulder width apart. At this point, your thighs should be bent at a 90 degree angle from both your hips and knees. **This is your starting position.** Begin exhaling and curl your hips to the right side as high as possible (the object is to get your thighs parallel to the floor). Once you're as high as you can get, pause and squeeze your right side obliques as hard as you can while forcing all the air out of your lungs. Inhale for a 3 count as you lower your hips back toward your starting position. Perform 10-15 repetitions on the right side then repeat for an equal number of repetitions on the left side. Take 60 seconds of rest between each of the 3 sets.

16. SEATED UPPER BODY ROTATIONS
(Obliques – Beginner)

Place two dumbbells (heavy enough to anchor your feet) perpendicular in front of a flat bench. Sit on the edge of the bench with your feet secured under the dumbbells for support. Rest a weightlifting bar (9 pounds or lighter) on your shoulders with a wide overhand grip and lean back a few inches while slightly slouching to create spinal flexion. **Looking straight forward, this is your starting position.** Keeping your hips in place, from your waist, use your oblique muscles to twist your torso from side to side. *Do not twist from your shoulders; rather originate each twist from your waist.* Also, your chin should be aligned with your sternum (your breastbone in the center of chest) throughout this exercise, keeping your spine in neutral position at all times. Start twisting slowly until you feel your lower back is loose. Then twist quicker, but in a controlled motion throughout this exercise. Twist slowly and carefully with this exercise if you have or had back problems. One twist to each side equals one repetition. Perform 30-60 repetitions (60-120 total twists) with 30 second rests between each of the 3 sets.

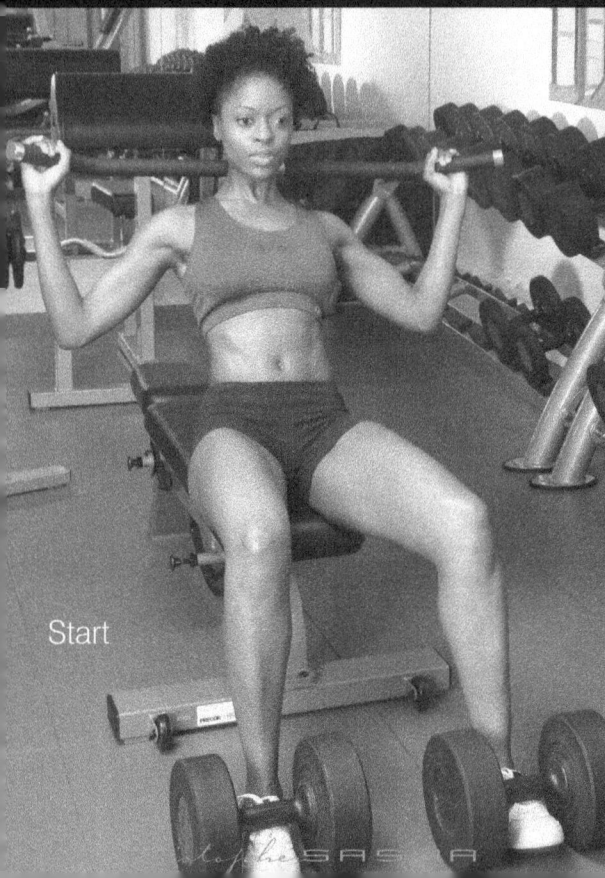

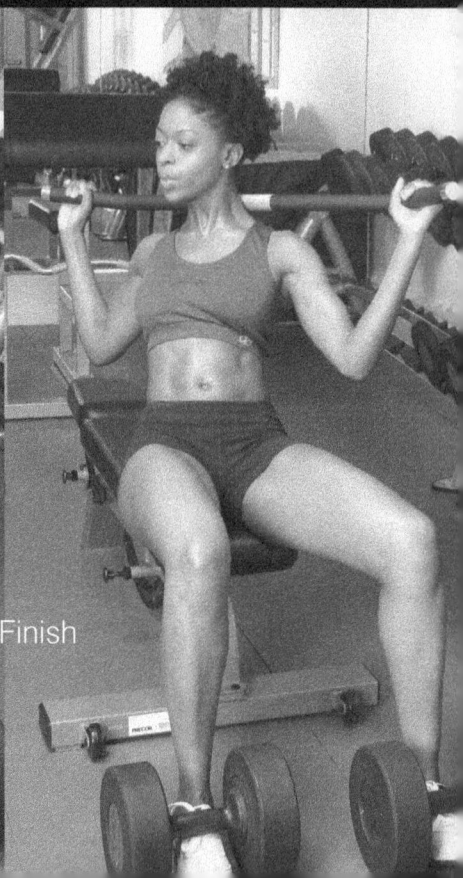

Start

Finish

Start

Finish

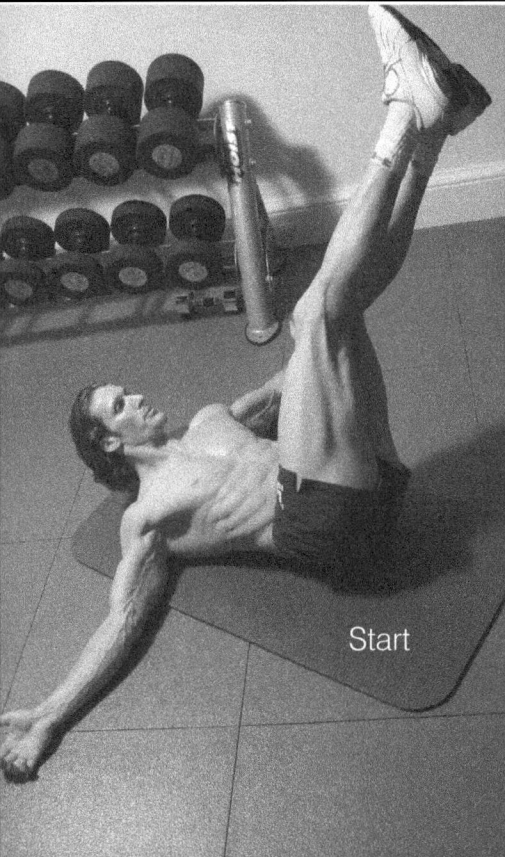

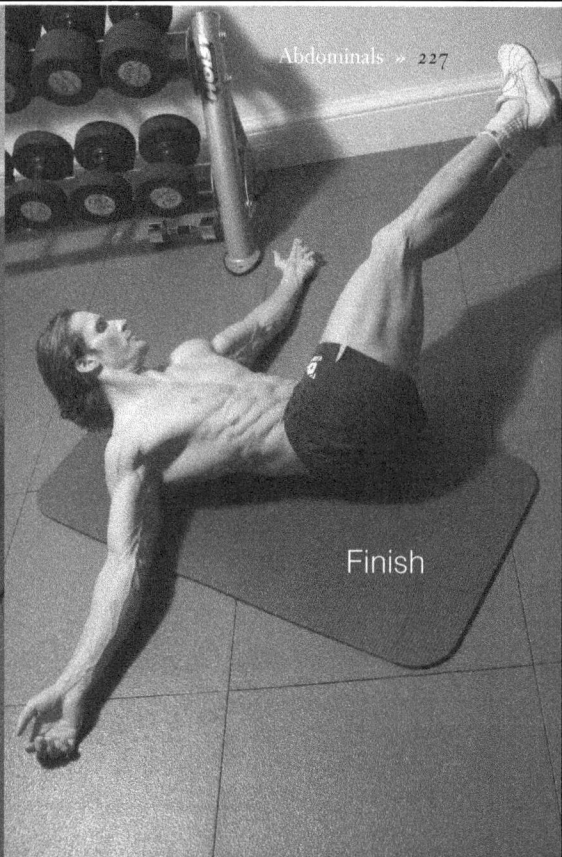

17. LYING LOWER BODY ROTATIONS (Obliques – Moderate)

Lie supine on the floor with your arms extended to either side so that your body forms a 'T' shape. Raise your shoulders a few inches off the floor until you feel your lower back is firmly pressed into the floor. With your legs together, knees slightly bent, raise them so your thighs are perpendicular to the floor. **This is your starting position.** Inhale for a 5 count as you lower your feet to the left side toward the floor, stopping about 6 inches before touching the floor. Your legs should be at a 45 degree angle in correlation from your buttocks and the floor. From this point, exhale for a 5 count and pull your legs up perpendicular to the floor. Without a break, inhale for a 5 count as you lower your feet to the right toward the floor, stopping about 6 inches before touching the floor. Again, your legs should be at a 45 degree angle from your buttocks and the floor. Exhale for a 5 count and pull your legs up perpendicular to the floor. This is counted as one repetition. Perform 10-15 repetitions with 45-60 second rests between each of the 3 sets.

christopherSASHA

Start

Finish

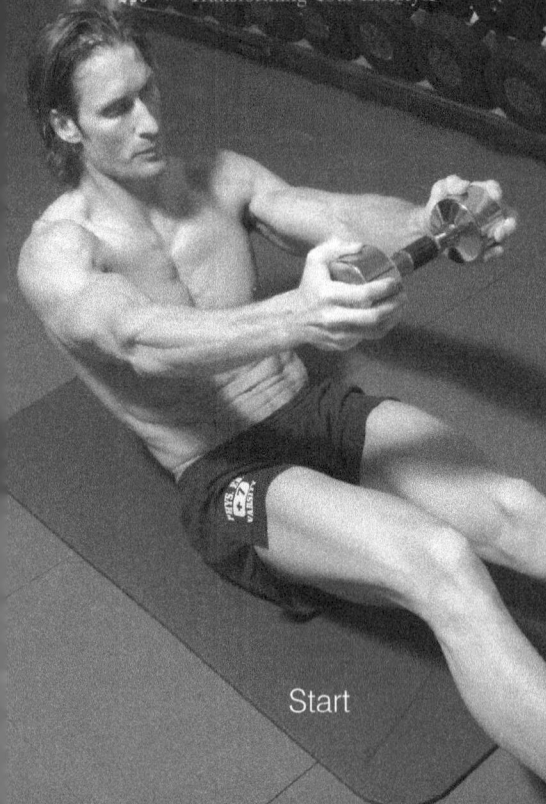

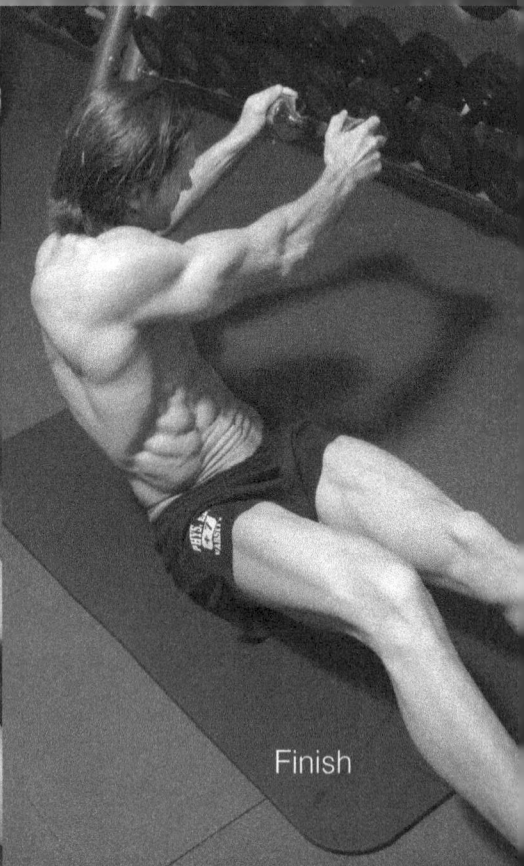

18. RUSSIAN TWISTS *(Obliques – Advanced)*

Sit on the floor with your legs in front of you and a slight bend in your knees. Lean your upper body back about 45 degrees and slightly curl to create spinal flexion. Holding both ends of a dumbbell, extend your arms in front of you so that they are parallel to the floor. **This is your starting position.** *From your waist*, slowly twist as far as possible to your left while exhaling. Your chin should stay aligned with your sternum throughout this exercise to keep your spine in neutral position at all times. Once you're as far as you can go, squeeze your right side obliques as hard as you can until all the air is out of your lungs. Your right side obliques will automatically work harder to balance your body due to the extra weight of holding the dumbbell to the left, and vice-versa. Inhale and slowly rotate to the center, which is your starting position. Repeat, twisting to your right side (from your waist) as far as possible and squeeze your left side obliques as hard as you can until all the air is out of your lungs. Once you're back to the center, this would be counted as one repetition. Perform 10-15 repetitions with 60 second rests between each of the 3 sets.

christopherSASHA

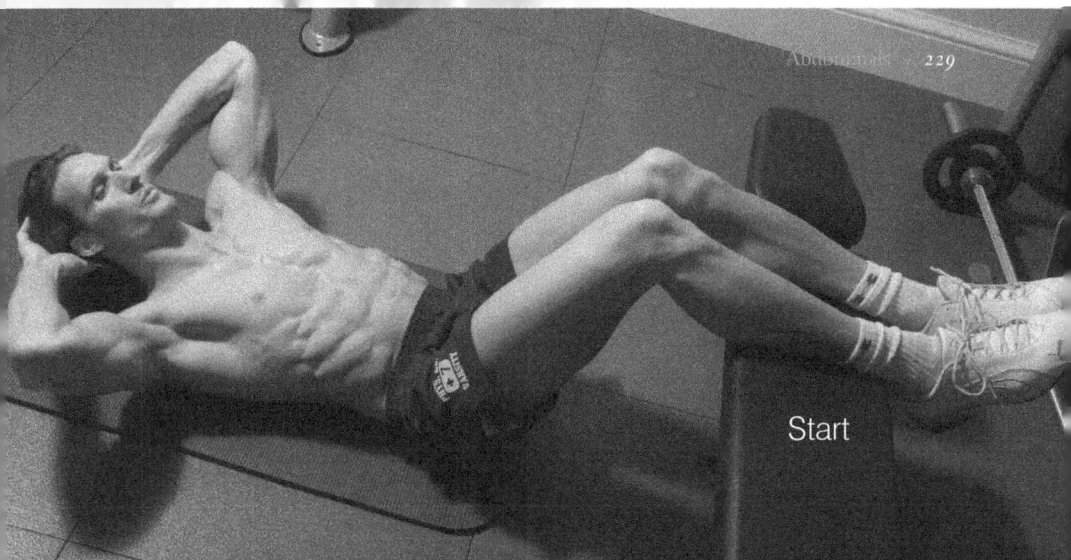

Start

19. SUPPORTED CRUNCH
(Upper Rectus Abdominis – Beginner)

Lie supine on the floor perpendicular to a flat bench. Place your calves on the bench so that your legs are bent at a 90 degree angle at both your hips and knees. Put the fingertips of both hands behind your head. Don't interlace your fingers behind your head because it will promote pulling yourself up by your head instead of using your rectus abdominis to pull your upper body toward your knees. Raise your shoulders slightly off the floor so the small of your back is firmly pressed into the floor, in spinal flexion. **This is your starting position.** Exhale for a 3 count as you curl your upper body toward your knees. At the top, continue to squeeze all the air out of your lungs then inhale for a 3 count as you lower your upper body toward the floor. Don't relax at the bottom. When you're at the bottom, your shoulders should still be slightly off the floor, which will promote tension in your abs the entire time you're performing this exercise. Perform 15-20 repetitions with 15 second rests between each of the 3 sets.

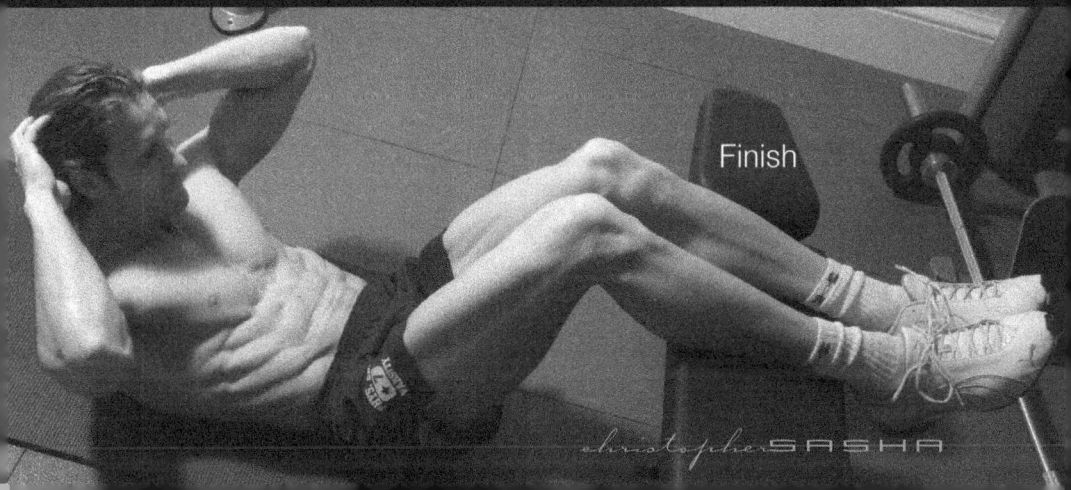

Finish

christopherSASHA

Start

Finish

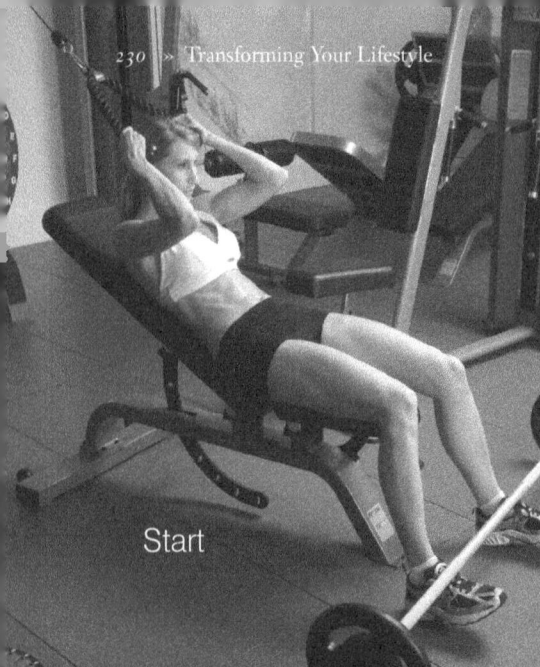

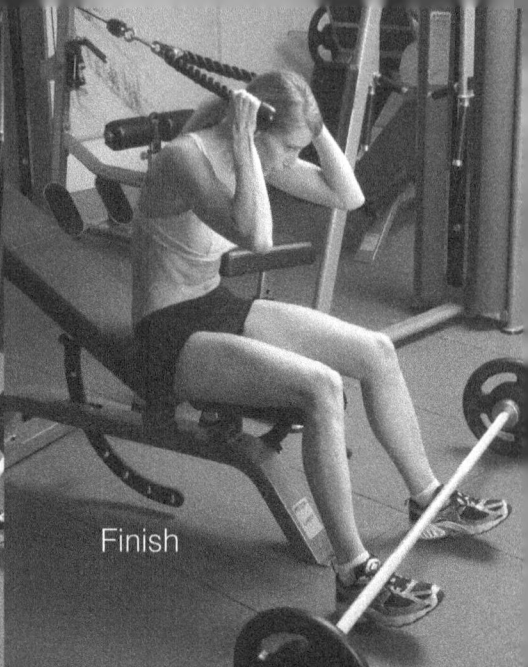

20. CROSS-CABLE CRUNCH *(Upper Rectus Abdominis – Moderate)*

Place an adjustable incline bench perpendicular to an adjustable pulley with the adjustable end of the bench facing the pulley. Set the angle of the bench at about 70 degrees. Place a weighted bar under the bench lengthwise so that you can anchor your feet under it for support. Attach a rope to the pulley so that it barely touches the high end of the bench. If the rope rests on the bench, adjust the pulley one position higher on the pulley bar. If the rope is one or two inches higher than the top of the bench, adjust the pulley one or two positions lower on the pulley bar. Sit on the bench (facing away from the pulley) and grasp the rope with both hands. Place both hands on the temples of your head and slightly round your shoulders forward while curling a little so that only the small of your back is firmly pressed against the bench – your upper back shouldn't be touching the bench. Position both feet under the weighted bar so they are firmly secured. **This is your starting position.** Exhale for a 5 count while you curl your spine forward as your elbows approach your knees. It's important that the angle of your arms remains constant throughout this exercise and the movement comes from curling your spine forward. Continue crunching forward until your elbows almost touch your knees. At this point, squeeze your abs as hard as possible while focusing on closing the gap between your belly button and spine. Suck in your stomach. Inhale for a 5 count as you slowly return to your starting point. Remember, you're not relaxed at the top because you should still be in spinal flexion. Repeat 10-15 repetitions with 60-90 second rests between each of the 3 sets.

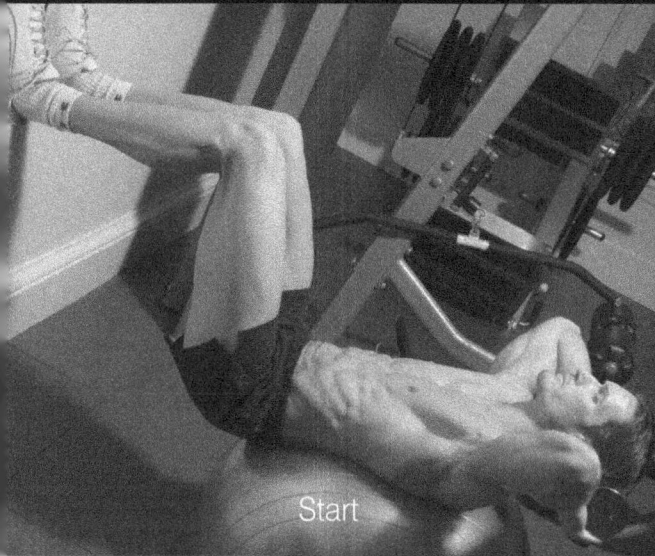
Start

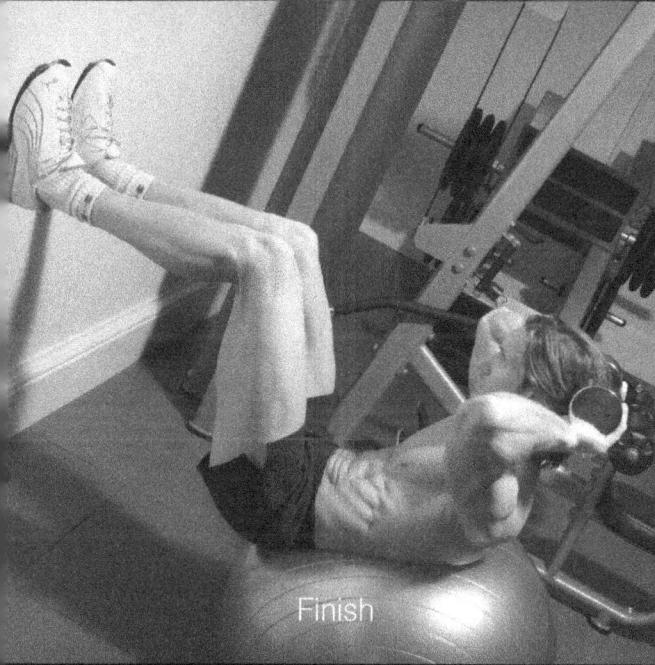
Finish

21. WEIGHTED SWISS BALL CRUNCH *(Upper Rectus Abdominis – Advanced)*

Place a Swiss ball about 3 feet away from the wall and lie back on the ball so that the small of your back is almost at the pinnacle of the ball. Position your feet slightly wider than shoulder width on the wall in front of you. This will require some balance to stabilize on top the ball. Hold the ends of a dumbbell with both hands behind your head. Slightly curl your upper body forward to create a 'C' shape, or spinal flexion. **This is your starting position.** Exhale for a 3 count while curling your upper body forward as your elbows approach your knees. If you curl too far forward, you'll lose the contraction and your abs will be relaxed. If this happens, slightly reverse your curl so that you feel the contraction in your upper rectus abdominis (just below your ribcage). This is your finishing point. From here, continue to exhale all the air from your lungs and squeeze your abs as hard as possible. Inhale for a 5 count as you lower your upper body back to the ball. Perform 12-15 repetitions with 60 second rests between each of the 3 sets.

Start

Finish

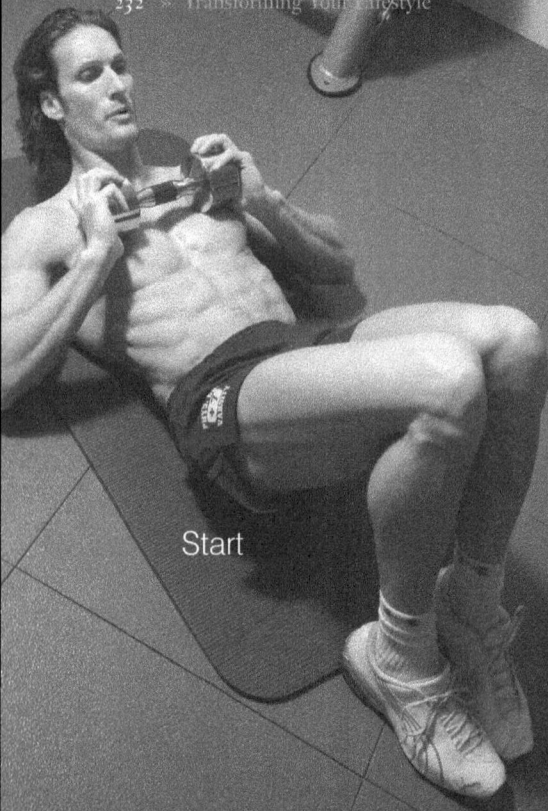

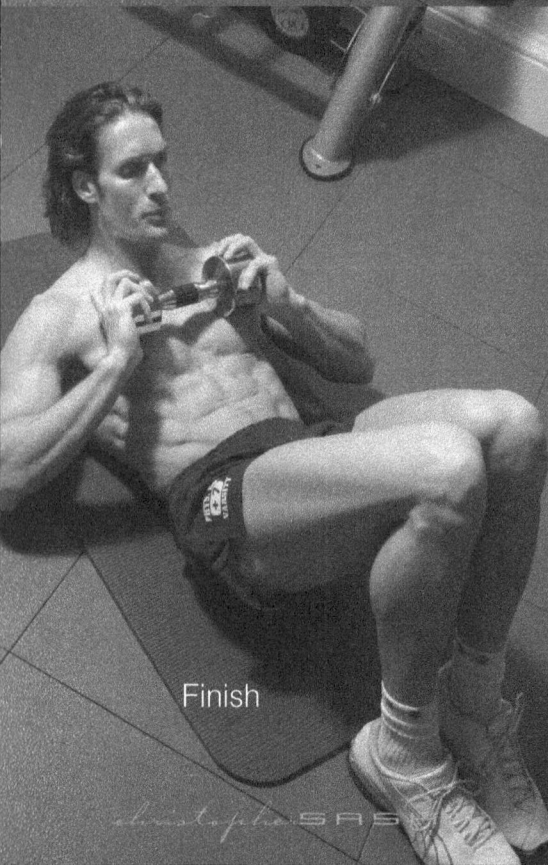

22. SUPINE WEIGHTED CRUNCH
(Upper Rectus Abdominis –Beginner)

Lie supine on the floor with your knees bent and feet flat on the floor. Grab a dumbbell on either end with both hands and place it on your upper chest. Raise your shoulders off the floor so that the small of your back is firmly pressed into the floor. **This is your starting position.** Exhale while curling your upper body up for a 3 count. Don't curl toward your knees; you should try to get your chest toward the ceiling. Once you're as high as you can go, squeeze your abs as hard as possible and continue forcing all the air out of your lungs. Inhale while lowering your upper body toward the floor for a 3 count. Remember not to touch your shoulders on the floor which will promote relaxation in your abs and bring you out of spinal flexion. Perform 10-15 repetitions with 30 second rests between each of the 3 sets.

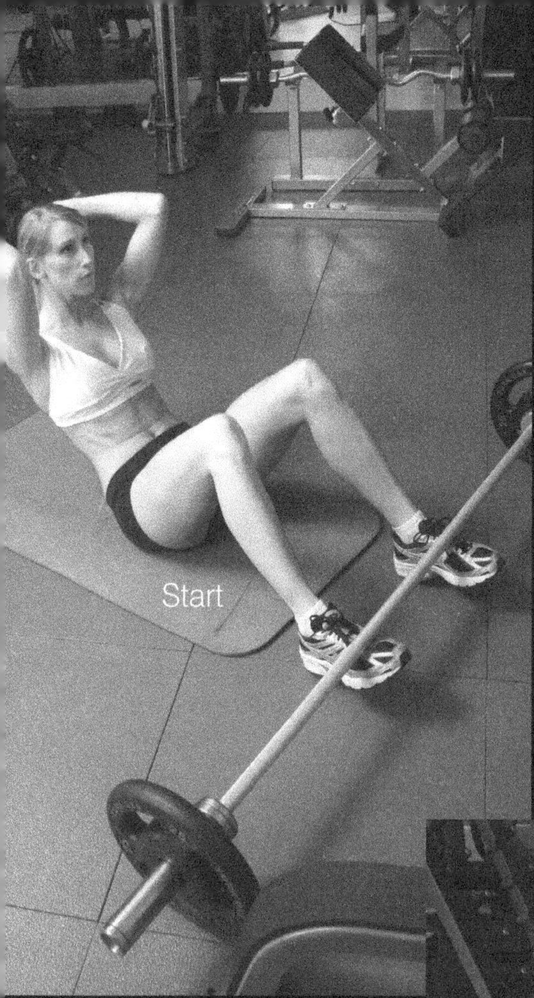

Start

23. TOUCH 'N GO WEIGHTED CRUNCH
(Upper Rectus Abdominis – Moderate)

Place a weighted bar on the floor and sit perpendicular with your knees bent and feet anchored under the bar. Grab a 10 pound plate with both hands and position it behind your head about midpoint of your cranial. Leaning back about 45 degrees, round your shoulders and curl your spine. **This is your starting position.**

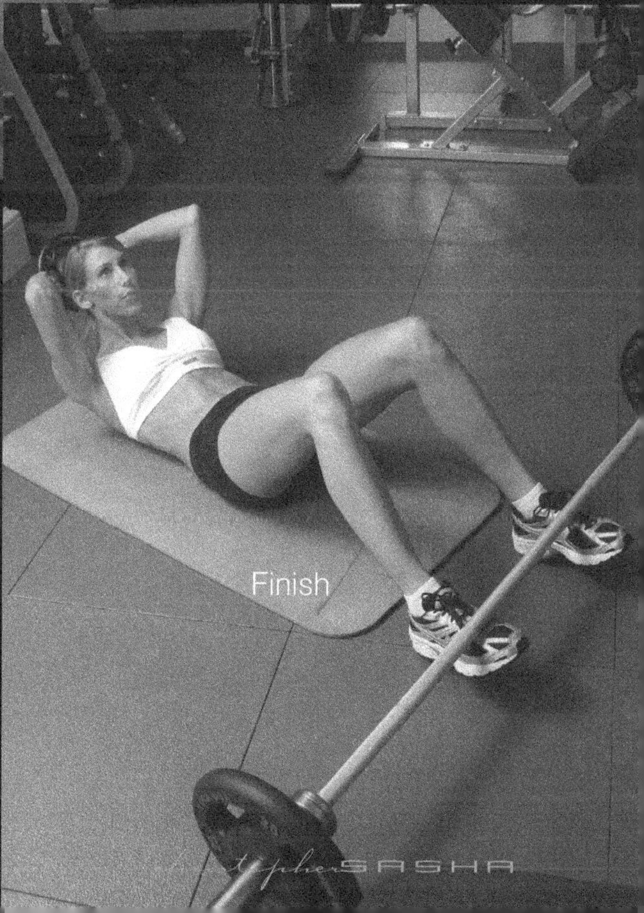

Inhale as you slowly lower your upper body toward the floor for a 3 count. Go to the point where the small of your back just touches the floor; this is your finishing point. This means that you should only go about ¾ of the way down and your shoulders are not touching the floor. Exhale for a 3 count while curling your upper body forward to your starting position. You should not rest at the top until the exercise is complete. Perform 10-15 repetitions with 60 second rests between each of the 3 sets.

Finish

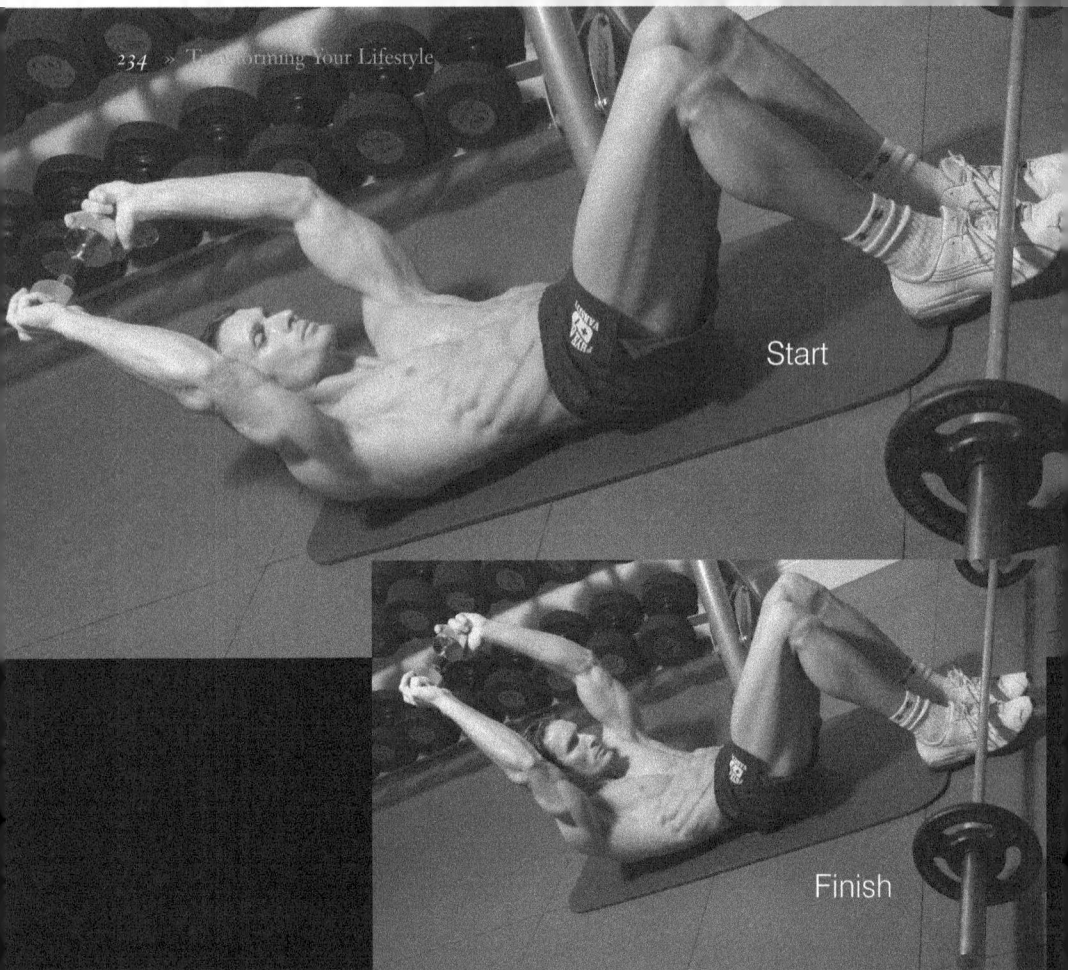

Start

Finish

24. LONG-ARM WEIGHTED CRUNCH
(Upper Rectus Abdominis – Advanced)

Place a weighted bar on the floor and lie supine and perpendicular on the floor with your knees bent and feet anchored under the bar. Grab a dumbbell on either end with both hands and extend your arms above your head so that your arms are beside your ears. Firmly holding the dumbbell, slightly raise your shoulders off the floor so the small of your back is firmly pressed into the floor. **This is your starting position.** Keeping your arms extended beside your head, exhale and curl your upper body toward the ceiling for a 3 count. When you're up as high as you can go, hold and squeeze your abs as hard as possible until all the air is out of your lungs. Inhale for a 3 count while lowering your upper body toward your starting position. Remember, your shoulders should not touch the floor when you're at the bottom so that you maintain spinal flexion. Perform 10-15 repetitions with 60 second rests between each of the 3 sets.

christopherSASHA

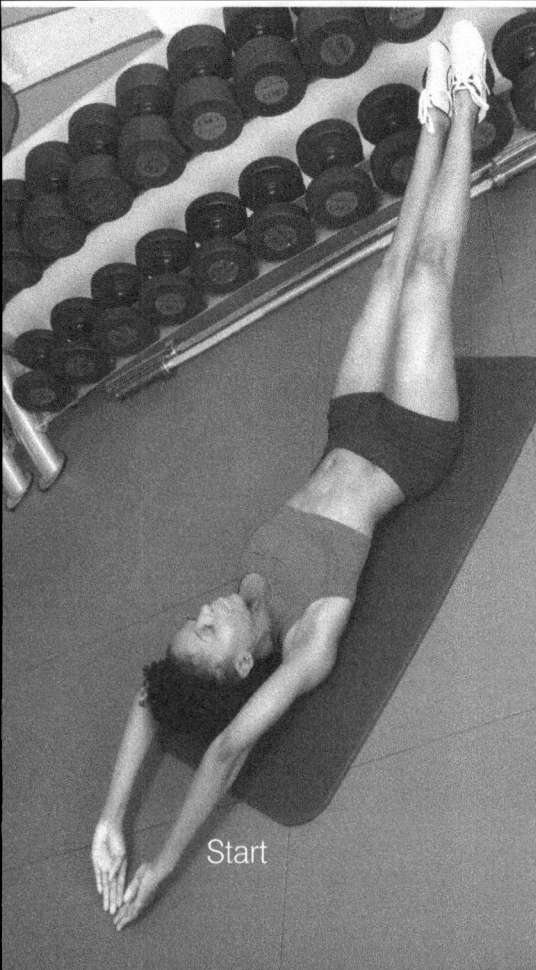
Start

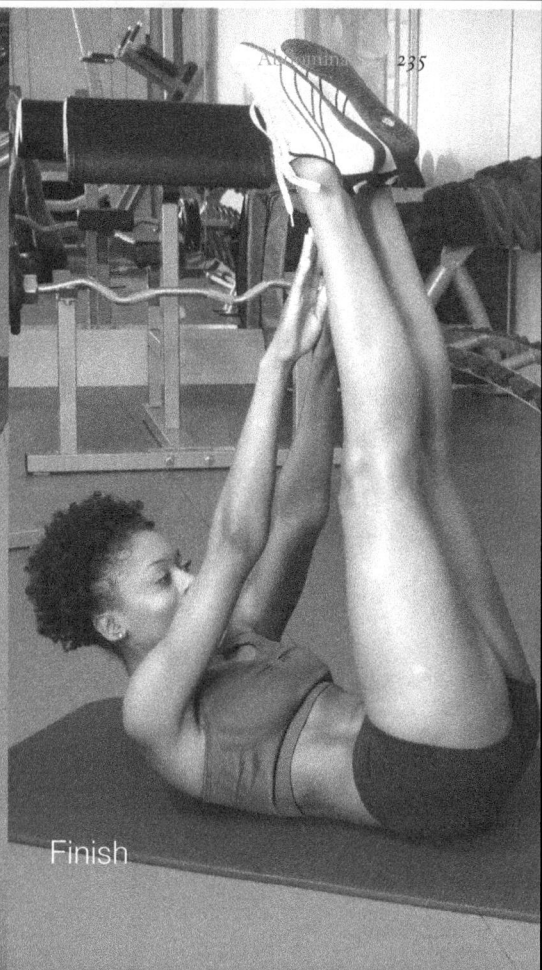

Finish

25. JACKKNIFE CRUNCH
(Upper Rectus Abdominis – Beginner)

Lie supine on the floor with your legs at a 45 degree angle to the floor. Extend your arms above your head so that your arms are beside your ears. Slightly raise your shoulders off the floor so the small of your back is firmly pressed into the floor. **This is your starting position.** Exhale for a 3 count while simultaneously curling your upper body and legs toward the ceiling. Continue reaching your hands and feet toward the ceiling as far as you can while forcing all of the air out of your lungs and squeeze your abs as hard as possible. Inhale for a 3 count as you simultaneously lower your arms and legs toward the floor. At the bottom, the small of your back should be pressed firmly into the floor while your shoulders remain slightly off the mat to maintain spinal flexion. Perform 10-15 repetitions with 60 second rests between each of the 3 sets.

26. ROPE CRUNCH *(Upper Rectus Abdominis – Moderate)*

Connect a rope handle to an adjustable pulley, placing the pulley at the high end of the pulley bar. Palms facing each other, grasp the rope handle with both hands and place them at the temples of your head. Facing the machine, kneel beneath the pulley and slightly curl your spine so that your torso is in a 'C' shape, or spinal flexion. **This is your starting position.** Exhale for a 3 count as you curl your upper body toward your knees. It's important to maintain the angle of your arms throughout this exercise and focus on the movement coming from curling your spine. If you don't feel a contraction at the bottom, you've gone too far. If this happens, slowly come up a little until you do feel a contraction in your abs. This is your finishing point. Once there, force all the air out of your lungs as you squeeze your abs as hard as possible. Inhale for a 3 count as your upper body returns to the top. Remember, at the top, your body should still be in a 'C' shape and you should still feel a contraction in your abs. If you don't feel a contraction in your abs at the top, you've gone too far. Perform 12-15 repetitions with 45 second rests between each of the 3 sets.

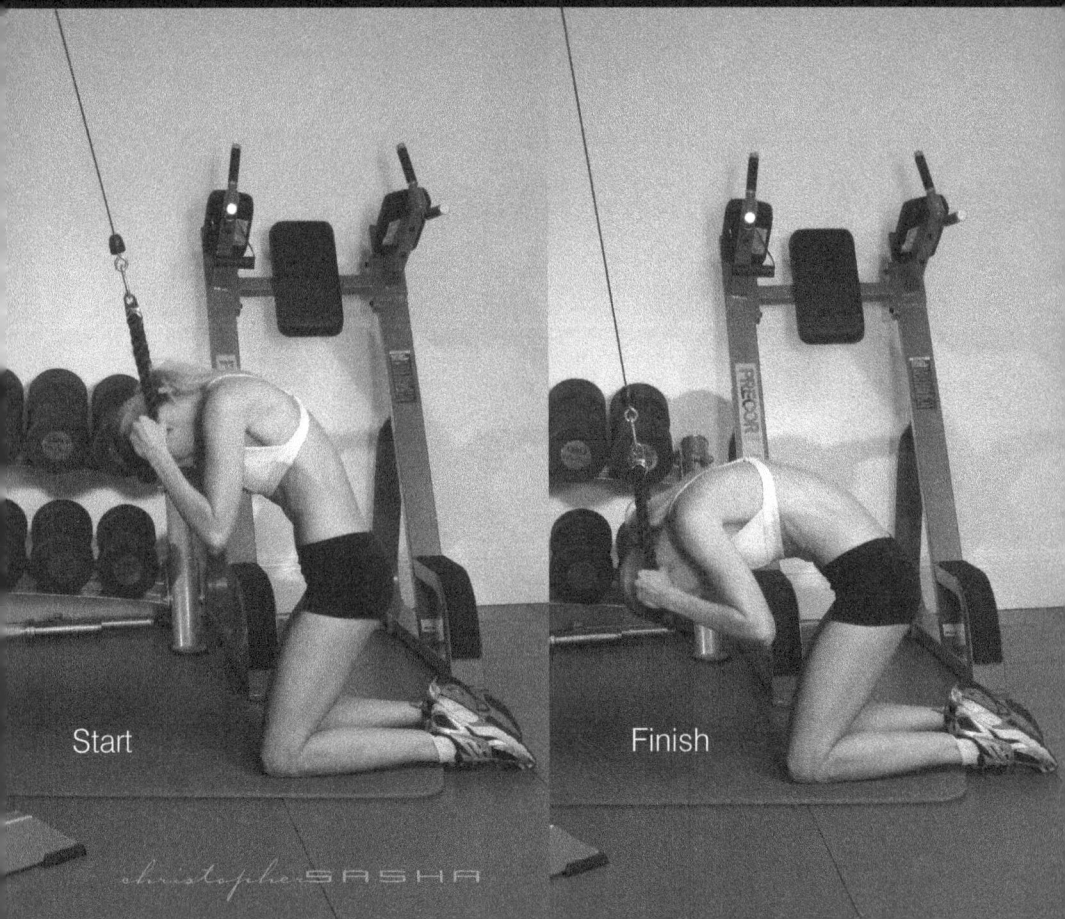

Start

Finish

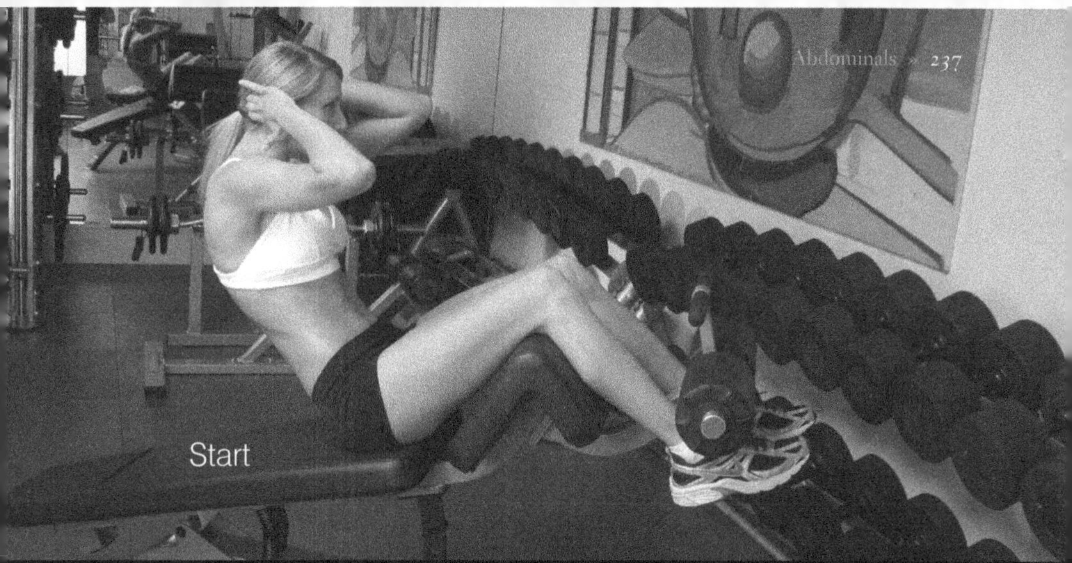

Start

27. DECLINE CRUNCH
(Upper Rectus Abdominis – Advanced)

Set an adjustable decline bench at a 30 degree angle. As you adapt to this exercise, increase the angle (making the decline steeper) to increase the difficulty level. Sit on the bench with your feet anchored under the rollers. Place just your fingertips behind your head but don't interlace your fingers (interlacing your fingers might promote pulling yourself up by your head). Lean back and curl your spine forward until you feel your upper abs (directly below your ribcage) contract. **This is your starting position.** Without changing the curl in your spine, inhale for a 5 count as you lower your upper body as low as you can without touching the bench. Your upper back and shoulders should not touch the bench at any time during this exercise. Once you're as low as you can go, exhale for a 5 count and curl your upper body to your starting position. Your abs should not relax at the top during this exercise. Be careful not to straighten your back during this exercise which may put too much pressure on your lower back. Perform 10-15 repetitions with 30-45 second rests between each of the 3 sets.

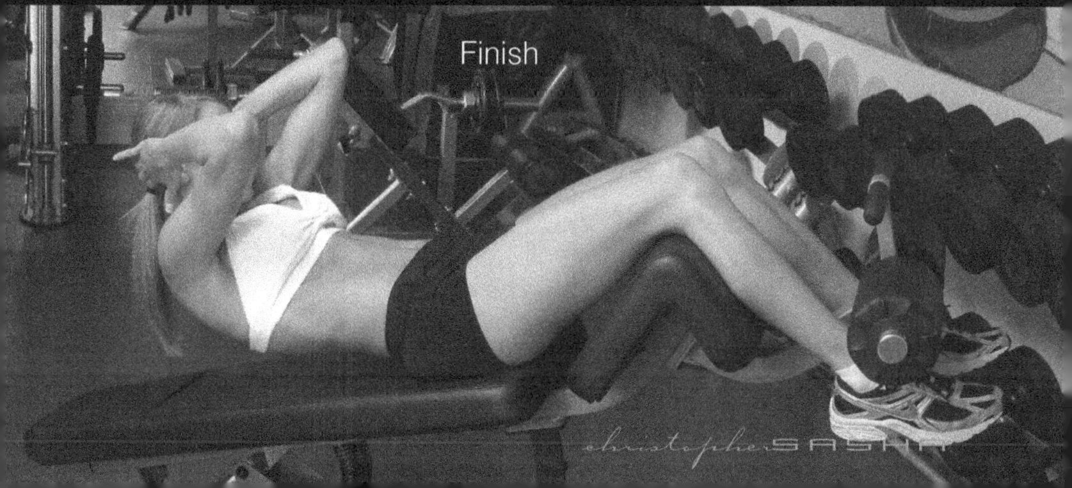

Finish

Start

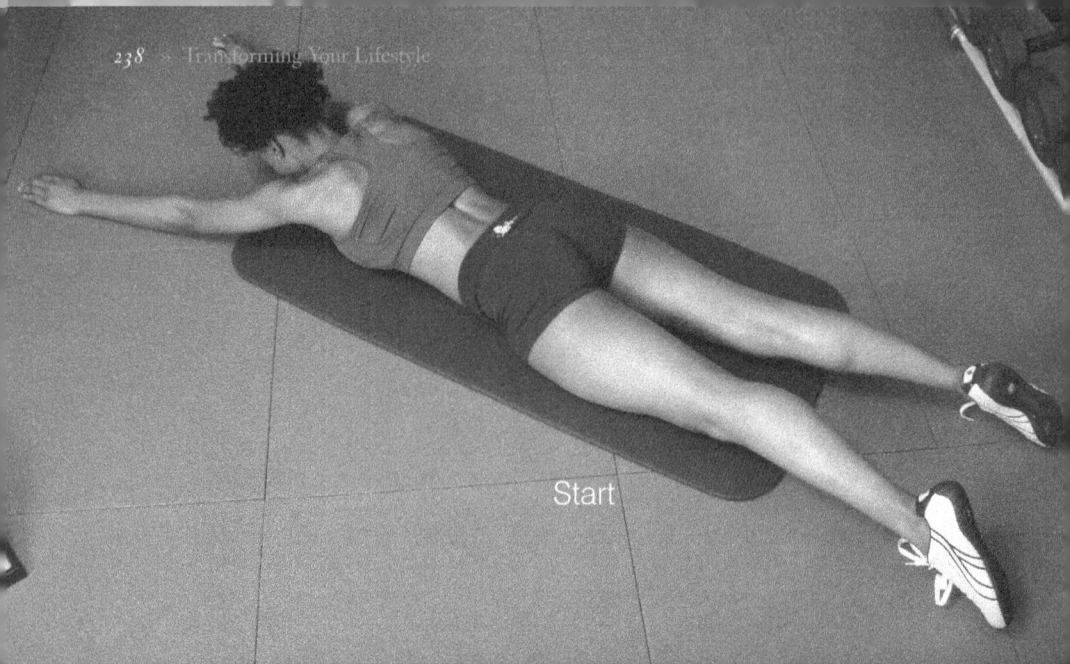

28. SUPERMANS *(Erector Spinae – Beginner)*

Lie prone (face-down) on the floor with your legs fully extended and arms directly above your head (your arms should be beside your ears). **This is your starting position.** Exhale for a 2 count while slowly raising all 4 limbs off the floor as high as possible. Hold the top position for a 2 count then inhale for a 2 count as you slowly lower all 4 limbs to the floor. There should be no rests throughout this exercise. Perform 10-15 repetitions with 15-30 second rests between each of the 2 sets.

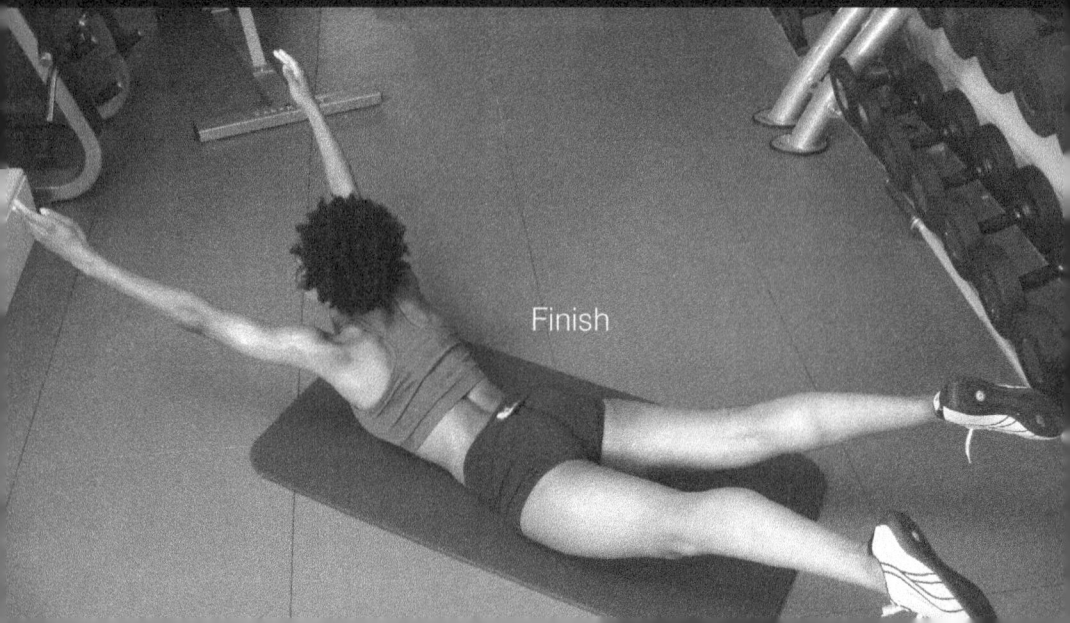

Finish

Start

Finish

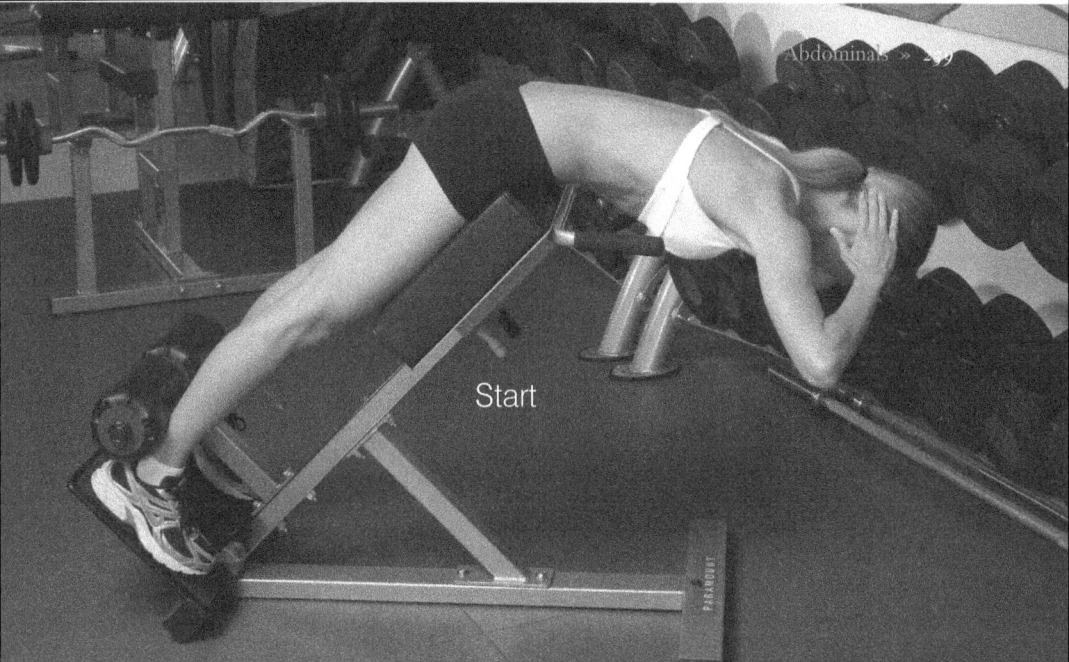

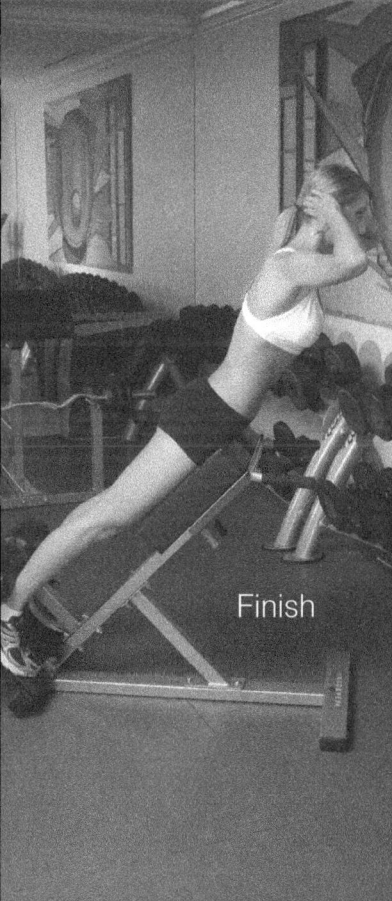

29. ROMAN CHAIR BACK EXTENSIONS
(Erector Spinae – Moderate)

Using a Roman chair, lie prone, with your waistline about 2 inches higher than the hip pad and your heels anchored behind the ankle pads for support. Lean over the hip pad so that your upper body is hanging toward the floor. Place the fingertips of both hands behind your head with your elbows bent and pulled back as far as comfortably possible. **This is your starting position.** Exhale for a 5 count while pulling your upper body up toward the ceiling from your waist by curling your spine backward until your entire body is linear, or at a 45 degree angle. There's no need to go beyond this point. Hold the top position for a 2 count then inhale for a 5 count as you slowly bring your upper body toward the floor. If you feel any pinching or strain in your lower back, stop immediately. Otherwise, perform 10-15 repetitions with 60 second rests between each of the 2 sets.

christopherSASHA

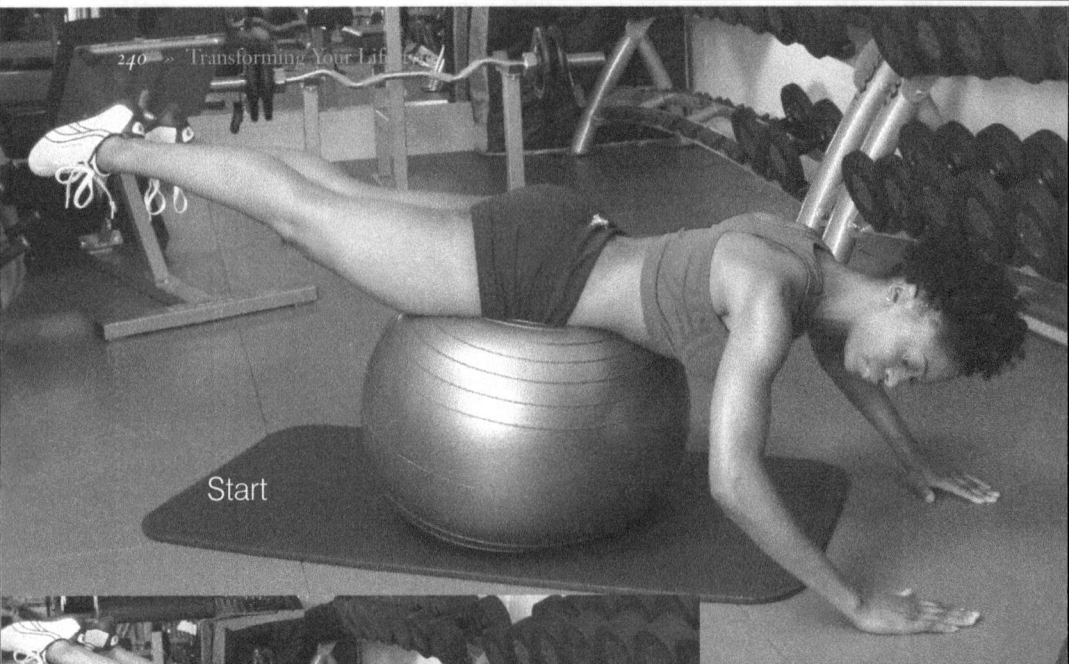
Start

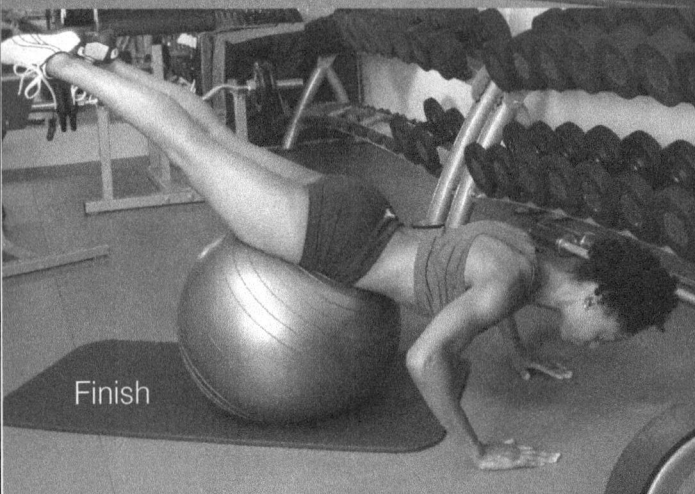
Finish

30. SWISS BALL PRONE LEG LIFTS
(Erector Spinae – Moderate)

Lie prone on a Swiss ball placing your hands shoulder width on the floor in front of you. Pull yourself forward until your waist is on the pinnacle of the ball. You should be in a push-up position with your feet together about 2-3 feet off the floor behind you. **This is your starting position.** Exhale for a 5 count as you pull your legs up toward the ceiling from your waist by curling your spine backward. Your entire body should be at a 45 degree angle. Hold the top position for a 2 count then inhale for a 5 count as you slowly bring your feet toward the floor. Again, if you feel any pinching or strain in your lower back, stop immediately. Otherwise, perform 10-15 repetitions with 60 second rests between each of the 2 sets.

christopherSASHA

31. GOOD MORNINGS
(Erector Spinae – Advanced)

With an overhand grip slightly wider than shoulder width, grab a weighted bar and place it behind your head on your shoulders. Stand erect with your knees slightly bent, feet shoulder width apart and toes pointed straight ahead. **This is your starting position.** Inhale for a 5 count as you slowly bend at your waist and lower your upper body parallel to the floor. You'll feel tension, *never pain*, not only in your lower back but also in the back of your legs – your hamstrings. Exhale for a 5 count as you pull your upper body upward, perpendicular to the floor by curling your spine backward. Perform 10-12 repetitions with 60 second rests between each of the 2 sets.

*CAUTION:

It's extremely important to keep your back straight throughout this exercise. I've seen people pull their backs because they didn't have proper form by arching their backs like a cat during this exercise. Lower your upper body only as far as your body allows while keeping a straight back. Some people may only lower a few inches before their back begins to curl. Others may be able to lower their upper body parallel to the floor while maintaining a straight back. Whatever your range may be, the most important focus is to maintain a straight back. You may only be able to lower a few inches at first, but with practice, you'll be able to increase your range.

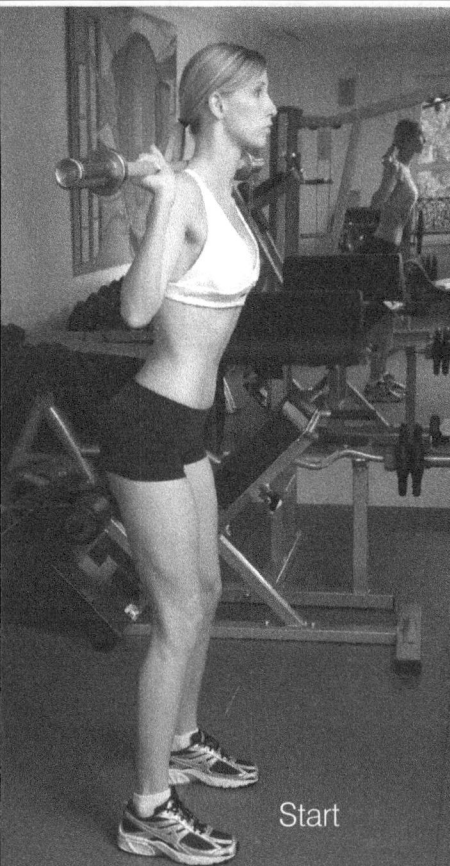

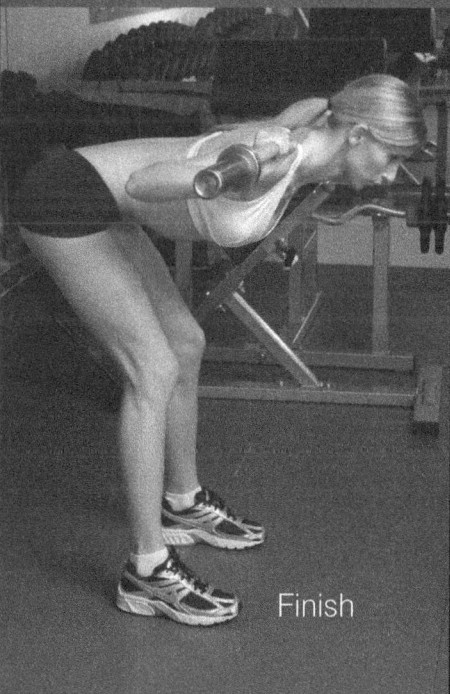

Start

Finish

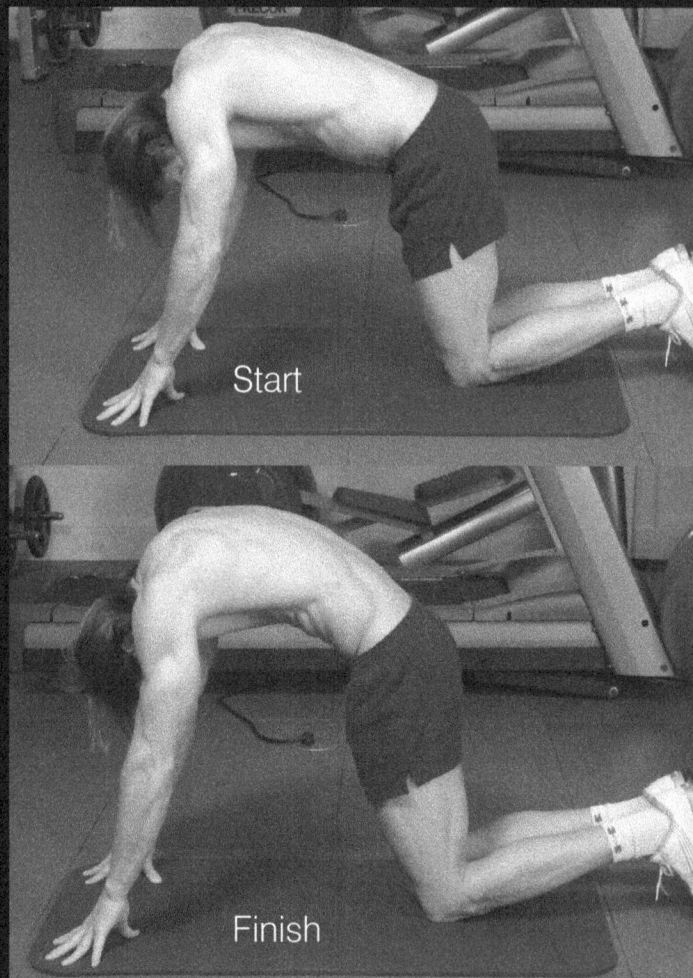

Start

Finish

32. CATS
(Transverse Abdominis)

Each of the aforementioned abdominal exercises work the transverse abdominis, which is the horizontal muscle that acts as a girdle holding your organs together and assisting in the support of your upper body for proper posture. There's a belief that you can decrease the girth of your waist by tightening the transverse abdominis. For this reason, a couple times each week I do an exercise called "cats" which focuses directly on taxing this muscle. **Begin by kneeling on your hands and knees.** As you exhale for a 10 count, round your back by curling your spine as high as possible. After you exhale all the air out of your lungs, slightly tilt your hips forward and pull your belly button in toward your spine as you force even more air out of your lungs. There's always just a little more air you can get out by really forcing it out. Inhale for a 2 count as you release the tension from your midsection. Don't rest between repetitions. Perform 10 repetitions with 30 second rests between each of the 3 sets.

Resistance training has many health benefits including increasing muscle mass to increase your metabolism and burn more body fat, keeping your joints aligned to help alleviate body pain, and helping maintain/improve bone density to help dodge the bone disease, osteoporosis. But we also need to keep our *hearts and lungs* strong by including a cardiovascular routine in our new and improved lifestyle. There are different cardio intensity levels which produce different results. Are you getting the results you want from your current cardio workout? If not, let's explore why you may not be.

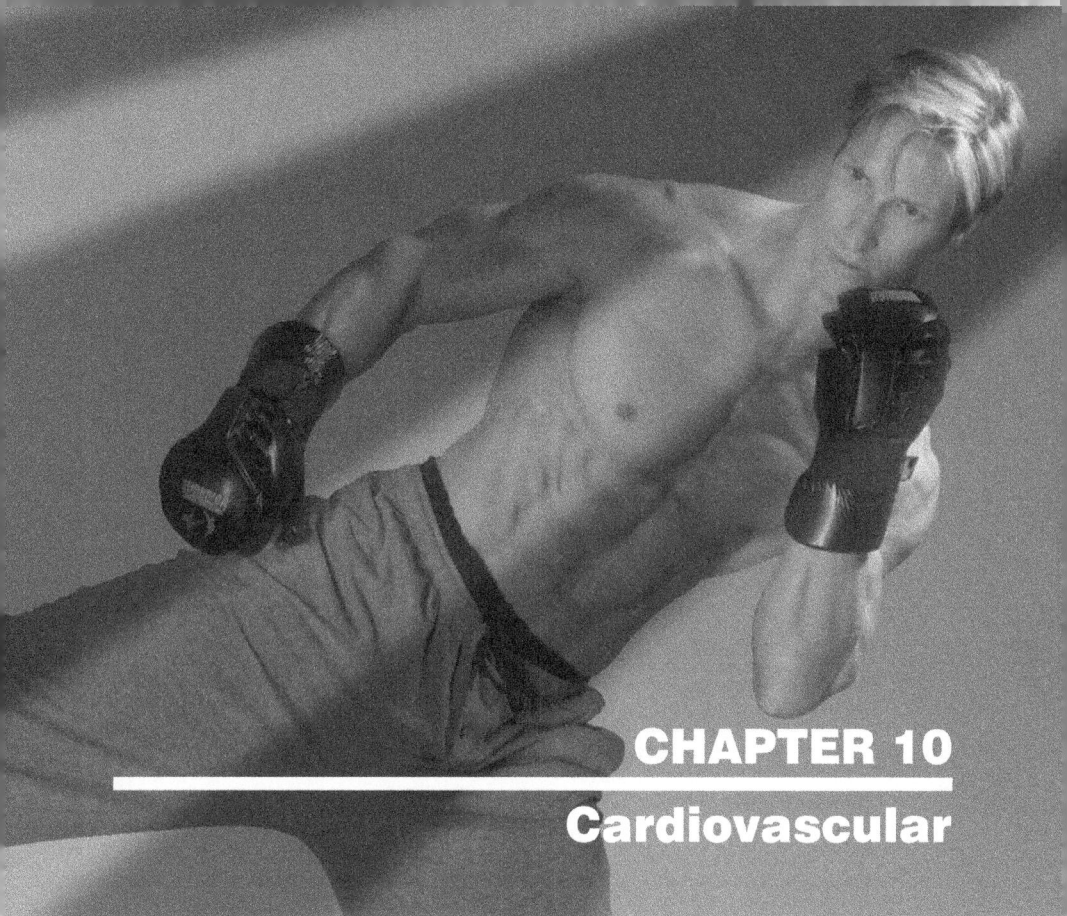

CHAPTER 10
Cardiovascular

One of the most important contributors to a healthy body, both inside and out, is a cardiovascular regimen. Cardio workouts burn body fat, strengthen the heart and lungs, and lower the resting heart rate. There are a variety of different activities that can be classified as "cardio." If you're one of those people who get bored easily and feel like a gerbil on a wheel getting nowhere fast doing traditional routines, get creative and get away from the rowing machines, ellipticals, treadmills, and stationary bikes. Instead, dance, take the stairs instead of the elevator, or buy a dog so you're forced to take a couple of walks every day. Maybe try jumping rope with your child – you'll burn approximately 135 calories in 10 minutes just jumping over that silly little string. Since the movie *Million Dollar Baby*, boxing has become very popular and many women have explored this sport as an option for their cardio workouts.

Let's face it. If you dread the walk towards any cardio machine, chances are you'll start looking for

> You don't have to work out on a piece of stationary equipment to increase your heart rate and burn calories and fat.

excuses to eliminate this essential aspect of weight management. No one ever said that you had to work out on a piece of stationary equipment to increase your heart rate and burn calories and fat. A lot of people do like using these cardio monsters, and that's great – for them. The point is to move however you like – and make physical activity a part of your lifestyle.

Benefits of Cardio

The advantages of cardio aren't limited to just burning fat and increasing the heart rate to help improve circulation. Other extras include improving "good" cholesterol (HDL) levels, increasing blood flow to the brain for alertness, increasing the metabolic rate, and reducing the everyday stress and anxiety which is commonplace in our fast-paced world. Cardio also increases the size and number of blood vessels which are the highways for oxygen and nutrients as they make their way to organ tissues, including muscles. Aerobics, cardiovascular exercise, or just plain "cardio" all have the same meaning. (If you use the word "aerobics", however, you just might be showing your age. That term hasn't been popular since the '80s!)

By sticking with a cardio program, you build the strength of your lungs to process more oxygen more efficiently, which means your heart will pump more blood with less beats, leading to an increase of blood supply to your muscles so they can work longer without becoming fatigued. Learning to do this process properly takes time. Your endurance may be low when you first embark on a cardio workout but it will increase with perseverance ...*I promise*. At first, you might feel exhausted while doing the exercise and immediately afterward, but it won't be long before your stamina increases and you benefit from the endorphins (hormones in the brain that help you relax and reduce pain, stress, anxiety, and depression) your body releases from regular cardio exercises.

> Your endurance may be low when you first embark on a cardio workout but it will increase with perseverance.

When I first included cardio in my training schedule, I decided to start with the StairMaster. In the early '90s, a friend of mine suggested I do a workout with him, which consisted of 30 minutes on this beast of a machine. As much as I wanted to impress him with my strength *and* stamina and determination, I could only muster enough energy to keep up with him for 3 minutes. After that, I laid curled in a little ball on the floor sucking wind for about 10 minutes. I thought I was a failure … until he told me that he respected me for trying my hardest. That day, I learned that everyone has to start somewhere. A few months later I had increased my endurance and was able to keep up with him for the full 30 minutes.

As the years passed, I've also realized that I don't catch colds or the flu as often. This is probably not coincidence. There are studies showing that regular cardio exercises help the immune system to fight off infections.

Aerobic vs. Anaerobic

One of the most frequently asked questions I get from fledgling exercisers is: "What's the difference between aerobic and anaerobic?" Aerobic activities are any exercises that coerce the heart and lungs to work harder for an extended period of time. In general, cardio involves large muscle groups (legs and arms). Exercising large muscles causes you to breathe harder, which makes your heart work harder to pump blood throughout your body. Cardio, therefore, improves the efficiency of your heart.

Here's the BIG BONUS associated with cardio…when keeping your heart rate between 60%-70% of your maximum heart rate (discussed on pages 248-251), fat becomes your body's primary fuel source (with carbohydrates and proteins being used to a lesser degree). Burning fat requires oxygen, so if you're breathing deeply and getting more oxygen delivered to your muscle cells, the cells will burn more fat to perform the exercise. Think of how a fire grows   it requires oxygen. The more oxygen, the bigger the fire. And without oxygen, the fire goes out. Our bodies also require oxygen to burn fat.

Anaerobic literally means "without oxygen." Anaerobic activities work against the force of gravity and promote strong bones which help

Aerobic activities are any exercises that coerce the heart and lungs to work harder for an extended period of time.

prevent osteoporosis and bone fractures. These activities last for less than a minute and do not require oxygen. Therefore these types of exercises (heavy weightlifting, short sprints) will not utilize fat as the primary fuel source. Rather, glucose and glycogen (carbohydrates stored in muscles and the liver that convert to glucose to be used as energy) are the driving forces in these activities. Benefits of anaerobic exercises include agility, muscle strength, and toning.

Maximum Heart Rate (MHR)

"Low-intensity," "moderate-intensity," "high-intensity" – what *do* these terms mean?

There are different levels of aerobic activities that utilize varying amounts of fat as a percentage of total calories burned during an exercise. "Low-intensity" exercise (walking, for example) would be if you could do the exercise while singing and talking without any effort. "Low-intensity" involves using somewhere between 50%-65% of your maximum heart rate (MHR) – more on this in a moment. "Moderate-intensity" (jogging, for example) requires a little more exertion on your part and brings your heart rate between 66%-79% MHR. This level of activity means that you won't be able to sing your favorite tunes or speak aloud without forcing the words out of your mouth. Finally, "High-intensity" (sprinting at full throttle, for example) can range between 80%-90% MHR. This level of intensity requires experience and is obviously not recommend for anyone just embarking on an exercise regime.

Each method, or intensity level, has benefits that work best for different people with different personal goals. For example, I use the low-to-moderate level for beginners and obese individuals because it's easier on the joints and can be done for a longer period of time. The elliptical is the perfect piece of cardio equipment because it mimics walking or stair climbing with little or no impact on the joints. Also, if you have access to a swimming pool, try swimming because it has no impact on the joints. I'm a huge fan of using a low-intensity cardio program as an *active recovery exercise* after an intense weight training workout. I mentioned before that aerobic activities require oxygen and encourage blood flow throughout the body. When oxygen is carried through the body, the size of the blood vessels increase. They carry the oxygen and nutrients to the muscles, promoting muscle growth and repair.

For more athletic and capable clients, I like to use high-intensity interval activities which require coordination and endurance. My favored cardio equipment for this is the treadmill, with a 15 degree incline and a top speed of 10 miles per hour. Occasionally I also use the elliptical and stationary bike. The goal is to get the heart rate in the 80-90 percent range. This method will increase your metabolic rate, will burn more fat by burning more total calories in a shorter period of time, and, in the long run, will help prevent osteoporosis.

Your Maximum Heart Rate (MHR) is 220 minus your age.

Let's calculate your personal MHR. As a very general rule of thumb, you can derive your MHR by subtracting your current age from 220. There's a more detailed formula which includes your resting heart rate but most people don't know what their resting heart rate is. So, for the sake of simplicity, let's use the general rule of thumb. The MHR for a person who is 38-years-old would be 182, for example. Then, to determine the desired intensity level, multiply your MHR by the percentage of each method. For quick heart rate zone calculations, go to www.fitbodiesbysasha.com.

Example:	220 – 38 (age) = 182		
Low-intensity	182 x .50 = 91	182 x .60 = 109	182 x .65 = 118
Moderate-intensity	182 x .66 = 120	182 x .75 = 137	182 x .79 = 144
High-intensity	182 x .80 = 146	182 x .85 = 155	182 x .90 = 164

Basically, the maximum heart rate is the highest amount of times your heart can safely beat in one minute. The calculation was formulated to help people exercise at a safe level. In the above chart I used the general and widely-used formula for tabulating an individual's maximum heart rate. But there can be a differentiation of plus or minus 15 points due to the fact that not everyone at the same age has the same-sized heart, blood pressure, stroke volume (the amount of blood ejected from the left ventricle of the heart in a single beat), etc. However, this calculation gives a good general estimate. Remember also that the maximum heart rate will decrease with age.

I use a relatively new high-intensity cardio method called High Intensity Interval Training (HIIT) in which I work to get my heart rate up to 95% of my maximum heart rate. For me, the easiest way to do this is by using the treadmill, but you can use the elliptical, rowing machine, stationary bicycle, or anything else you feel comfortable using. I warm up for five minutes by walking for two minutes, jogging for two minutes, and then walking again for another minute. This assures me that I have gradually increased my heart rate and heated the muscles thoroughly and I'm now ready for the "real" workout.

According to the American College of Sports Medicine (ACSM), both a warm-up and cool-down period is recommended for all aerobic training sessions. Warm-up periods prepare the body for exercise by gradually increasing the heart rate, heating the muscles for better flexibility which will decrease the risk of injuries like muscle strains and tears, and increasing blood flow to the muscles. Remember, oxygen and nutrients are carried via blood throughout the body, helping fuel energy in our muscles. Likewise, a cool-down period is necessary after a vigorous workout. While you're exercising, your muscles become fuller with blood and oxygen. If you abruptly stop exercising, the blood in the muscles could accumulate, blocking oxygen, which could result in a heart attack.

I put a 3 degree incline on the treadmill to reduce shock to my joints and run 10 miles per hour, which equates to a 6-minute mile. A cycle consists of running at this speed for one minute, then walking at 3 miles per hour for two minutes. It doesn't sound like much but try it! This gets the heart pumping in no time and I get both anaerobic *and* aerobic benefits. While sprinting I'm forcing my muscles to work harder and I don't get much oxygen in my lungs, so I'm doing an anaerobic workout. Then I walk at 3 miles per hour, at which time I'm able to breathe to let the oxygen carry the nutrients to my muscles. So I'm also getting the benefits of an aerobic workout at the same time. I repeat the cycle for 20 minutes …and am exhausted beyond belief. Then I walk for 5 minutes to get my heart rate down to about 100 beats per minute.

Make a game of it and increase the intensity each week.

This method is strenuous and requires common sense and caution. Please be smart and responsible by starting at a sensible pace. Make a game of it and increase the intensity each week. As always, consult with your family physician before starting any type of exercise program.

HIIT differs from traditional cardio in that your body never hits a "steady state." With a traditional cardio workout, you stay

Staying at a steady state while performing cardio allows your body to adjust itself to the energy you're exerting while conserving calories at that pace.

christopherSASHA

at a constant pace, allowing your body to adjust itself to the energy you're exerting, and then conserving calories at that pace. HIIT utilizes different exertion levels, preventing your body from going into the steady state. This forces your body to use the maximum amount of calories to sustain its energy needs.

Benefits from the HIIT cardio method include:

- burning more calories (including fat) due to increasing your metabolism for a longer period of time than with traditional cardio,
- increasing your VO_2Max (maximal oxygen consumption) so fat can utilize more oxygen to burn itself.

If you try this method, set the speed at a pace which helps get your heart rate to at least 85% of your maximum heart rate and do it for a shorter duration. For instance, if a speed of 4 miles per hour gets your heart rate up to 85% and you can only perform this exercise for 5 minutes before being completely exhausted, then this would be your starting point. Then slowly increase the speed and time to bump up your heart rate. Remember, it takes time to build endurance and stamina.

Preparing for the Underwear Advertisements…

In the modeling world, your booker only gives you a day or so to get ready for a go-see (audition) for the hiring client. I usually get a phone call from my agency in the afternoon a day or two before a go-see for either underwear or swimsuits, which always stresses me because I always think I can be in better shape than I am whenever these auditions arise. The busy time for modeling in Chicago is from April until September. I usually start a strict cardio regime in March so all I have to do is fine-tune my body when the go-sees start.

I know that in order to benefit the most from cardio, you need to mix and match low-and-moderate-intensity with high-intensity cardio. This strategy has proven itself time and again for me – and for my clients.

Starting in March, and for the next 8 weeks, I get to the gym early, before eating anything, and ride the stationary bike for 30 minutes. I'm still half asleep as I pedal at a pace that resembles slow-motion. I have a half gallon of water with the juice of a medium-sized lemon squeezed in it with me which I drink constantly while I'm pedaling. I don't want to dehydrate because that causes the metabolism to slow down. Every 5 minutes I drink some water which will help burn my body fat.

I specifically go slow to keep my heart rate around 65% of my MHR so I can breathe and get oxygen to my muscles. The theory is that I've been fasting while sleeping the past 8 hours. So my body should be low on glucose, glycogen, and insulin, forcing it to use fat as the main energy source. *CAUTION: Be very careful at this point. Your body is in a catabolic state (starvation mode) first thing in the morning. It's performing a biochemical process called gluconeogenesis. Your liver converts protein (muscle tissue) into glucose to survive. If you hit the cardio too hard, you won't get the oxygen your body needs and it'll use less fat and more glucose as energy. And the glucose that your body uses at this point is not from carbohydrates but from muscle tissue that's being converted to glucose. In essence, you'll be burning muscle – exactly what we don't want to do.*

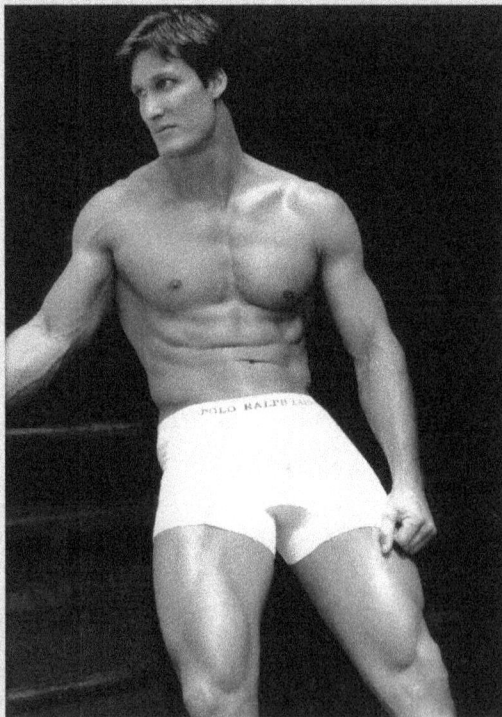

At night, I do another 30-minute cardio session. This time it's the high-intensity aerobic exercise that I explained earlier.

Within 8 weeks, I can drop 15 pounds and get my body fat around 3.5%. Now I'm ready for the auditions and just have to do a little fine-tuning when my booker calls me.

Estimated Calories Burned Per Hour

Everyone burns calories at a different rate, depending upon certain variables. For example, a male who weighs 190 pounds, with a large percentage of muscle mass, a high metabolism, and a high-intensity workout is going to burn more calories than a 120-pound female doing a low-intensity workout. The purpose here is to give a rough estimate of the amount of calories burned per hour for a variety of exercises. I've chosen to use a "moderate-intensity" level for a male weighing 170 pounds. If you weigh more than 170 pounds, you're more likely to burn more calories, and vice versa. Generally, women have less muscle mass than men, so the amount of calories burned during an hour of moderate-intensity exercise for a woman who weighs 170 pounds is still going to be a little less than a male weighing the same.

EXERCISE	CALORIES PER HOUR
Bicycling, stationary	549
Boxing (punching heavy bag)	470
Dancing (general)	353
Elliptical Trainer	668
Fencing	470
House Cleaning (general)	274
Jumping Rope	788
Rowing, stationary	549
Treadmill, running (5 mph)	627
StairMaster	646
Swimming (breaststroke)	784
Walking (3 mph)	274

Cardio Before or After the Workout?

Is cardio better to do before or after the workout? As with most controversial questions, the answer depends. If your primary goal is to gain muscle or maintain the muscle you already have, I would suggest doing cardio after your workout. Here's why. Your body is freshest before your workout and you have an abundant amount of glucose in your bloodstream just waiting to be put to use. You'll be able to take advantage of

A low-intensity cardio exercise after your workout should burn mostly fat.

christopherSASHA

this by working out at a higher intensity level to obtain the best results. As you continue your routine, you exhaust the amount of glucose and glycogen stored in your muscles. When you hit a low-intensity cardio exercise after your workout, you should be burning mostly fat.

Human Growth Hormone

Besides glucose and glycogen, the other factor to consider when planning your workout is human growth hormone (hGH) levels. Human growth hormones are produced in the pituitary gland in the brain. Everyone has different amounts of this minuscule protein substance that is generally abundant in our youth but wanes as we age. Human growth hormone is a critical contributor to growth, cell reproduction, lowering the amount of body fat, and metabolism which may be why it's plentiful in our youth.

Growth spurts and a high metabolism are associated with adolescence,

> Growth spurts and a high metabolism are associated with adolescence when larger amounts of growth hormones are produced.

when larger amounts of growth hormones are produced. Growth hormones are generated shortly after the onset of deep sleep and after exercise, then dissipate within a few moments. During this timeframe, they trigger the liver to secrete Insulin-like Growth Factor (IGF-1), which may be the catalyst to the more direct effect in muscle growth. Generally speaking, growth hormones activate protein synthesis (building of proteins) which forces fat to be burned and used as energy. Variables like sleep, exercise, nutrition, and stress all play a role in the production of growth hormones.

I feel growth hormone levels also play a role in deciding the best time to do cardio. A study in Japan concluded that growth hormone levels increased a fair amount after a cardio session but *increased three times more after a resistance training session.* Since human growth hormone is a dynamic anabolic hormone, it makes sense to do cardio *after* your lifting routine when you undertake both on the same day – especially if your primary goal is to maximize muscle growth.

Intensity Levels

The type of cardio and the amount of time you spend doing it depends on your personal goals. Whatever your objective may be, I believe preserving muscle should be imperative. Muscle increases your metabolism which forces your body to burn more calories and gives it less chance to store calories as fat. Let's keep this short and sweet by working with the three cardio intensity levels I mentioned earlier….low, moderate, and high.

1. Low-intensity

I use this method for obese individuals or those who are just beginning an exercise regimen. It's very easy on joints and can be done for a long period of time. It won't burn as many total calories as the other methods, but it will help burn fat at a slow and steady pace. I also use this method for my clients who compete in amateur bodybuilding. They do a low-intensity cardio workout first thing in the morning before having anything to eat. As I stated earlier, the body has been fasting overnight. By the time the person wakes up in the morning, glucose and insulin levels should be low, causing the main source of fuel to be fat.

Ideally, your heart rate should be in the 50%-65% range of your maximum heart rate (MHR), which will make you burn more total calories from fat without stressing the body. Although any aerobic activity will do, I would recommend either walking on the treadmill or riding the stationary bike. Both are in a controlled environment where it's easy to maintain a constant pace. About 30 minutes will suffice.

This early cardio session doesn't mean that you can't benefit by doing another 30-minute session later during the day, however. In general, low-intensity cardio will make you healthier and help you recover from workouts quicker because it boosts blood flow and augments the size of blood vessels to help repair muscles.

2. Moderate-Intensity

This level is a little more stressful and will burn more total calories than the low-intensity level. The bad news is that it won't burn as high of a percentage of calories of fat from total calories. The good news is that it doesn't consume as much time. I try to limit moderate-intensity cardio sessions to between 20-30 minutes jogging on the treadmill with a 3 degree incline to reduce the impact on joints. While in this zone, try to keep your heart rate between 65%-75% MHR; otherwise, you start to venture into the anabolic zone. The moderate-intensity level utilizes more carbohydrates and protein than fat as a main energy source. Moderate-intensity will increase your stamina as well as your metabolism for a longer period of time than the low-intensity level.

3. High-Intensity

I categorize this zone of intensity between 80%-90% MHR. Others argue that this percentage is too high, putting you in the anabolic zone, which is the complete inverse of the aerobic zone – and defeating the purpose of using cardio to burn fat. The lower your intensity level, the more *percentage* of fat from *total* calories will be burned. I believe this, but I also believe when your heart rate is between 80%-90% MHR you burn many more calories – *including more fat.*

I use a myriad of activities with this type of cardio training … the StairMaster, rowing machines, stationary bikes, and boxing. My most frequent method is hitting the heavy bag for 3 minutes. That brings my heart rate to 90% MHR, then I do reverse crunches (page 217) for 3 minutes to decrease my heart rate to 70% MHR. I would suggest no more than 20-30 minutes with any of these activities. Believe me, you'll be ready to hit the shower by then.

With high-intensity cardio you benefit by:

- getting your cardio done in much less time while burning more total calories,
- draining glycogen that needs to be replenished, giving your body less chance to store new fat,
- greatly increasing your metabolism – estimated to last a few hours after the workout, referred to as the "after burn."

Our bodies are constantly alternating between anabolic (building) and catabolic (breaking down) phases. It's called protein turnover and it's a normal part of life. During our workouts, our bodies are breaking down then rebuilding to make us stronger and healthier. This is why it's so important to eat right after a workout – to put our bodies back into an anabolic state.

It's called protein turnover – relax, it's a normal part of life.

Our bodies will utilize the calories to replace muscle glycogen and repair themselves. Unless you go crazy and stuff yourself to the point of blowing up, I wouldn't worry about new fat being stored. Of course we're also talking about eating healthy foods (lean protein and good carbs and fats), not hot dogs, beer, and chips. Just because you did a workout, doesn't mean it's open season to eat junk food as a means to refuel the body!

Timing and Duration

Whatever your goals may be, the most important thing to remember is to have fun. If you're having fun while doing any type of activity, you're more apt to do it often. And this is the goal: making physical activity a part of your everyday life. Right?!

The other consideration is that you don't have to do an hour workout all at one time. In our hectic schedules, few of us have a "spare" hour to set aside. Break your workout into two sessions. If you only have 30 minutes in the morning before heading off to work, squeeze another 30 minutes in after work or during your lunch break. Split your routine by doing cardio in the morning and resistance training after work. The advantage is that you'll actually benefit more from the split because you'll fire up your metabolism for some time after each workout, burning more calories than if you did a one-hour session alone.

I'm a strong advocate of doing cardio first thing in the morning before you have anything to eat. Study upon study has found that people who work out in the morning, usually stick to a routine and work out the majority of days during the week. Also, as the day progresses, responsibilities tend to pile up and exercise gets put on the backburner. More often than not, it never gets the attention it deserves. Don't forget about the endorphins like serotonin that are released to make you feel like a million bucks or that your metabolic rate increases for hours after you're done with the workout...meaning that you'll burn more calories afterwards. If that isn't enough, a study at Kansas State University found that when cardio is done in the morning after a 12 hour fast, 67% of total calories burned are from fat compared to when the same exercise is performed later in the day and/or after eating when food is still being digested.

Does Cardio Metabolize Muscle?

Of course there's the whole controversy as to whether or not cardio metabolizes muscle. In my opinion, formed both scholastically and through 13 years of experience, cardio can, *in certain circumstances*, metabolize muscle. I've experimented with a myriad of diet and exercise programs. I've had tremendous results with some programs; others, not so much. *Transforming*

Too much cardio at a high-intensity level will metabolize muscle.

Your Lifestyle has gotten me down to 3.3% body fat. I have consistently hit the 3.5% body fat range every time I've employed my strategies. In general, *under normal conditions*, cardio should not metabolize muscle. However, there are negative conditions (poor diet, too much cardio) that, when combined on a frequent basis, can cause cardio to metabolize muscle.

To avoid this, keep in mind the advantages of morning cardio, when the physiological environment is at its most perfect to metabolize mostly fat. The two major rules to remember at this point are to keep your heart rate between 50%-65% of your maximum heart rate (low-intensity range), and keep your session about 30 minutes. As we've learned, while sleeping, your body has been in a starvation mode, not having been fed any nutrients for 8 hours. It's been converting muscle tissue into glucose in order to perform its many functions to keep you alive. By keeping your cardio session short and at a low intensity, you'll be breathing in plenty of oxygen so your body will use less glucose and more fat as energy.

Cardio exercise can metabolize muscle if:

- performed at a high-intensity level for too long of a period,
- you have a poor diet,
- you perform cardio too often.

As an example, when I get ready for any modeling photo shoot, I get my body fat measured before I bump up my cardio. The results of my body fat measurements show too much cardio at a high-intensity level will metabolize muscle tissue. I started weighing in at 190 pounds with 7.5% body fat. I wanted to get into the 3% range so I bumped up my cardio by riding my bike to and from work twice each day, every day. It was a 35-minute bike ride in each direction, for a total of 2 hours and 20 minutes every day. My average heart rate was 156 beats per minute, or 85% of my maximum heart rate. Within 6 weeks I weighed 178 pounds with 3.3% body fat. **I lost over 3 pounds of muscle in 6 weeks.** I also increased my caloric intake by the amount of extra calories I was burning from the additional cardio. Cardio can metabolize muscle!

Rehydrate

Whether you're playing a sport or doing cardio, remember to drink approximately 5 ounces of liquids every 15 minutes to rehydrate your body. By imbibing smaller amounts more frequently, your body will process and utilize fluids more efficiently, keeping you fully hydrated. Wolfing down a half gallon at one time compels your body to expel what it can't utilize. As discussed in Chapter 8, try drinking cold water whenever possible. Research suggests the body absorbs cold water into the system more rapidly than tepid water.

Drink approximately 5 ounces of liquids every 15 minutes.

Which is better, sports drinks or water? Unless you're a marathon runner or some other type of high-endurance athlete practicing for hours on end, I would stick to drinking plain water during your exercise sessions. Although it's true that our bodies are depleted of electrolytes (chloride, sodium, potassium) through our sweat, a healthy diet should easily replenish any lost electrolytes.

Also, if you're trying to lose weight, know that sports drinks come with a hefty price of excess calories … translation: unwanted body fat.

Many exercisers understand the importance of being physically active in maintaining a healthy body. But they forget to take time to rest and get enough sleep. In our chaotic world, having to juggle work, family, friends, personal interests, and everything else, many of us don't leave enough time for sleep and rest. It's during these peaceful moments that our bodies build and repair themselves from all the damage stress, toxins, and injuries caused on a daily basis. Not getting enough zzz's will result in more damage than you may think.

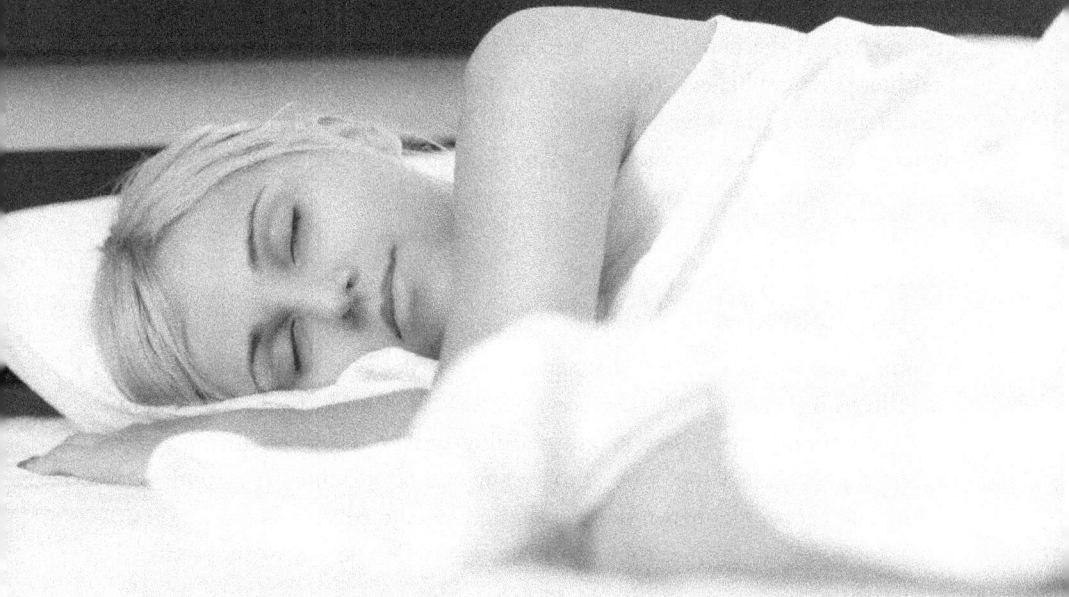

CHAPTER 11

Sleep and Rest

Rest: the frequently unexpressed basic necessity for building a stronger and healthier body. I've been in the fitness arena since the age of 21 and never have I heard any personal trainer emphasize the necessity of rest. As a matter of fact, hardly any fitness or health books utter a single word about the importance of rest. We won't make that same mistake here.

I cringe when I hear people say that they only need 4 hours of sleep per night. There are different stages we go through when we sleep (when combined, these create a cycle). Our bodies and minds repair themselves within these various stages. Four hours of sleep doesn't allow ample time for the body to go through enough cycles to repair itself on a daily basis.

I know that in today's competitive world, a person has to work 25 hours a day, 8 days a week to stay ahead of his/her competitors. Plus we have family obligations, personal activities, and the list goes on. I actually know people who become vexed at even the thought of sleeping ...in case they miss something. What they're

> Our bodies and minds repair themselves within the various stages of sleep.

christopher SASHA

missing are all the benefits that sleep and rest offer to make them happier, healthier people. I believe many of us (including myself) take for granted that we will always be healthy, both inside and out. But in order for our bodies to become and/or remain healthy, we need sleep. Why else do you think the doctor tells you, "Get plenty of rest" after your sick visit?

Immune System

Although there is no hard evidence that sleep rejuvenates the immune system, research does suggest that a good night's sleep strengthens it and will help thwart infections (such as viruses) and disease. A healthy immune system is of paramount importance in safeguarding our bodies from illnesses and preserving our well-being. The primary purpose of our immune system is to distinguish between our own body's cells and foreign cells. When the system zeroes in on foreign cells and toxins, it produces white blood cells. These specialized cells identify the invaders and annihilate the little buggers in order to protect us from illness and disease. A healthy immune system is perpetually on guard to attack any foreign cell at a moment's notice.

A healthy immune system is perpetually on guard to attack any foreign cell at a moment's notice.

Our body's number one line of defense is vulnerable if not treated well. Even though it's believed that exercise improves the immune system, an overabundance of high endurance and/or high-intensity exercising may produce too many stress hormones (cortisol, etc.), which may weaken the system making us more susceptible to colds, the flu, and even premature aging. I said it before and I'll say it again: *moderation is the key*. Stress isn't the only guilty party jeopardizing the functions of the immune system. A sedentary lifestyle, smoking, and unhealthy diets all contribute as well.

Sleep occurs when our bodies are free from moving, thinking, and worrying. Scientists believe it's a time when our bodies repair and rebuild. Think of sleep as a daily vacation from the worries of the world. Take advantage of it and allow the body to perform one of its natural functions. We've all heard that oxygen, food, and water are life's essentials, but have you ever heard anyone say that sleep is also one of life's necessities?

When we sleep, our bodies effectively focus on producing new blood and repairing skin and muscles. That's right. For all the avid exercisers who are struggling to put on some muscle, your body repairs the damaged muscle fibers *after* your workout. For the longest time, I thought that I was building muscle with every laboring repetition. Later I found that the contrary was true.

When exercising you need to make the resistance harder than what your muscles are capable of performing so that you actually cause microscopic tears in the muscle fibers. Only *after* this self-punishment will your body begin to repair the muscles you have marred. And it's during *sleep* when our skeletal muscles relax and immobilize, allowing our bodies to truly renew the injured fibers to make them bigger and stronger.

Human Growth Hormone (hGH)

While the immune system is responsible for building a healthier body, human growth hormones are largely accountable for building a stronger body. As discussed in Chapter 10, human growth hormones (hGH) are naturally produced in the anterior pituitary gland in the center of the brain, and they're discharged in 6-12 distinct pulses throughout the day – especially during the deep sleep stage of the sleeping cycle. It's estimated that two-thirds of growth hormones are released during deep sleep, leaving the remaining to be set free during the day when we're awake. If you exercise, most of these growth hormones will be released *after* your workout.

Growth hormones are responsible for a myriad of functions:

- height growth in children and adolescents,
- energizing the immune system to repel infection and disease, including cancer,
- increasing calcium retention for strong bones,
- repairing tissue and regenerating muscle cells to increase lean body mass,
- regulating fat metabolism by assisting the production of lipase (the enzyme that breaks down fatty acids),
- helping regulate glucose levels.

The levels of these fascinating hormones vary in people depending on their gender, age, and amounts of body tissue. Our bodies are most abundant with growth hormones when we're children and the amounts wane as we age. The rate of decline, too, is dependent on several factors, such as gender,

> The decline in the production of growth hormones might be the predominant reason for weight gain and muscle mass loss as we age.

diet, and level of physical activity. Until recently, scientists believed there were no functions for hGH in adults and that hGH stopped being produced after puberty. Now, they know growth hormones play a large and important role during a person's entire lifetime and researchers speculate that the decline in production of growth hormones might be the predominant reason for weight gain and muscle loss as we age. Maintaining lean body mass (muscle, bone, and organ density) prolongs life. Muscle weakness, organ failure, and death are direct results of lean body mass loss. *If you want to live a healthier, longer life, exercise is a must.*

Three Ways to Increase hGH

You might ask, "If human growth hormones are responsible for so many functions, how might we maximize our body's full potential of producing these invaluable players?" I'm glad you asked! So far, experts suggest we can increase growth hormone bursts through diet, exercise, and sleep patterns.

First, a few research experiments have indicated that avoiding food three hours before going to bed can assist your body with the production of growth hormone. And if you remember, approximately two-thirds of hGH is released during the first couple hours of sleep. Your body will be able to focus on repairing itself and not waste precious energy digesting food. To maximize the production of hGH, make your final meal of the day low in fat and simple carbohydrates and high in protein. Fats have been found to diminish growth hormone secretion. And simple carbs raise insulin production which inhibits the release of human growth hormone leading to depressing the immune system.

Second, exercise is well recognized as a potent catalyst in the fabrication of growth hormone. Intense, heavy physical activities increase the output of growth hormones. But be careful to limit these types of activities to 45-60 minutes. Beyond that amount of time, stress hormones increase, which decreases growth hormone output. Our bodies are in a constant battle between anabolic and catabolic states. Anabolic hormones build tissue, while catabolic hormones destroy tissue. The amount of anabolic hormones which are naturally produced in our bodies is one determinant of how muscular each individual is capable of becoming. (Other factors in musculature build are listed in Chapter 9.)

When we work out, our muscles prepare anabolic hormones. Muscular people have higher amounts of anabolic hormones in their blood. I can't count how many times I hear, "Why aren't my arms bigger than Tom's arms when I can arm curl heavier weight?" or "Why does Jennifer have better developed shoulders even though I train my shoulders harder?" One reason is because some lucky individuals have higher levels of anabolic hormones in their blood. But don't be fooled into believing professional bodybuilders are naturally built like they are, because there is no way on God's green earth that our bodies are designed to get as big as these behemoths. The only way – *the only way* – to achieve looks like theirs is through the use of anabolic steroids. They help the body grow bigger by increasing the amount of anabolic hormones in the blood. But with that, of course, comes an enormous amount of perils.

Third, sleep is crucial in the production of human growth hormone. In fact, it's not only the *amount* of sleep that is critical but the *quality* of sleep (continuous and uninterrupted) seems to be just as important. A study at the University of Chicago concluded that a lesser amount of deep sleep leads to a lower production of human growth hormone. The largest volume of hGH is secreted during the first deep sleep stage, which is usually about an hour after the onset of sleep. It's during this deep sleep that tissue grows and repairs and the supply of blood increases to the muscles. It's during this stage when growth hormones are most produced and utilized.

> Sleep is crucial in the production of human growth hormone.

The quality of sleep is critical if you want to optimize production of growth hormones, or, even more importantly, your overall well-being. The deeper you sleep, the more hGH is released. I have clients with newborns who don't get quality sleep because they're up sporadically throughout the night, which breaks the sleep rhythm. After a few weeks they begin to get sick very easily and they have a hard time concentrating. After a few months of broken sleep patterns, they gain a few pounds and lose strength and stamina during their workouts.

Napping! It's not just for kids any more…

Have you ever noticed that you seem to get tired by mid-afternoon? You sit at your desk trying to focus on work, but all you want to do is close your eyes for just a few minutes to catch a power nap.

You're not alone. About eight hours after we wake up in the morning is when our body temperature drops and our metabolism slows down. This is the lowest biorhythm point of the day… and our bodies, like everything in nature, love rhythms. After an hour or so, you typically get a second wind. But what are the possible side effects of pushing yourself through this time period?

Statistics show that this is when most industrial and traffic accidents take place because alertness, concentration, and reaction times decrease. Productivity is also diminished during this time.

If you're creative, you should be able to give your body what it needs … rest. Even if you can only afford five minutes for closing your eyes and relaxing, you'll feel better. Ideally, experts suggest that a nap should be around 20 minutes long. Just 20 minutes later you'll feel refreshed and ready to tackle the rest of the day. Some of the benefits of a nap include reducing stress, being more alert, and improving your mood. I'm one of those people who gets really cranky when I'm tired, and if I'm tired and hungry…

Now you might say, "I can't afford to take a nap! Not even for five minutes. I have way too much work to do!" I mentioned earlier that I used to be an auditor. I would find myself struggling to keep my eyes open around 1 o'clock. At the time, I worked in a cubicle with my back facing the opening of my workstation. I'd rest my head on my hand as if I was reading something on my computer monitor and close my eyes for 10 minutes or so. Afterwards, I felt better, became more productive, and could easily get through the rest of the workday. I did that almost every day.

I'm not advocating that you cheat your company out of work time. I took my naps during legitimate lunch breaks. I just needed a quiet place to rest and relax for a few minutes. But I am saying that you need to be creative sometimes to give your body what it needs. If this idea doesn't work for you, go to your car and take a power nap during your break. I used to do that one, too. Try anything … just close your eyes for a few minutes and I promise you'll feel much better and ready to conquer whatever comes your way for the rest of the day. Studies show a person becomes more focused, energized, and productive after a short nap mid-afternoon.

There are two things to take into consideration before you begin your quest for the perfect napping environment:
1. don't take a nap too close to bedtime because it could interfere with your normal sleeping pattern at night, and,
2. If you're suffering from insomnia, napping could be one of the guilty parties contributing to your lack of sleep at night.

Sleep Deprivation

Studies with totally sleep-deprived rats have shown that the rats die after two to four weeks. Sleep deprivation and sleeping disorders are serious problems in the United States. Long-term lack of sleep has been linked to increased risk of stress, heart disease, obesity, and type 2 diabetes. We seem to be the only culture that doesn't believe sleep is an essential element in a healthy life. In our high-powered, vigorous lives, dealing with the stresses of work obligations, family responsibilities, and personal activities, when can we find the time to get the much needed sleep our bodies demand? If you don't want to fall victim to the chain reaction of sleep deprivation, I'd suggest that you come to grips with the fact that more often than not, you're not going to be able to get everything done in 24 hours. It's a hard lesson to learn and I find I often have to remind myself of this.

Stress is the body's assailant, triggering diseases like diabetes and cancer by weakening the immune system. Stress increases your heart rate, blood pressure, glucose levels, and other health-threatening factors. Your blood pressure and heart rate drop during sleep, but stress hormones like cortisol and adrenaline increase your heart rate and blood pressure and may be more abundant when you're robbed of sleep which could increase your risk for heart disease. A report from the Harvard University Nurses'

> Stress is the body's assailant that triggers diseases like diabetes and cancer by weakening the immune system.

When our bodies are bereft of sleep, the appetite hormone ghrelin increases making us crave food.

Health Study found that women who consistently slept 5 or less hours per night had a 39% greater risk for a heart attack than women who slept the recommended 8 hours per night.

Usually lack of sleep makes you lose energy and leaves you with a feeling of lethargy. More than likely, to make up for the loss of energy, you'll eat, hoping it will satisfy your fatigue. Sleep helps balance the levels of two hormones (leptin and ghrelin) responsible for our feelings of fullness and hunger. While sleeping, our bodies increase the production of the appetite suppressor leptin and lower the production of the appetite stimulant ghrelin. But when our bodies are bereft of sleep, ghrelin increases, making us crave food.

Research indicates that people who are sleep deprived are more likely to eat foods high in carbohydrates and calories. A study at the University of Chicago found that people who sleep only 4 hours per night have more complications processing carbohydrates due to increased levels of insulin and cortisol. Loss of sleep hinders the body from processing glucose (carbohydrates) and weakens the metabolism, thereby increasing your risk of type 2 diabetes. A current study with participants who were young and healthy and slept less than 6 ½ hours per night on a regular basis had greater insulin resistance than their counterparts who received 7 ½ to 8 ½ hours of sleep per night. Type 2 diabetes is often the aftermath of prolonged insulin resistance.

Type 2 diabetes is often the aftermath of prolonged insulin resistance.

How Much Sleep Do I Need?

Now that we understand the importance of rest, the next logical question is how much is the right amount of sleep for me? If you've heard it once, you've heard it a thousand times – 8 hours. Right? Wrong! The truth is that 8 hours is merely a benchmark. Different people require different amounts of sleep. Newborns sleep the most – somewhere between 10½ and 18½ hours per day. As we age, we need less sleep. Children between 5 and 12 generally need 9-11 hours, teenagers require a little less and as we become adults we plateau somewhere between 7-9 hours for a full night's sleep. Again, this is just an average. I know people who get less sleep than average and function just fine, while others I know are dragging all day if they get less than 9 hours of rest.

Age is just one of many factors to take into consideration in determining the amount of shut-eye you need. Your genetic make-up, the activities you perform while awake, and your amount of exercise all play a role in how much sleep your body requires. There have been plenty of weekends when I had errands to run all day and, even though I slept for more than 8 hours the night before, I still needed a nap in the afternoon. When I was an auditor, I sat at a desk all day which didn't require much energy, so I was fine with only 7 hours of rest at night. All that changed when I became a wellness coach. Now I'm lifting weights all day with my clients, running from one client to the next, working out 75 minutes a day for myself, and working 12-14 hour days. Currently I get about 7½ hours of sleep, including a nap in the late morning or early afternoon. Sometimes I need two naps to get me through the day. It all depends on what my body is telling me.

You're likely to need more rest when you're sick. When you're under the weather, your immune system secretes hormone-like proteins called cytokines. These hormones act like mediators, signaling cells and coordinating a cellular immune response to fight the infection. If you don't get enough rest, you'll probably find yourself feeling worse because your immune system is weakened and doesn't have the strength to work properly. By allowing your body the rest it desperately needs when you're ill, the immune system will be able to produce cells that make up cytokines, thereby annihilating infection.

A rule that's wise to follow is that if you're alert throughout the day, you're getting enough sleep. However, if you're dragging and can't concentrate, it's time to reevaluate your sleep requirements. Try going to bed one-half hour earlier and waking up at your usual time. If you're still tired, try another half hour earlier until you finally wake up feeling refreshed and rejuvenated. According to the National Sleep Foundation, nearly 60% of all Americans report having trouble sleeping at least a few nights every week. Statistically speaking, you'll probably have a night here and there when you don't sleep well due to stress or something of the kind. Just go to bed a little earlier the following night to adjust for it. Also, know that you'll require more sleep the longer you're awake and the more exertive you are during the day.

Sleep improves the quality of our lives. It's as much a priority as exercise and proper nutrition to maintain our well-being. Rest is essential to combat infections, viruses, and diseases. We need rest for our bodies to perform daily functions, to grow and develop, to repair tissue and regenerate muscle cells, to regulate fat metabolism – and so much more. To optimize your state of health, listen to your body and give it the rest it requires to properly perform its functions.

Sleep improves the quality of our lives.

Proper nutrition, exercise, and rest are necessities for health. Without your health, you'll eventually have nothing. I constantly hear people say that they don't have time to exercise, they don't have time to prepare nutrient-dense meals, and they don't have time to get enough rest. My clients own and operate multimillion and multibillion dollar corporations, yet they *make time* for their health. Now, I don't own a multibillion dollar corporation but I do have the same 24 hours in a day as everyone else, and the same responsibilities as the majority of American adults. I get up at 5 o'clock and usually don't finish my day until 9 o'clock at night. In Chapter 12, we'll see how I fit exercise somewhere in my hectic schedule every day. We'll also see how I make healthier food choices when I don't have much to choose from. You can do the same. You can make your health a priority... sometimes you just have to be a little creative!

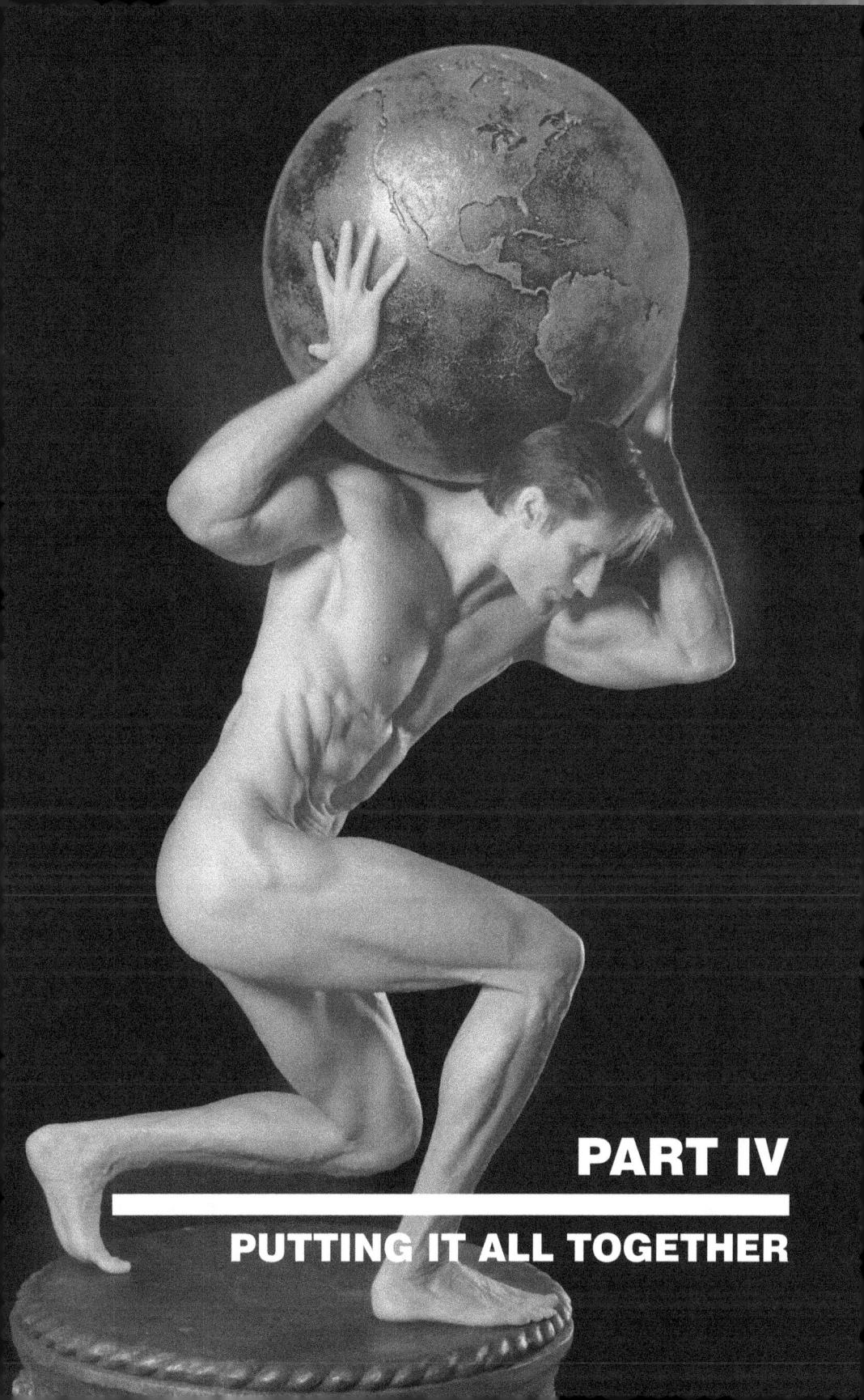

PART IV

PUTTING IT ALL TOGETHER

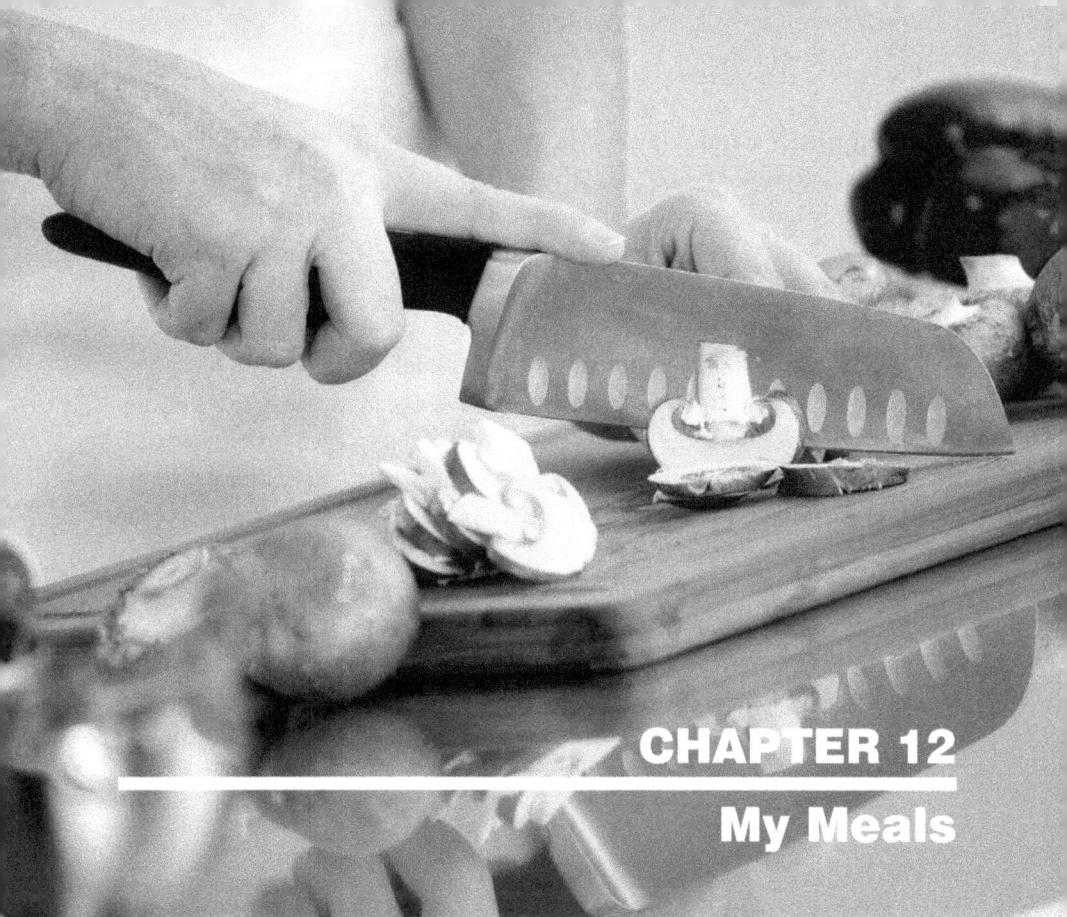

It doesn't seem very long ago that, like the typical American, I was eating the standard American diet (SAD). I imagined sitting down with Pop Tarts and Cap'n Crunch cereal was the only way to start a hectic day. Of course, that breakfast only happened if I had time to eat before I rushed out the door to catch the commuter train downtown for work.

By the time I could squeeze in lunch, it was usually 3:30 and the only dining establishments serving food between lunch and dinner were fast food joints. So I would order a "value meal," which usually consisted of a hamburger, fries, and a cola, which I would then proceed to wolf down usually in less than five minutes. Then it was time to run back to my desk and start work again.

I normally got home around 7:00, only to find myself crashing on the couch and watching television for a few hours before going to bed. Most of the time, I didn't even eat dinner because I wasn't hungry (having eaten at 3:30). I was baffled as to why I was getting fatter when I hardly ate during the day. Then

> I was baffled as to why I was getting fatter when I hardly ate during the day.

christopherSASHA

one of my friends started going to the gym because his girlfriend told him that he was starting to look like the Pillsbury Doughboy. It was true! She would push his belly button and he would giggle. I went to the gym with him initially for support – and (I admit) to watch his body jiggle as he attempted to jog on the treadmill. It was amusing. At first. But then I started to think that it was really sad for a young man to be so out of shape.

When I got home, I busted out my old modeling photos and began my own analysis as to how my body had changed between my early twenties and my early thirties. My 30-plus-year-old body was definitely a little fuller than my svelte 21-year-old body. I began wondering why we get fatter as we get older. Is it normal to gain weight as we age? Or is it lifestyle changes and the types of foods we eat that make us put on the poundage?

I began a quest to rediscover my younger body, and to find out what I did differently then. The only thing I could actually recall was that when I was in my twenties, I walked to work and did a mediocre workout a few days each week. That was it.

As I entered Corporate America, I became mentally active and physically lethargic.

Changing My Eating Habits

Over the course of about six months, I became diligent with my workouts and noticed palpable changes in my physique. I lost some weight and packed on some muscle. The girls were starting to notice me again, reassuring me that I wasn't dead yet. Physically, things were getting back to how they were 10 years prior. But I still couldn't develop that six-pack of rock hard abs, so I dove into all the muscle magazines that filled the bookstores. They all seemed to say the same thing: "If you want abs of steel, you need to consume more protein … and we have just the product you need."

I evaluated my diet. Because I was working out, I was eating more but my body wasn't developing the way I wanted. I wanted the Greek-god abdominals that most people yearn for. I was eating a lot of processed foods and knew I had to educate myself as to what a "healthy" diet really was. Being the genius I like to think I am, I came up with the idea that since protein bars and shakes were engineered by scientists, they should be exactly the nutrition that our bodies need. Right? The healthy diet research I did was completed with that single decision. Basically I stopped eating real food. I mainly ate only protein bars and protein shakes. I did this for almost three years. Even vegetables were completely banned from my house.

At the gym, I would consume two or three protein bars as I forced my way through a workout. People would tell me I was going to glow in the dark from all the chemicals I was eating, yet they always came to me asking which was the best tasting protein bar. Immediately after my workout, I would rush home to down a protein shake. I never calculated how much of my diet was protein, but I'm quite certain it was way above the U.S. Dietary Guideline recommendation. Even though I was working out and thought I had a healthy diet, I felt lethargic and sluggish during this phase of my life. I was tired all the time. I eliminated as many carbohydrates as possible because I thought that carbs wouldn't build muscle since muscle is made of protein, not carbohydrates. So why on earth would I want to consume carbs? It wasn't until later that I learned that glucose is the preferred source of fuel by the working muscle tissue. And the most efficient source of glucose derives from carbohydrates. Then the muscles perform properly and the brain produces a brain neurotransmitter called serotonin, which helps the body relax.

Following the rest of the sheep on these low-fat, high-carb diets was not giving me the results I wanted.

Obviously, I was as perplexed as the majority of the population as to what a healthy diet was. Following the rest of the sheep on these low-fat, high-carb diets was not giving me the results I wanted. In reality, just because a diet has worked in the past doesn't necessarily mean that it will always work. For instance, our body composition changes as we age because we start to lose muscle as early as our mid-twenties. The less muscle we have, the slower our metabolism will be.

We start to lose muscle as early as our mid-twenties.

Therefore, the fewer calories we need to consume. The problem is that we're used to eating a certain amount of calories per day and we don't take into consideration that we lose muscle without resistance training. So as we age, we don't require as many calories as we once did. The extra calories we consume, and don't burn off, are more than likely going to be stored as body fat. Remember, just 50 extra unused calories per day will become over 5 pounds of body fat at the end of the year. This is probably why we don't realize we're gaining weight. We gain the weight little by little, over a long period of time.

Gaining weight is always the mystery in clients' lives. Most clients tell me that they've been eating the same for years and never gained an ounce. Then, all of the sudden.... bam! – they've turned into pudgeballs. Unfortunately, losing the flab isn't as magical or mysterious – or as easy – as gaining it. Most people expect to lose the weight they've packed on in the past 5 or 10 years overnight without much effort. If this was the case, we'd all be fitness models and America wouldn't have an obesity epidemic.

KISS Method

When it comes to taking weight off, and keeping it off long term, the KISS Method seems to be the most successful method for most of my clients. KISS – *Keep It Simple Stupid* – is used in a myriad of training scenarios. Popular actors even use this technique when developing their characters on movie sets. It's based on the premise that if you maintain simplicity, you can accomplish your goals. In dieting, the big picture is to keep the foundation basically the same. Make only small changes to obtain the widest array of nutrients and to keep from getting bored. In the world of weight management, your daily caloric intake should be 30% good fats coming mainly from monounsaturated fats, 40% carbohydrates coming mostly from complex carbs, and 30% high-quality protein.

Although this may sound a little drab at first, it won't be long before you find foods that you enjoy eating and you learn to combine them with other foods you relish. For instance, a few of my clients are fans of turkey sandwiches and salmon, so they eat turkey sandwiches for lunch and salmon for dinner on most days. These are foods they savor and eating them easily keeps them within their daily caloric requirements. Planning is 90% of the caloric intake battle. When you keep things simple and make slight variations to keep from getting bored, you're much more likely to stay in control of your weight.

For me, I know I can have tuna (chunky light), salmon, and steak three times a week. So I rotate these foods every three days. I'm a sucker for steak so I choose lean steaks like top sirloin or eye of round steaks every other day.

There are some important factors to consider when making up your meal plan. First, breakfast is the most important meal of the day. Yet according to Technomic's *Breakfast Consumer Trend Report*, nearly 6 out of 10 people say they skip breakfast at least once a week. Not being hungry, not having the time, and **trying to lose weight** are among their excuses for neglecting the day's most important meal. And skipping breakfast will almost certainly lead to overeating by 10:00 a.m.

Breakfast is the most important meal of the day.

The reason for this is simple. Say the last thing you ate was at 8:00 p.m. the night before. The next day you wake up at 6:30 a.m. and run out the door to work by 7:30 a.m. without breakfast. By this time you haven't eaten for almost 12 hours and your body is in starvation mode and craving nourishment – of any kind. You start feeling hunger pangs because your blood sugar level is too low, and you want those pangs to subside. With modern conveniences, you're more apt to grab a couple of doughnuts and coffee, rather than sitting down with a couple of eggs, Canadian bacon, and sourdough rye toast. Because the appetite suppressant hormone, leptin, takes approximately 20 minutes to trigger your brain to realize that you've eaten something, during those 20 post-doughnut minutes, you probably devour more calories than you would have if you had planned your meals for the day. Not only do you eat more calories than expected, but the calories in those doughnuts are refined sugars, which will quickly spike your insulin levels and lead to a sluggish feeling, making you crave more carbohydrates to energize you. And the vicious cycle continues while you gain more and more weight.

So the next time you think you're saving calories by skipping breakfast or any other meal, remember that you will almost always sabotage yourself by overeating at the next meal.

Second, snacks are a must. I'm not talking about chips and cookies, but healthy snacks like raw berries, vegetables, and nuts. They're an excellent way to get extra nutrients, give you an energy boost in the middle of the day, and hold you over until your next meal. Be careful with nuts because they pack an enormous amount of calories. One serving of nuts (about a handful) should equal about 170 calories. Snacks are a low calorie way to put something in your stomach to ward off cravings, stabilize insulin levels, and keep your energy level up until your next meal.

Snacks are a must.

For the average business person, I would recommend a snack three hours after every meal. If you ate breakfast at 7 o'clock, then have a snack at 10 o'clock. If lunch was at 1 o'clock, your next snack would be at 4 o'clock, and dinner around 7 or 8 o'clock. Of course the more active you are, the more snacks may be required. In my case, running all over town from one client to the next and working out requires that I consume more food than the average sedentary person. My body generally needs five snacks throughout the day as opposed to the traditional two snacks.

Third, everyone's metabolism slows down by mid-afternoon. This is why it's wise to eat the majority of your nutrients at breakfast. If breakfast is your big meal for the day, your body has time to burn off those calories instead of storing them as fat. Remember… moderation is the key.

On page 279 is a food journal of my personal meals during a sample day. Remember, these are my personal likes – I do vary it slightly from day to day.

christopherSASHA

This is my blueprint for the week, except for that one special day during the week where I put my diet aside and eat whatever I want. For me, one off day means 24 hours, so I start my cheat day at noon on Saturday and end at noon on Sunday. The reason is because I work until noon on Saturday. Usually there's some kind of event happening Saturday night and/or those infamous Sunday brunches that I can't say "no" to. But then it's back to my diet by Sunday afternoon.

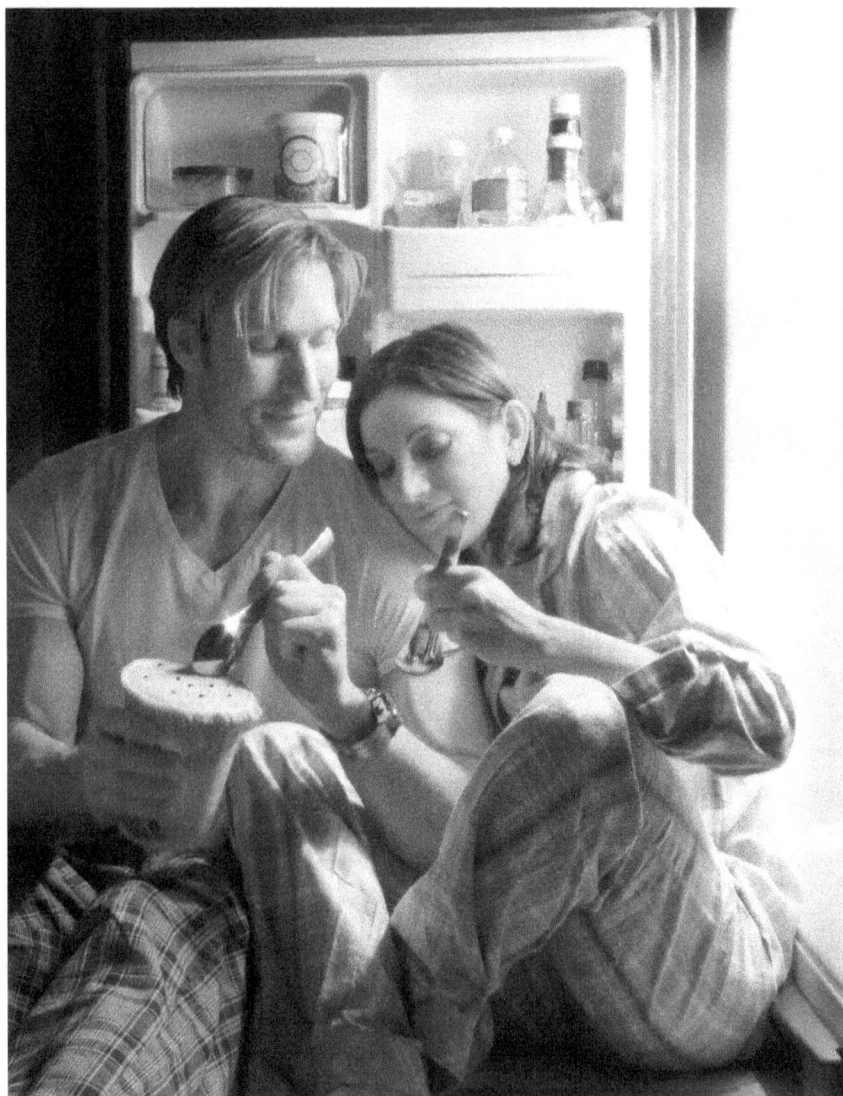

FOOD	CALORIES	FAT	SAT. FAT	CARBS	FIBER	SUGAR	PROTEIN	CHOLESTEROL	TIME
Kashi - Go Lean	140	1.0g	0.0g	30.0g	10.0g	6.0g	13.0g	0.0mg	
Soy Milk	100	3.5g	0.5g	9.0g	1.0g	8.0g	7.0g	0.0mg	
Whey Protein Shake	240	1.0g	0.6g	7.0g	1.5g	4.0g	50.0g	9.0mg	
Breakfast Total:	480	5.5g (10%)	1.1g	46g (36%)	12.5g	18.0g	70g (54%)	9.0mg	5:00 a.m.
Granny Smith Apple	90	1.0g	0.0g	21.0g	4.0g	17.0g	0.0g	0.0mg	
1 Serving of Almonds	160	14.0g	1.0g	6.0g	3.0g	1.0g	6.0g	0.0mg	
Snack Total:	250	15g (51%)	1.0g	27g (40%)	7.0g	18.0g	6g (9%)	0.0mg	7:00 a.m.
Low Fat Kefir Cultured Milk	120	2.0g	1.5g	12.0g	3.0g	14.0g	8.0g	10.0mg	
Dark Chocolate (73% Cocao)	180	12.0g	7.0g	15.0g	4.0g	14.0g	2.0g	0.0mg	
Snack Total:	300	14g (46%)	8.5g	27g (39%)	7.0g	28.0g	10g (15%)	10.0mg	9:00 a.m.
2 Slices of Whole Grain Bread	220	5.0g	0.0g	40.0g	8.0g	2.0g	10.0g	0.0mg	
4 Tbsp. Soy Nut Butter	340	22.0g	3.0g	20.0g	6.0g	6.0g	14.0g	0.0mg	
Snack Total:	560	27g (42%)	3.0g	60g (41%)	14.0g	8.0g	24g (17%)	0.0mg	11:00 a.m.
2 Servings of Brown Rice	340	2.0g	0.0g	70.0g	4.0g	0.0g	8.0g	0.0mg	
10 Egg Whites	170	0.0g	0.0g	3.5g	0.0g	0.0g	40.0g	0.0mg	
1 Tbsp. Canola Oil	120	14.0g	1.0g	0.0g	0.0g	0.0g	0.0g	0.0mg	
3 Tbsp. Soy Sauce (Lite)	30	0.0g	0.0g	3.0g	0.0g	0.0g	3.0g	0.0mg	
Lunch (Pre-Workout) Total:	660	16g (22%)	1.0g	77g (47%)	4.0g	0.0g	51g (31%)	0.0mg	1:00 p.m.
½ Serving Whey Protein Shake	120	0.5g	0.3g	3.5g	0.75g	2.0g	25.0g	4.5mg	
During Workout Total:	120	0.5g (5%)	0.3g	3.5g (12%)	0.75g	2.0g	25g (83%)	4.5mg	4:30 p.m.
2 Servings 1% Cottage Cheese	180	3.0g	2.0g	10.0g	0.0g	6.0g	24.0g	20.0mg	
1 ½ Servings Blackberries	112	0.5g	0.0g	28.0g	9.0g	19.0g	3.0g	0.0mg	
Post-Workout Total:	292	3.5g (11%)	2.0g	38g (52%)	9.0g	25.0g	27g (37%)	20.0mg	6:00 p.m.
4 Slices Whole Grain Bread	440	10.0g	0.0g	80.0g	16.0g	4.0g	20.0g	0.0mg	
2 Servings Turkey Breast	220	2.0g	0.0g	0.0g	0.0g	0.0g	52.0g	140.0mg	
1 Roma Tomato (sliced)	17	0.5g	0.0g	3.5g	0.5g	0.0g	0.5g	0.0mg	
Dinner Total:	677	13g (16%)	0.0g	84g (45%)	16.5g	4.0g	73g (39%)	140.0mg	8:00 p.m.
DAILY TOTAL:	3339	94g (25%)	17g	362g (42%)	71g	103g	286g (33%)	184mg	

I'm not suggesting candy bars with caramel and nuts – rather just plain dark chocolate.

You might have noticed that I eat dark chocolate every day. I wouldn't recommend this for everyone, but if you can limit your intake of dark chocolate to only one serving (approximately 180 calories), it's a great way to trick yourself into feeling like you're cheating. I'm not suggesting candy bars with caramel and nuts – rather just plain dark chocolate bars. If you do decide to allow yourself a serving of dark chocolate for the day, remember that *moderation is paramount and you must deduct an equal amount of calories from another food(s) in your diet.* The reason I include dark chocolate (not milk chocolate, not white chocolate) in my diet regularly is because it contains flavonoids which have been proven to help lower blood pressure and prevent clogged arteries by increasing HDL cholesterol levels. It also boosts glutathione, a detoxing molecule within each cell that neutralizes free radicals that damage healthy cells.

I wouldn't recommend going on a dark chocolate binge. Although there's evidence that dark chocolate has some health benefits, there's still that little obesity-related nutrient called *sugar.* So be wary, and try dark chocolate that's at least 60% cocoa.

Everyone worries about the amount of fat they're consuming, but we fail to recognize that sugar is the worst culprit of all. Everything tastes better with sugar added, and it gives you a quick jolt of energy. But with this hellacious ingredient comes consequences.

The average American consumes 22 pounds of candy annually.

In Chapter 5, we discussed how sugar is extremely addictive and how insulin levels cause your body to store these unwholesome calories as body fat. Some sugar is fine, but a lot of sugar is just opening a Pandora's box.

Here's a fantastic Chicken Spinach Salad some friends and I created….

SASHA'S CHICKEN SPINACH SALAD

4 small grilled boneless, skinless
  chicken breasts (sliced)
1 pound fresh spinach
  (triple washed)
1 cup mushrooms (sliced)
1/4 cup walnuts (chopped)
1 medium avocado
½ cup blue cheese (crumbled)
1 cup cherry tomatoes
½ cup raspberries

DRESSING:
4 Tablespoons Extra Virgin
  Olive Oil
8 Tablespoons Balsamic Vinegar

Serves 4

NUTRITION FACTS:
Per Serving: 424 calories,
24g fat*, 4g saturated fat,
22g carbs, 30g protein.

*This salad contains approximately 50% fat, which might concern some. The important thing to realize is that almost all of the fat is monounsaturated fat, the "good" fat that improves cholesterol levels and helps prevent certain types of cancer.

Five Days Following Me Around

While I'm on the topic of my daily meals, I thought it might be beneficial to see how healthy a person can be, even with a hectic schedule. Good health is about making choices and what's most important to you. Challenge yourself and you won't be disappointed. I promise!

During the week, my days usually begin at 5 o'clock in the morning and end around 9 o'clock at night.

MONDAY

5:00 A.M.

Slowly waking up by smashing the snooze button… twice. Mondays are always hard for me to get back into the swing of things, hence the glorious snooze button. (I deliberately bought an alarm clock with the most vexing alarm buzzer to coax me out of bed. The first morning I used this monster, I thought I was going to have a heart attack. It served its purpose.) Kashi cereal and a whey protein drink are my breakfast staples.

They give me enough carbs and protein to last a few hours until I have my first snack. I read the *Wall Street Journal* to see where the market is and what's going on in the financial world.

6:00 A.M.

I run (as usual) out the door to my first client. It doesn't matter what time I get out of bed, I'm always running late. In the car, I listen to a talk radio show to stay informed about what's going on in the world. This news helps me carry on conversations with clients during the cruel and unusual exercise hours they endure with me. In between clients, I set 15 minutes aside to have a snack – a cup of strawberries and a handful of almonds.

10:30 A.M

I have a half-hour break before my 11 o'clock client so I do an abdominal workout (explained in Chapter 9) consisting of 4 sets of 60 crunches with 15 second breaks, 4 sets of 60 knee bends with 30 second breaks, 3 sets of 60 twisting crunches on each side with no break between, and 2 sets of 15 lower back extensions with 45 second breaks between the sets. It takes 30 minutes to complete this ab workout, but it hits the entire "core." I feel great when it's done. "Anyone ready for an ab contest?" is my usual response to the next person who says good morning to me.

12:00 P.M

I'm done with my morning clients and it's time to eat lunch. I'm currently writing a business plan to open my own gym so I meet with my real estate broker to show me possible locations for the facility during my lunch break.

By the time I look at three locations, I'm ready for a 20 minute power nap. I don't care where I am. I sit down, close my eyes and relax for 15-20 minutes. I might be in my car in which case I pull into a shopping mall parking lot and close my eyes. If I'm at a gym looking for ideas for my gym, I go into the locker room and sit on a bench with my head against the wall. Where I am doesn't matter to me.

It's amazing how refreshed I feel for the rest

> It's amazing how refreshed I feel for the rest of the day because of those few minutes spent with my eyes closed.

*christopher*SASHA

of the day because of those few minutes spent with my eyes closed. Don't underestimate the power of a nap. Give it a try and you'll be astonished at how much better you'll feel and how much more productive you'll be the rest of the day. A word of caution… studies have indicated that 20 minutes is the optimal amount of time for a nap. After 20 minutes, you usually begin to fall into a deep sleep and you'll probably feel more exhausted than before the power nap. So set your alarm on your cell phone for 20 minutes, just to recharge *your* batteries.

3:30 P.M

It's time for my workout. Leg Day! I'll take in a higher amount of carbs about three hours before the workout to make sure I have enough energy to get through the routine. Three hours is long enough for my insulin level to drop back to a normal level so my body can burn fat as energy – high levels of insulin prevent fat from burning by suppressing the hormone glucagon. High levels of insulin also suppress growth hormone which is responsible for building new muscle mass. This is my longest workout – a little over an hour. By the time I'm done, I'm ready to torture my next client.

> Three hours is long enough for my insulin level to drop back to a normal level so my body can burn fat as energy.

I always get some protein back into my system immediately after the workout. I mean immediately – within 15 minutes. I wait 15 minutes after my workout because the body needs a little time to get back into a state of digestion after a workout. I usually consume one half of a whey protein drink with BCAAs (Branched Chain Amino Acids), which are fast-acting proteins that are metabolized in the muscle (as opposed to the liver where all other amino acids are metabolized) to rebuild the muscle tissue I stressed. Also, it "theoretically" suppresses protein catabolism. Don't forget to have some real food with carbohydrates too. The carbohydrates are necessary to deliver the protein to the muscles, so include them between 30 and 45 minutes after your workout. While exercising, most of the blood goes to the muscles (periphery) leaving little in the visceral area to digest food. I also have one cup of 1% cottage cheese and one serving of blackberries or blueberries approximately 2 hours after my workout. Cottage cheese is a casein protein, which is a slow-acting protein that takes 3-4 hours to digest. So it leaves you feeling satisfied for a longer period of time and slows the rate of protein breakdown, which is exactly what we want. Furthermore, cottage cheese has CLA (Conjugated Linoleic Acid) that research has proven to build muscle and reduce body fat.

8:00 P.M.

I finish with my last client for the day, and go home and have dinner. A serving of wild sockeye salmon and a spinach salad do the trick and I start a fitness assessment report for one of my new clients. I end my day at 9 o'clock by sitting on the back deck gazing at the city lights, the illuminated Chicago skyline. It's relaxing for me and sets the mood for sleep.

TUESDAY

5:00 A.M

It's a sunny day and I decide to ride my bike to my first client today. I start every workday with my usual Kashi cereal and whey protein shake because I know this will carry me over until my first snack. However, since I decided to do a cardio workout first thing this morning (the bike ride), I won't eat until I get to my client's house. This way I can take advantage of a low insulin level and burn mostly fat as energy. It takes about 40 minutes to get to my client's place, so I should burn about 450 calories. Chicago is one of the best places to be in the summer. The lake view, the people, the restaurants – it can't be beat. And best of all, the sunrise over Lake Michigan is breathtaking on a clear, sunny day. It makes all the sweat and effort worth every grueling pedal stroke.

11:00 A.M.

I attend a seminar about the best home improvements to increase the value of your house. I own a few rental properties that are in up and coming areas of Chicago, and want to take advantage of improvement ideas to compete in that area. As usual, the lunch provided by the organization hosting this seminar is Subway sandwiches, chips, and soda. Have no fear. We can still have a healthy meal by being creative and using a little imagination.

The staples are always turkey, ham, and roast beef sandwiches. You've seen them – one razor-thin slice of meat, a half pound of lettuce, and a tomato slice stuffed into a small loaf of bread they call a

Some food is better than no food.

christopherSASHA

bun. Then they have the individual sized bags of regular potato chips and baked potato chips, regular colas and diet colas. Wait a minute! They actually have bottled water in the back, so I quickly grab two bottles and wander over to the sandwich table. I don't mean to be greedy, but I'm trying to make the best of the situation. I take four turkey sandwiches and sit down at the conference table. Everyone near me starts to stare. I begin creating my sandwich, hollowing out one bun and plopping all the deli meat from the four sandwiches into my hollowed out bun. Then I add a meager amount of lettuce and the tomato slices. In this way I get rid of most of the refined carbs in the bread. It's not the healthiest meal – but some food is better than no food. My goal is to keep my metabolism and energy levels up.

3:00 P.M

I have clients to train with a 30 minute break in between another series of clients. I can't get an entire workout done in 30 minutes so I split my chest/back routine by doing all of my chest exercises in the 30 minutes I have. Again, 15 minutes after I'm done with my chest workout, I chug down my protein drink with Branched Chain Amino Acids (BCAAs) to help rebuild the muscle tissues I just attacked. And it's time to greet my next victim.

6:30 P.M.

I finish my clients for the day, and now it's time to conclude my workout. Though I didn't train both body parts consecutively, I'll still benefit from the workout hours later because my body will use energy to rebuild the muscle tissue I destroyed instead of storing body fat.

9:00 P.M.

I have a black tie charity event for a boys and girls club in Chicago. The mayor of Chicago, among other political figures, is mingling. One lesson I've learned is to always give back to the community. It makes me feel good that I can help. If you don't have time, then donate money. If you don't have extra money, then donate time. Of course, they're serving hors d'oeuvres and cocktails at this event. I sample two or three hors d'oeuvres and a glass of red wine while I inquire about any other charity functions where I can donate some time or money. I'm a part of my community and I'm a big believer in contributing to make it a little better place.

11:00 P.M.

I'm home and I listen to some jazz to help ease me into a relaxed mode so I can sleep. I reflect on the things I could have done differently throughout the day and how I can make tomorrow better.

WEDNESDAY

5:00 A.M.

I do my morning ritual …reading the *Wall Street Journal* and *New York Times* while I eat my Kashi cereal and protein drink. I knew that I had an extra hour to sleep in this morning so I took advantage of it. Instead of waking up at 6 o'clock, I needed to get my thoughts together for a very important meeting. I'm putting together an exercise regime for the police department. Currently, Chicago is one of the fattest cities in the country and observing the physiques of those on our police force validates that statistic.

11:00 A.M.

After training my last morning client, I bolt out of the gym, heading to police headquarters. As I drive, I imagine how many people are going to be present to listen to my pitch for a healthier police force, wondering if I missed any details that need to be presented, and I plan where I'm going to position myself at the conference table.

Positioning is more important than you might think. Have you ever noticed when you're called in to your manager's office for your annual review, your manager has a higher chair than you and sits with the sun behind him or her? Your manager's higher and bigger chair represents the fact that you're an inferior in the office hierarchy. The sun behind your manager ensures that he or she isn't distracted by anything and can completely focus on communicating. At the same time, you sit in this little chair trying to see your manager's face while squinting into the sun and trying to remember all the ways you helped the company profit this year.

This is why I will sit at one of the ends of the conference table if it's a rectangular table. I want to let them know that I'm in charge during this meeting because I'm the expert. If the table is round, I won't sit. I'll give my presentation standing and walking around the people sitting at the table. I'll tell them that I think better on my feet or something like that. I want to be above them to make them feel less superior to me. People in an inferior position don't say "no"; they say "yes". This isn't a power trip for me. It's a method I've used for years that works, so I wanted to share it with you.

2:45 P.M.

The pitch to the police department is done. I was there longer than I had expected, which indicates it went well. They peppered me with questions, letting me know that they're interested in the proposal. I felt very positive after leaving the conference room, which is another good indicator for me. I had a vision – how many people were going to be in the discussion, what questions they were going to ask – and I envisioned them telling me they wanted to go ahead with the proposal. I had a vision of winning. And I felt like I accomplished my goal. I felt like I won the proposal.

4:00 P.M.

I used to work seven days a week and felt guilty if I took time off for fun. I burned myself out after a few years, and lost out in relationships with some people who were very important to me. So I've recently taken steps to learn how to balance my life with work and personal time.

I always wanted to compete in the Mackinac Island Race, a sailing race from Chicago to Mackinac Island, Michigan. It's an excursion that tests your physical abilities for four straight days while you sail the choppy waters of Lake Michigan.

Every Wednesday night in the summer, the Chicago Yacht Club has a sailing race called the "Beer Can Race." This is a chance to test your sailing skills before the "big" race to Mackinac Island. It's a lot of fun and I have never seen so many beautiful sunsets over the Chicago skyline as I have sailing this past summer.

Sailing makes me stop and actually see some of the beauty God put on earth for us to enjoy. This makes all the bruises and line burns I accumulate during the race worth the pain.

11:00 P.M.

I'm finally home from sailing and hungry from all the energy I used during the race. It's late and I'm going to bed shortly, but I know that it's better to eat something to replenish my body with nutrients than to not eat at all. I have to be

> The glycogen stores need to be replenished before glucose will be stored as fat.

christopher SASHA

smart, so I decide on a whey protein shake. Whey protein is a fast-acting protein that my body will utilize immediately. It shouldn't store as fat because my body has used most of its glycogen stores during the physical activities of sailing. The glycogen stores need to be replenished before glucose will be stored as fat. The protein drink is down and so am I.

THURSDAY

5:00 A.M.

I'm a little tired today because I didn't get much sleep last night but I have to train a client at the Four Seasons Hotel in downtown Chicago. As I walk through the lobby, rapper/actor Ice Cube passes me on his way out of the elevator. He's a lot shorter than he looks in the movies but he has a pleasant face. I go to the gym and the owner says "Good morning" to me as he always does. As I walk toward my client, who's warming up in a corner of the gym, I see Anthony Hopkins walking on a treadmill. He seems to be on a promenade in his own little world, wearing gray sweats and a red baseball cap with the brim pulled down to his nose. I read that he and Julia Roberts are in town making a movie. After I train my client, my jaunt down the staircase leads to the locker rooms and Julia Roberts scurries past me for her morning workout. I didn't recognize her until I was in the locker room and a few members asked if I had seen her in the gym. It's always entertaining for me to train at the luxury hotels downtown because I get a chance to see what celebrities truly look like … without all the make-up and lights. It's fun!

9:30 A.M.

My booker at my modeling agency left me a message to be ready for a go-see tomorrow afternoon. I've been modeling off and on for various agencies since I was 21 years old. Most of the time I was too big to model "high fashion" clothes because I'm a size 46 Long, whereas the established size for those types of shows is 40 Regular. I've been branded in the "fitness" arena in modeling, which is great for me because this branding encourages me to stay in shape. I usually go on underwear and swimsuit auditions in the Chicago market. For whatever reason my booker never lets me know about auditions until the day before, so I have to slam my cardio into high gear for the next 24 hours. In between clients I ride the stationary bike, jump rope, hit the heavy bag, and power-walk on the treadmill with an incline set at 30 degrees. I believe the 30 degree incline with a pace of 3 miles per hour is the Herculean of all cardio exercises. Most treadmills are equipped with only a 15 degree incline, but the Nordic Trak 9100 series has a 30 degree incline that kicks butt. Instead of running, I try walking as fast as I can. While running, you're in the air half the time. On the other hand, you remain on the ground for the entire time when you walk, thereby exerting more effort and burning more calories. Try it for 10 minutes. You'll see this is no sissy exercise.

3:00 P.M.

I have an hour for my workout before my next protégé. *Arms Day!* For the first time this week I have time to focus on my workout so I take full advantage of it by going extremely heavy with my weights. The heavier the weights, the more time I need to recuperate between sets. I'll start with 10 repetitions for each exercise to warm up my arm muscles and go through these muscles full-range by

> Glutamine is the most copious amino acid in our bodies that helps our bodies maintain muscle tissue.

doing a full contraction and going to full extension. Some people don't go all the way up and all the way down (full-range) which, in time, may cause muscles to shorten, resulting in less flexibility and shorter range of motion. The next three sets of each exercise will consist of only 4-6 repetitions. If I can't do at least 4 reps, I know the weight is too heavy and needs to be lightened.

7:00 P.M.

I finish training my last client and need to burn some more calories before the day is over. Interval training is a cardio exercise I do when I want to get my heart pumping. I decide to use the treadmill at a top speed – 10 miles per hour for the treadmills at my gym. I put the incline at 3 degrees to soften the shock to my joints. Then I run for 30 seconds, jump off to either side of the treadmill track for 60 seconds, jump back on the treadmill track to run for 30 seconds, jump off to either side of the treadmill track for 60 seconds, and so on. The logic is that this exercise pushes the heart rate to its limit. Then I rest to bring my heart rate back down – right before it's time to run again to jack the heart rate back up. By keeping the heart rate up, the body burns more calories. I get both an anaerobic and aerobic workout with this type of interval training. I do this for about 20 minutes. By this time, I'm exhausted. I down a whey protein shake and go home so I can get to bed early. I don't want bags under my eyes for the audition.

FRIDAY

4:00 A.M.

I get up early so I can get some cardio in before my first client arrives at the gym. During the night, all the carbs and protein I ate at my last meal were utilized to keep my body functioning while asleep. After glycogen (glucose stored in the liver and muscle tissue) burns off, bodies switch to fat as a main source of energy until we eat again. In theory, if body fat is the main source of energy available, then the amount of fat should diminish as it's being burned as an energy source. For this reason I don't eat anything until after my early morning cardio. I want to burn body fat, so I ride my bike to work this morning. I make sure to keep my heart rate low (approximately 121 bpm, or 65% MHR) and finish the ride in 30 minutes. By keeping my heart rate low and finishing the cardio workout in 30 minutes, I minimize the risk of muscle tissue being used for energy. This has been a method I've used for years to drop my body fat to 3.3%. When I arrive at the gym I take a shower and eat my usual breakfast, Kashi cereal and a whey protein drink.

> For years, early morning low-intensity cardio before eating anything has proven to drop my body fat to 3.3%.

10:00 A.M

I finish my last morning client and run off to the modeling go-see. When I get there I sign in and wait in a 1,500 square foot room along with 30 other guys. In the end, over 100 male models audition in the hopes of getting this one job. Competition is fierce in the world of professional modeling. To pass the time, some of the models talk about their experiences modeling in Europe. For some reason, American models fare better in Europe and European models do better in America. All the same, we pass our "books" (portfolios of previous work in magazines torn out, called tear-sheets) and admire the models who have done work for Armani, Gucci, and all the other high fashion designers.

12:15 P.M.

My name is finally called. After two hours of waiting in the cattle herd, I'm greeted by the assistant of the photographer who will shoot the advertisement. The assistant tells me they're looking for someone who has a chiseled jaw, high cheek bones, and a set of six-pack abs. I possess all of those qualities …but so do the other 100 models! I walk into the room where the photographer sits behind a colossal black desk with covers of magazines framed on the wall surrounding him – his prior work. He doesn't even look at me when I introduce myself. I'm just a number to him.

The first words out of his mouth are, "get undressed, down to your boxers." Then he asks for my book, still without looking at me. I hand it to him and strip down to my boxers. He proceeds to tell me to stand on the tape about 15 feet away from the camera. While I stand almost buck-naked, he directs me into the positions he wants. After a few shots, five other people walk in the room and start whispering. I don't know who they are …maybe the magazine owners or other assistants? What I do know is the pressure is on. The photographer shows the test shots we just took to these people and tells me to put on one of their swimsuits. At this point, I'm thinking that I got the job and my confidence soars. Everyone is behind the camera and the assistant dims the lights. The overhead lights are turned on and the photographer tells me to move around "like I'm on the beach." Between 5 and 10 shots are taken in this swimsuit, and then the lights are turned back on. The assistant tells me to put my clothes back on, and the audition is over without another word … from the photographer or the other five people.

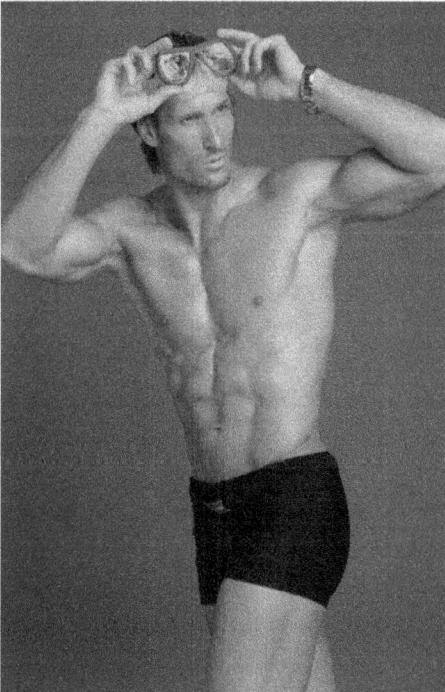

As I walk out with the photographer's assistant, I ask her name and the exact address of the location where the audition took place. As I walk back to my car to head back to the gym for my next client, I notice a flower shop. I order a bouquet of flowers for the assistant, in gratitude for auditioning me. I've learned that little things like this make a difference. Even if I don't get this job, she'll remember me for the next one.

2:00 P.M.

I haven't eaten since 6 o'clock this morning and I'm starved. My first instinct is to stop at a pizza parlor on the way to the gym. The shop I'm passing has the best pizza in town. But the rational side of my brain tells me that that's not a very good idea. The worst time to order food or grocery shop is when you're hungry because everything in abundance looks good. The last time I grocery shopped when I was famished I spent almost double my usual food bill… and I ate doughnuts while I shopped! Instead, I now go to McDonald's and order a side salad with low-fat balsamic dressing, a Chicken McGrill sandwich, and a bottled water. If you have self-discipline, you can still frequent fast food joints and order fairly healthy food. You just have to be a little savvy like we discussed in Chapter 4. By taking a moment to think about what's better for me, I saved myself from bingeing on refined carbs that would have jacked up my insulin levels and been converted directly into sugar, leading to more body fat.

7:00 P.M.

I'm done with work for the day. I meet some friends at North Avenue Beach on Lake Michigan. They've scheduled a volleyball game for us, an opportunity to catch up on each others' lives and to bring out the competitive side in each of us. After the game, we limp off, with all of our aches and pains, to Castaways, an outdoor café on the beach. We reminisce about our glory days in college and how our bodies used to immediately rebound from all the torment we endured. That's when it hits me… we have to take care of our bodies (both inside and out) if we want to live long and functional lives, or even just functional lives. I've seen too many people in their forties and early fifties with arthritis and other ailments that they shouldn't have at such a young age. Most of these ailments could have been avoided if these people had taken care of their bodies when they were younger. It's never too late, though. Start today to have a better tomorrow. I promise you, you'll have a more fulfilling life.

My Main Foods That Keep My *Transforming Your Lifestyle* Physique

Here are the main foods that have gotten me into bodybuilding competition, modeling, and all-year general *transforming your lifestyle* shape. Whether preparing for a photo shoot or competing in bodybuilding, I still eat these foods and I calculate each macronutrient to ensure I'm consuming fewer calories than I expend.

Meats/Poultry/Fish Per 3 ounces, cooked (85 Grams)	Calories	Total Fat	Saturated Fat	Protein	Carbs.
Eye of Round Roast	160	6g	2.5g	24g	0g
Top Round Roast	130	3.5g	1g	31g	0g
Top Sirloin Steak	150	4.5g	2g	26g	0g
Ground Beef, extra lean	100	3.5g	1g	18g	0g
Veal Loin Roast	150	6g	2g	22g	0g
Veal Sirloin Roast	140	5g	2g	22g	0g
Veal Leg Roast	130	3g	1g	24g	0g
Pork Tenderloin	140	4g	1.5g	24g	0g
Boston Butt Roast	180	7g	2.5g	26g	0g
Loin Chops	170	7g	2.5g	26g	0g
Ham, fresh	130	4.5g	1.5g	21g	0g
Lamb Tenderloin	160	7g	3g	23g	0g
Loin Chops	170	8g	3g	23g	0g
Chicken Breast, skinless	140	3g	1g	26g	0g
Turkey Breast, skinless	110	1g	0g	26g	0g
Turkey Tenderloin	130	2.5g	1g	25g	0g
Turkey Drumstick	140	4.5g	1.5g	24g	0g
Cod	90	0.5g	0g	19g	0g
Flounder	100	1.5g	0g	21g	0g
Mahi Mahi	90	1g	0g	20g	0g
Monkfish	80	1.5g	0g	16g	0g
Crab, King	80	1.5g	0g	16g	0g
Lobster, Rock	120	1.5g	0g	22g	3g
Clams	130	1.5g	0g	22g	4g
Mussels	150	4g	0.5g	20g	6g
Oysters	70	2g	0.5g	6g	6g
Octopus	140	2g	0g	25g	4g

Grains/Breads/Pastas	Calories	Total Fat	Saturated Fat	Protein	Carbs.
Whole Grain Cereals, Kashi (Go Lean) 1c	140	1g	0g	13g	30g
Oatmeal, Quaker Old Fashion, ½ c dry	150	3g	0.5g	5g	27g
Whole Wheat Bread, Natural Ovens 1 slice	120	2g	0g	4g	21g
English Muffin, Sourdough, 1 muffin	130	1g	0g	4g	26g
Whole Grain Brown Rice, Texmati, 1 c cook	170	1g	0g	4g	35g
Couscous, Texmati, 1 c cook	150	0g	0g	4g	31g
Whole Wheat Angel Hair Spaghetti, 1 c dry	210	1g	0g	7g	44g
Whole Wheat Rigatoni, 1 c dry	210	1g	0g	7g	44g

Vegetables	Calories	Total Fat	Saturated Fat	Protein	Carbs.
Asparagus, 5 spears	18	0g	0g	2g	4g
Broccoli, 1 medium stalk	28	0g	0g	3g	5g
Bell Pepper (Green, Red), 1 med., Raw	40	0g	0g	1g	10g
Cauliflower, 1 cup	25	0g	0g	2g	5g
Eggplant, Purple, 1 c diced	22	0g	0g	1g	5g
Mushrooms, Button, 5 med	20	0g	0g	3g	3g
Onions, (Red, Yellow) 1 med	60	0g	0g	2g	14g
Romaine Lettuce, 1 ½ c	4	0g	0g	1g	2g
Spinach, 1 ½ c	40	0g	0g	3g	10g
Squash, Acorn, 1/4 med	40	0g	0g	1g	10g
Squash, Spaghetti, 1 c	31	1g	1g	1g	7g
Squash, Zucchini, sliced ²/₃ c	12	0g	0g	1g	3g
Sweet Potato, 1 med	56	0g	0g	2g	14g
Tomato (Roma, Vine) 1 med	35	1g	0g	1g	7g

Fruits	Calories	Total Fat	Saturated Fat	Protein	Carbs.
Apples (All), 1 med w/ skin	90	1g	0g	0g	24g
Blackberries, 1 c	75	1g	0g	1g	19g
Blueberries, 1 c	78	1g	0g	1g	20g
Boysenberries, 1 c	73	0g	0g	2g	18g
Cranberries, 1 c	25	0g	0g	0g	6g
Gooseberries, 1 c	70	0g	0g	2g	16g
Raspberries, 1 c	61	1g	0g	1g	15g
Strawberries, 8 med	44	1g	0g	1g	10g
Hass Avocado, 1/5 med	55	5g	1g	1g	3g

Dairy/Egg Products	Calories	Total Fat	Saturated Fat	Protein	Carbs.
Milk, skim, 1 c	86	0g	0g	8g	12g
Cultured Milk (Kefir), 1 c	120	2g	1.5g	14g	12g
Cottage Cheese (1% fat), ½ c	81	1g	1g	14g	3g
String Cheese, 1 stick	60	3.5g	2.5g	8g	1g
Egg (Whole), 1 large	70	5g	2g	6g	0g
Egg (White), 1 large	17	0g	0g	4g	0g

Legumes/Nuts	Calories	Total Fat	Saturated Fat	Protein	Carbs.
Green Beans, ¾ c (cut)	25	0g	0g	1g	5g
Green Peas, ½ c	65	0g	0g	4g	11g
Kidney Beans, ½ c	110	0g	0g	8g	20g
Almonds, approx. handful (1 oz)	180	14g	1g	7g	7g
Black Walnuts (1 oz)	173	17g	1g	7g	3g
Pistachios (1 oz)	160	13g	2g	6g	8g

Good Oils	Calories	Total Fat	Saturated Fat	Protein	Carbs.
Canola Oil, 1 Tbsp	120	14g	1g	0g	0g
Flaxseed Oil, 1 Tbsp	120	14g	1g	0g	0g
Olive Oil (extra virgin), 1 Tbsp	120	14g	2g	0g	0g

After skimming through the list of foods you should notice that this diet has all the food groups and that it isn't boring or monotonous. There are plenty of foods to choose from for you to create your favorite dishes – dishes that will help keep you eating a healthy diet and maintaining a healthy weight for life.

Supplements

I also wanted to make a quick note about the supplements I take on a daily basis. Some people are opposed to supplements because they're not regulated by the Food and Drug Administration (FDA). I'm certainly not mandating that you include supplements in your diet. I'm only being as honest as possible about how I maintain my body, both inside and out. If you feel like any of these supplements might be beneficial to your health goals, please consult your physician before adding any of them to your diet.

1. Whey Protein with Branched Chain Amino Acids (BCAAs)

A "fast-acting" protein that is metabolized in the muscles (rather than the liver) so it gets into the bloodstream much quicker to be utilized by the body. I drink a whey protein shake first thing in the morning and immediately (within 15 minutes) after my workout. First, the body needs nutrients, especially protein (amino acids) as soon as you wake up because you haven't eaten since your last meal the night before. The longer you go before eating, the higher the risk of your body cannibalizing itself. Not good.

While we're sleeping, our bodies aren't getting the amino acids from foods that they need to perform bodily functions. Instead, the amino acids are coming from our muscles, leading to a catabolic response. Our bodies utilize these amino acids from our muscles as part of a biochemical process called gluconeogenesis – "gluco" means sugar, "neo" means new, and "genesis" means to create. Even while sleeping, our bodies need glucose for energy. In fact, glucose is the only form of energy our brains can use to function. Since we can't eat while we sleep, our livers create glucose from the amino acids robbed from our muscle tissue.

Second, during your workout, you're putting tremendous amounts of stress on your muscles and you're actually destroying the muscle you currently have. Your body craves protein so it can start rebuilding your muscles into stronger, thicker muscles. The quicker it receives protein, the quicker it can repair the damaged muscle tissue you broke down during your workout.

2. Creatine Monohydrate

Helps with better muscle contractions by producing more energy, which leads to bigger muscles and more strength.

3. Glutamine

Aids in storing glycogen in the muscles, helping to keep muscle tissue from breaking down. My goal is to slow the breakdown of my muscle in order to keep my metabolism revving and my body from storing fat. Cells in the immune system and gut use glutamine as their primary fuel source. Also, glutamine increases the secretion of human growth hormone which is involved in processes like the regulation of fat metabolism and the turnover of muscle, bone, and collagen.

Caution: Diabetics are strongly advised to consult their primary physician before supplementing glutamine in their diets as diabetics metabolize glutamine abnormally.

4. Digestive Enzymes

Assists in the digestion of the foods I eat so that other types of enzymes don't have to be utilized to digest my food. When we eat, enzymes are needed to turn food into energy. But during this process, our energy levels ebb (this is a reason why people fall asleep on the sofa right after Thanksgiving dinner – they're in a food coma) while free radicals and oxidative stress increases. So there's a breakdown with the enzymes when our food is being turned into fuel our bodies can use for energy. By supplementing my diet with digestive enzymes, the other types of enzymes are able to perform their specific jobs to keep my body healthy and strong.

5. Fish Oil (EPA/DHA)

I use fish oil primarily for the huge amounts of Omega-3s it contains. The benefits of preventing heart disease, lowering blood pressure and cholesterol levels, reducing inflammation, and helping prevent osteoporosis and rheumatoid arthritis is enough to get me on the bandwagon. Omega-3s are essential for building and repairing cell membranes. Also, it helps balance out the high amount of Omega-6s in our Western diets.

6. Multivitamins and Minerals

Most people are deficient in many vitamins and minerals. So as a precaution, I add a multivitamin and mineral supplement with plenty of the complex vitamin Bs to my diet. Also, research suggests that multivitamins taken before a workout will help speed the recovery of your muscles.

7. Coenzyme Q10 (CoQ10)

An antioxidant that also strengthens the immune system and helps produce adenosine triphosphate (ATP), or energy.

NOTE: individuals taking statin drugs might want to discuss with their primary physician about supplementing CoQ10 in their diet because statins deplete CoQ10 levels in the body.

8. Calcium

Needed for muscle contractions, helps our blood to clot, transmits nerve impulses, and is responsible for absorbing fat. Calcium also neutralizes acids our bodies release while digesting protein.

9. Magnesium

Responsible for over 300 different enzyme reactions in the body; by relaxing muscle contractions, it's the opposing mineral to calcium. Magnesium is crucial for producing energy. It also boosts serotonin levels which makes you feel happy and reduces stress. It's the stress antidote, meaning that stress depletes magnesium from our bodies.

10. Probiotics (Good Bacteria)

When your immune system is out of balance, you start to get chronic diseases. Sixty percent of your immune system is in your gut. Probiotics help keep your PH balanced in your gut to keep you healthy. They also help make vitamins, detox the poisons we eat (mercury, lead, pesticides, herbicides, PCBs, etc.), regulate cholesterol metabolism, and help produce energy.

Well, now we've seen how I do it. But wait – isn't there an easier way? At least when it comes to losing weight, in this day and age of scientific know-how, isn't there some kind of pill or something? Well, if you look at the diet ads you'll find *plenty* of them. Fat-burning pills with all kinds of different brand names are available everywhere. Let's see if we can find one that works!

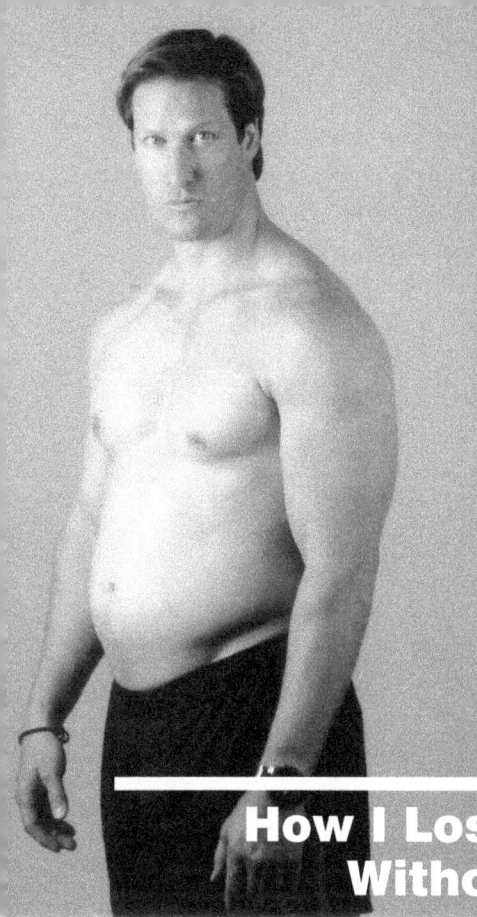

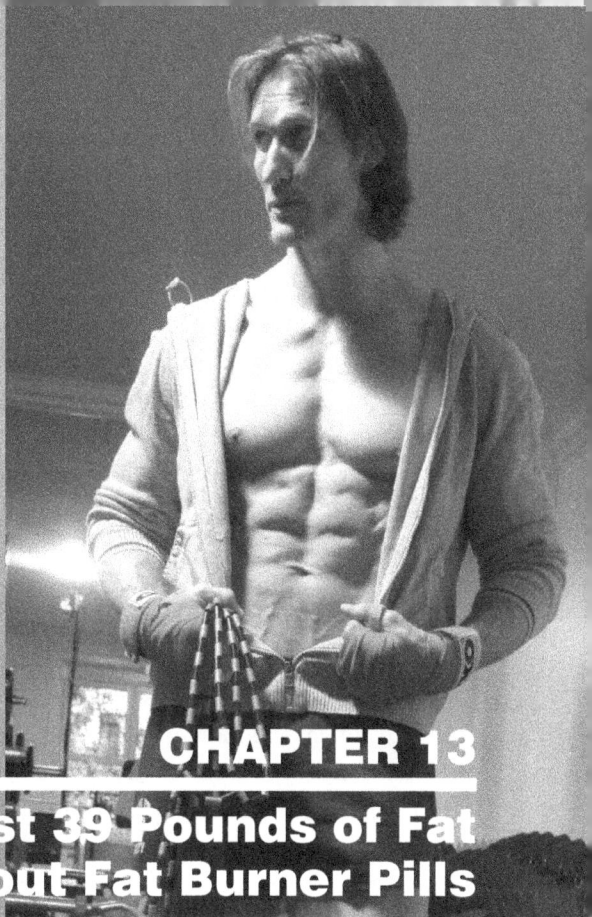

CHAPTER 13

How I Lost 39 Pounds of Fat Without Fat Burner Pills

Fat burner pills promise to make you lose extraordinary amounts of weight in a short period of time. Unfortunately, the main loss you're most likely to incur is financial. No supplement burns fat exclusively. If these advertisements were true, wouldn't you think everyone would be fashion-model material – without lifting a weight or stepping on a treadmill?

Thermogenics, better known as "fat burning pills," have recently been under attack by the FDA which has been questioning the safety of the ingredients used to produce these pills. First, "thermogenics" is the science of heat production and has nothing to do with fat burning. Yes, a calorie is a unit of heat (the amount required to raise the temperature of one kilogram of water by one degree Celsius), but any physical activity, food, beverage, or supplement that can increase heat production can burn calories, including calories from fat.

> If these ads were true, everyone would be fashion-model material – without lifting a weight or stepping on a treadmill.

*christopher*SASHA

Some of the ingredients in these pills are stimulants (much like coffee or caffeine) that stimulate your central nervous system. As you may know, stimulants speed body functions, ultimately burning calories. There are other ingredients in thermogenic supplements that suppress your appetite and still other ingredients that act as diuretics, causing water to leave your body. When combining stimulation, appetite reduction, and the expulsion of water from your body, you're certain to lose weight – *water weight.* In no way is the weight loss coming solely from fat as the marketing ploys lead you to believe.

Fat burning pills are effective at first but their effects wane after a couple of weeks. At that point, you're probably disappointed because the initial results jazzed you. So then you might think, "Increasing the dosage will increase my results!" Think twice. Thermogenics are addicting for some people who enjoy the rush from the stimulants. The problem is that your body develops a tolerance for these stimulants (just like coffee) and more is required to maintain the same rush. The irony is that as you increase the dosage, you get fewer results while you increase your risk for side effects.

> As you increase the dosage, you get fewer results while you increase your risk for side effects.

Make no mistake: every "miracle drug" has negative side effects and thermogenic supplements are no exception. Some adverse effects include irregular heartbeat, increased blood pressure, headaches, nervousness, dizziness, insomnia, tremors, stroke, and even death. These aren't common, but they *are* documented side effects that people have experienced after taking these pills. Unfortunately, more desperate individuals, in need of losing weight quickly, are often people who have pre-existing conditions, such as high blood pressure and cardio-respiratory and thyroid problems. These conditions put them at high risk right off the bat.

> Some adverse effects from fat burner pills include irregular heartbeat, increased blood pressure, stroke, and death.

Also, when you finally decide to stop using fat burning pills, you might experience atrocious headaches – just like when going cold turkey drinking coffee. Your body actually goes through withdrawal from these substances. Other symptoms include a depletion of energy and feelings of weakness. Basically, you'll feel like you just got hit by an 18-wheeler. Worst of all, don't be surprised when you see the numbers on the scale go back up once you stop taking these supplements. What's more, your basal metabolic rate (BMR) plunges, putting you at risk of gaining fat at twice the rate as before you decided to use a thermogenic. The body is an amazing machine. It maintains homeostasis by returning to its original state.

Although the short-term results achieved with fat burning pills might be apparent for some, there's no evidence of long-term success. You'll spend a lot of money only to discover what the research on these pills is indicating: the maximum benefit is the burning of an additional 150-200 calories per day. I know I can burn an additional 200 calories by jumping a rope for 15 minutes, and it won't cost me a cent. The more heat I create, the more calories I will burn. I guarantee if I jump rope for 15 minutes, I'll generate more heat than if I swallow a pill.

> Don't be surprised when you see the numbers on the scale go back up once you stop taking fat burner pills.

Miracle Drug or Miracle Waste of Money?

On May 1, 2009 the FDA warned consumers to immediately stop using Hydroxycut products (a brand of fat burning pills) and announced a recall of 14 types of Hydroxycut products that were audaciously labeled as made with "natural" ingredients. Cocaine is natural as well. Is it safe? Some very poisonous substances are natural, so beware of labels with statements like "all natural" or "made with natural ingredients." A few of the reported adverse effects of these Hydroxycut pills include cardiovascular disorders, seizures, jaundice, liver disease, liver failure … and the death of a 19 year old.

> On May 1, 2009 the FDA warned consumers to immediately stop using Hydroxycut products (fat burner pills).

There is no miracle drug that will make you lose fat and keep it off without exercise. The best and healthiest method by which to lose fat and total weight – and keep it off – is proper diet, exercise, and rest. Instead of dropping massive amounts of money on short-term solutions, wouldn't it be wiser to drop by a local gym? The bonus of working out at a club, other than exercising, losing weight and building a stronger, healthier body, is you'll very likely meet some new friends who also value exercise. You'll have common ground. All the friends I've amassed from gyms I've trained in have been exceptional motivators for me to stay in shape. They're essential in my maintenance plan – to remain healthy.

The FTC alleged that the weight-loss and weight-control claims were not supported by competent and reliable scientific evidence.

In January 2007, marketers of four weight control pill products – Xenadrine EFX, CortiSlim, TrimSpa, and One-A-Day WeightSmart – settled with the Federal Trade Commission (FTC), surrendering cash and other assets worth at least $25 million and agreeing to limit future advertising claims. The FTC alleged that the weight-loss and weight-control claims of these companies were not supported by competent and reliable scientific evidence.

According to the U.S. Federal Trade Commission:

*1. **Xenadrine EFX:*** had to pay between $8 million and $12.8 million to settle FTC allegations that Xenadrine EFX's weight-loss claims were false and unsubstantiated. Xenadrine EFX has not been scientifically proven to cause rapid and substantial weight loss. According to the FTC complaint, consumer endorsers were paid up to $20,000 for their testimonials. These "endorsers" actually lost weight by engaging in rigorous diet and/or exercise programs.

These "endorsers" actually lost weight by engaging in rigorous diet and/or exercise programs.

*2. **CortiSlim and CortiStress:*** had to surrender at least $12 million to settle FTC charges for false and unsubstantiated claims that their products can cause weight loss and reduce the risk of, or prevent, serious health conditions. CortiSlim's claims to cause rapid, substantial, and permanent weight loss in all users were false and unsubstantiated. CortiStress's ability to reduce the risk of osteoporosis, obesity, diabetes, Alzheimer's disease, cancer, and cardiovascular disease were also false and unsubstantiated.

*3. **TrimSpa:*** (former endorser was celebrity Anna Nicole Smith) had to pay $1.5 million to settle FTC allegations that marketers had inadequate scientific evidence to support TrimSpa's claims of rapid and substantiated weight loss and that one of its ingredients, HOODIA gordonii, enabled users to lose substantial amounts of weight by suppressing appetite.

*4. **One-A-Day WeightSmart:*** the Bayer Corporation will pay a $3.2 million civil penalty to settle FTC allegations for violating an earlier Commission order requiring all health claims for One-A-Day brand vitamins to be supported by competent and reliable scientific evidence. Claims of Bayer Corporation's One-A-Day WeightSmart include that the pills will increase metabolism, enhance metabolism through EGCG (epigallocatechin gallate – a green tea extract), help prevent some of the weight gain associated with a decline in metabolism in users over the age 30, and help users control weight by enhancing their metabolism.

Faithfully, the FTC chairman said, "You won't find weight loss in a bottle of pills that claims it has the latest scientific breakthrough or miracle ingredient. Paying for fad science is a good way to lose cash, not pounds."

Losing Weight Without Thermogenics

When I began writing this book in May, 2006, the very first issue I wanted to address was the public's misconception about these fat burner pills that were so popular. I believe the pills' popularity derive from their ability to offer a quick-fix, short-term solution to a long-term problem. I see these advertisements as often as you. I can't pick-up a fitness magazine without seeing pages flooded with guarantees to lose massive amounts of weight within a very short period of time by using fat burner pills.

I wanted to argue two points concerning these advertisements. My first point was to prove that you can lose all the weight you want without paying obscene amounts of money on these pills. Secondly, the photographs taken of these "endorsers" use lighting angles, body postures, and other tricks of the photographic trade that can make the endorsers appear worse or better than they actually look in person.

My first goal was to pack on 20-30 additional pounds. I started this weight-gain quest in March, 2006, at 198 pounds and took a little over two years to end at 218 pounds. I couldn't squeeze into my clothes anymore and was wearing t-shirts and sweatpants with elastic bands. Once, I had to wear one of my suits to a wedding. I couldn't sit so I had to stand the entire time because my pants were ripping at the seams and I couldn't suck my gut in while I was sitting. I was miserable. So I know that weight gain puts an emotional strain on overweight and obese people. I felt unattractive, uncomfortable, and unfit.

christopherSASHA

By May 26, 2008, I was fluctuating between 218 and 221 pounds. At that time, my body fat was 20.8%, which means I was carrying over 45 pounds of fat. Again, your body needs some fat to function properly ... but not *that* much.

The next day was the beginning of my adventure to prove that it's possible to drop just as much weight, and in the same short amount of time, as these fat burner pill advertisements claim, without the use of fat burner pills. I also wanted to take my experience one step further than the advertisements by recording my body fat percentage progress from the first day of my *transforming your lifestyle* program to 7 weeks into it, and then on the final day – 10 weeks total. Here are the results:

WEEK	BEFORE - WEEK 0	DURING - WEEK 7	AFTER - WEEK 10
Total Body Weight	218 lbs.	193 lbs.	180 lbs.
Body Fat	20.8%	7.5%	3.6%
Body Fat Weight	45.34 lbs.	14.47 lbs.	6.48 lbs.
Lean Body Mass	79.2%	92.5%	96.4%
Lean Body Mass Weight	172.66 lbs.	178.53 lbs.	173.52 lbs.
Waist Size	37 1/2"	31 1/2"	29 1/2"

In 7 weeks, I was able to lose 25 pounds (total body weight) without the use of any fat burner pills. But when you take a closer look at my weight-loss regime for the first 7 weeks, you'll see in the chart above that I lost 31 pounds of fat, gained 6 pounds of muscle, and dropped 6 inches from my waist – without fat burners!

You know by now that I'm an adamant proponent of losing no more than 1-2 pounds per week. Yet in 7 weeks I lost 25 pounds. So what gives? The reason I lost 25 pounds instead of only 7-14 pounds in the first 7 weeks is due to all the pounds lost during the initial first 2 weeks. I cut my total amount of daily calories, including calories from carbohydrates. As discussed in Chapter 5, each gram of carbohydrate holds about 3 grams of water. Decreasing carbohydrates leads to water loss and total weight loss. After the first few weeks, my body adjusted by excreting water it didn't need. This is why dieters who practice the Atkin's Diet and South Beach Diet, among other diets, lose an amazing amount of weight during the first few weeks. Many diets that provide meal plans put meals with very low

> I lost 31 pounds of fat, gained 6 pounds of muscle, and dropped 6 inches from my waist – without fat burners!

carbs in the first phase so water will drain out of the body. So it's no surprise that dieters see a decrease in weight on the scale. The scale can't distinguish whether the weight loss came from fat, muscle, or water. The only way to make sure the weight you're losing is unwanted fat weight is to test your body fat percentage before, during, and after your weight loss program.

The scale can't distinguish whether the weight loss came from fat, muscle, or water.

The fourth week I was right on target … only to fall short in the fifth week by losing only one pound. After reviewing my food diary and exercise log, I found that I had increased my total calories (including carbohydrates) and cut a few of my cardio sessions short. So I decreased my calories a little and increased my cardio sessions by a few minutes. The following week, I was back on track.

During the seventh week I measured my body composition. I found that I had lost 31 pounds of body fat and gained 6 pounds of lean body mass (muscle). My progress was worthy of a Kodak moment, so I captured it (on page 308). At this point, I got a little overzealous. I decided to get back to my college weight and strayed from my own exhortations about losing 1-2 pounds per week. I added another 30 minutes of cardio to my workout regime and cut back on my daily caloric intake. A combination of both decreasing my calories too much and increasing my activity level too much caused my body to start cannibalizing muscle tissue. I wasn't consuming enough total daily calories for my body weight and activity level.

I decreased my calories a little and increased my cardio sessions by a few minutes. The following week, I was back on track.

As you can see in the chart (on page 304), in the final 3 weeks I lost another 8 pounds of body fat. But with that greedy decision, I also lost 5 pounds of the very muscle that helps keep my metabolism revving and fat storage at bay. This is exactly the opposite of the *transforming your lifestyle* way. The final 3 weeks of my experiment reinforced the theory of losing weight slowly (1-2 pounds per week) to discourage losing muscle tissue. Again, we want to lose the body fat and preserve the muscle tissue to keep the metabolism high and keep the weight off.

christopherSASHA

I kept a record of my weight loss once per week:

Week	Weight
Week 1	8 pounds
Week 2	7 pounds
Week 3	3 pounds
Week 4	2 pounds
Week 5	1 pound
Week 6	2 pounds
Week 7	2 pounds
Week 8	4 pounds
Week 9	5 pounds
Week 10	4 pounds

Now, if I didn't break down my total body weight loss into two important categories (lean body mass and body fat weight), I wouldn't be impressed with losing 38 total body weight pounds in 10 weeks. Remember, the scale can't distinguish between muscle weight and fat weight. The muscle I lost during the final three weeks of my experiment made my metabolism slow down a little, which inevitably allowed my body to store more fat, increasing my risks of chronic illnesses. And this is why most people who lose weight too quickly, and/or don't exercise (resistance training and cardiovascular exercise), gain all their weight back within 1-5 years. Most of these people will even gain more weight than before they started their fad diet.

In the end, my scale showed me that I had lost 38 pounds of total body weight. However, by breaking my weight loss into lean body mass and body fat weight, I found that, though I did lose 38 pounds of total body weight, I also lost 39 pounds of body fat. The difference of 1 pound being what I gained in muscle.

> Most people who lose weight too quickly, and/or don't exercise (resistance training and cardiovascular exercise), gain all their weight back within 5 years.

I'm now in a much better position by losing 39 pounds of body fat. My risks for diseases like lipid disorders, high blood pressure, type 2 diabetes, cardiovascular disease, and other chronic illnesses have been drastically reduced. Oh, I also eradicated my sleep apnea, acid reflux, and lower back pain problems. Let's not forget the psychological effect losing a chunk of weight has on the ego. I became more confident, felt better about myself, and loved going to the beach without wearing a baggy t-shirt and worrying if people were going to either harpoon me or roll me back into the water before I died. Here is the accumulation of my progress:

Week 0
218 lbs. 20.8% Body Fat

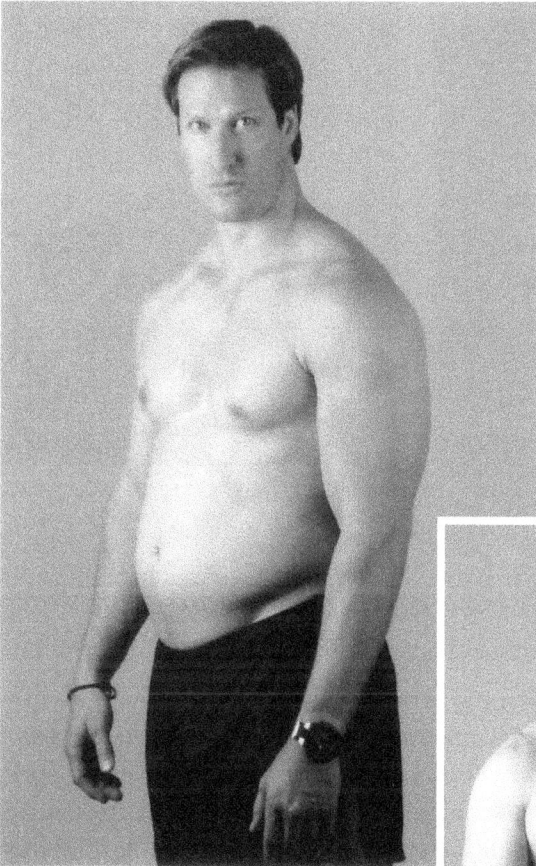

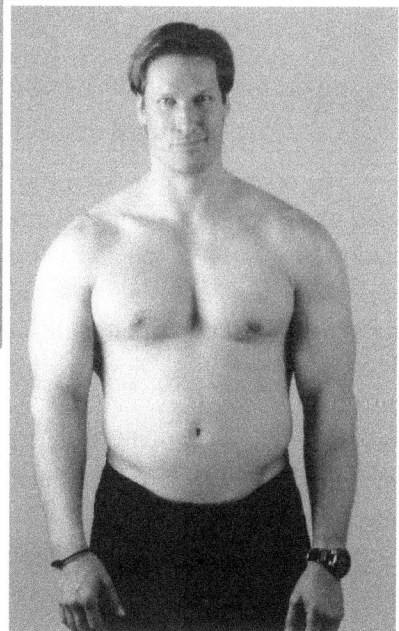

christopherSASHA

Week 7
193 lbs. 7.5% Body Fat

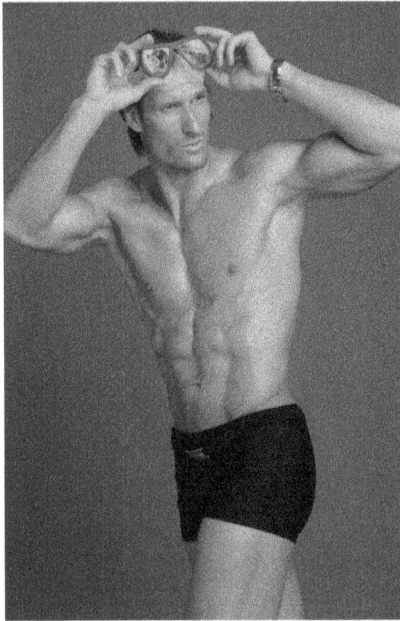

Week 10
180 lbs. 3.6% Body Fat

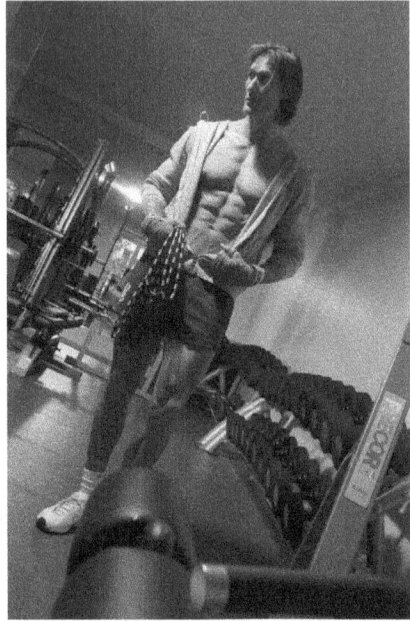

Tactics Used by Fat Burner Advertisement Photos

The other objection I want to bring to your attention is the before and after photographs fat burner pill marketers use to really *WOW* the consumer. As I'm sure you've noticed, the "before" picture is an average looking guy or girl who appears overweight. Taking a closer look at the picture, you'll notice a few additional things. First, the person is pale and has no tan. If the person had any color at all, shadows would form and give the person definition which would show muscle separation. Secondly, a light is placed parallel to the person's midsection to drown out any possible muscle definition this person may have. In doing so, the person appears to be overweight and with no muscle tone.

Another tactic used is having the model position him/herself in a bad posture position, tilting the pelvis forward and rolling the shoulders forward.

This position creates the illusion of a flat chest and a round belly, making him/her appear fat. These are just a few of the ploys used to create an illusion that the model in question has a weight problem.

Then there's the "after" photo which shows an impressive physique worthy of fitness model material. In a short period of time, the participant has lost an amazing amount of weight, displaying six-pack abs and defined shoulders, chest, and arms. While vetting the after photo, you might notice that the lighting is different due to angles used to create shadows. This creates the illusion of a better definition of muscle separation. Also, you might notice that the participant has a tan and better posture, pulling his/her shoulders back a little which helps the body appear taller and more svelte. Another reason the after photo looks good is because the individual has dehydrated him/herself to excrete excess water retention from beneath the skin. The skin then lies flatter on the muscles and shows separation between muscle bellies (the individual muscles from the bone to the joint) and muscle groups.

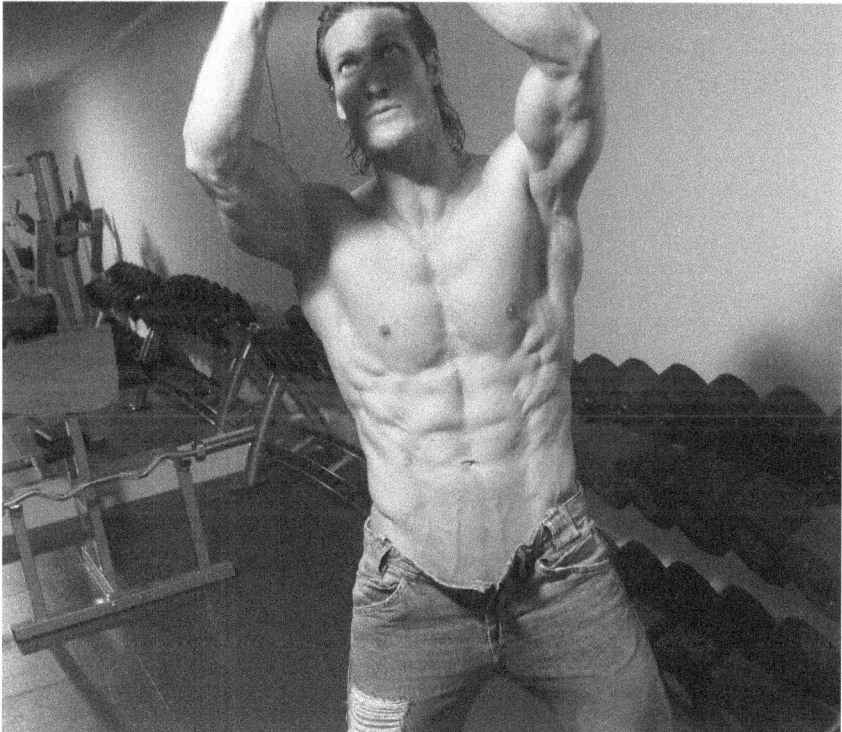

The after photo is a byproduct of weight loss, lighting angles, tanning, proper posture, dehydration, and flexing of the abdominals. As a fitness expert, I know the body cannot sustain this condition for an extended period of time.

christopherSASHA

Read the fine print at the bottom of these ads... "Results are not typical and will vary."

One final thought ...please read the fine print at the bottom of these ads. Most state: "Results are not typical and will vary." Before succumbing to these staged, fat burner pill ads and losing more money than pounds, allow me to be your coach. Allow me to help you achieve a *transforming your lifestyle* body through proper nutrition, exercise, and rest.

I've explained in great detail exactly how I lost an incredible amount of body fat, and continue to keep it off. I've given you the same strategies I use to help you achieve the same results that I've achieved. I've given you the knowledge you need to change your body and health – and your life!

Now it's your choice as to what you'll do with all this newfound information. The *transforming your lifestyle* program is mere information until you put it into action. You can either put this book on the shelf with the other diet program books you've read, or you can put what you've read here into action to help you transform into a healthier, happier you.

Together, we can win the war of health management!

christopherSASHA

NOTES

NOTES